W9-CBA-897

Serono Symposia Publications from Raven Press
Volume 87

"REDO" VASCULAR SURGERY
Renal, Aorto-Iliac and Infrainguinal Areas

Serono Symposia Publications from Raven Press

Vol. 87: "Redo" Vascular Sugery - Renal, Aorto-Iliac and Infrainguinal Areas, *C. Spartera, R. Courbier, P. Fiorani and A.M. Imparato, editors;* 332 pp., 1992.

Vol. 86: Stress and Reproduction, *K.E. Sheppard, J.H. Boublik and J.W. Funder, editors;* 375 pp., 1992.

Vol. 85: Nutritional Aspects of Osteoporosis, *P. Burckhardt and R.P. Heaney, editors;* 380 pp., 1991.

Vol. 84: Advances in Surgery *F.G. Moody, W. Montorsi and M. Montorsi, editors;* 496 pp., 1991.

Vol. 83: Hereditary Tumors, *M.L. Brandi and R. White, editors;* 220 pp., 1991.

Vol. 82: The Status of Differentiation Therapy of Cancer, vol. II, *S. Waxman, G.B. Rossi and F. Takaku, editors;* 152 pp., 1991.

Vol. 81: Growth Disorders: The State of the Art, *L. Cavallo, J.C. Job and M.I. New, editors;* 372 pp., 1991.

Vol. 80: Ovarian Secretions and Cardiovascular and Neurological Function, *F. Naftolin, J.N. Gutmann, A.H. DeCherney and P.M. Sarrel, editors;* 320 pp., 1990.

*Vol. 79: Progress and Perspectives in Chemoprevention of Cancer, *G. de Palo, M. Sporn. and U. Veronesi, editors.*

Vol. 78: Papillomaviruses in Human Pathology. Recent Progress in Epidermoid Precancers, *J. Monsonego, editor;* 531 pp., 1990.

Vol. 77: Plasminogen Activators: From Cloning to Therapy, R. Abbate, T. Barni and A. Tsafriri, editors; 204 pp., 1991.

Vol. 76: Horizons in Endocrinology, vol. II, *M. Maggi and V. Geenen, editors;* 360 pp., 1991.

Vol. 75: Comparative Spermatology 20 Years After, *B. Baccetti, editor;* 1112 pp., 1991.

Vol. 74: The New Biology of Steroid Hormones, *R.B. Hochberg and F. Naftolin, editors;* 360 pp., 1991.

Vol. 73: Major Advances in Human Female Reproduction, *E.Y. Adashi and S. Mancuso, editors;* 410 pp., 1990.

Vol. 72: Computers in Endocrinology: Recent Advances, *V. Guardabasso, D. Rodbard and G. Forti, editors;* 207 pp., 1990.

Vol. 71: Reproduction, Growth and Development, *A. Negro-Vilar and G. Perez-Palacios, editors;* 439 pp., 1991.

Vol. 70: Hormonal Communicating Events in the Testis, *A. Isidori, A. Fabbri and M.L. Dufau, editors;* 296 pp., 1990.

Vol. 69: Diabetic Complications: Epidemiology and Pathogenetic Mechanisms, *D. Andreani, J.L. Gueriguian and G.E. Striker, editors;* 361 pp., 1991.

Vol. 68: Cytokines: Basic Principles and Clinical Applications, *S. Romagnani and A.K. Abbas, editors;* 370 pp., 1990.

Vol. 67: Developmental Endocrinology, *P.C. Sizonenko and M.L. Aubert, editors;* 252 pp., 1990.

Vol. 66: Establishing a Successful Human Pregnancy, *R.G. Edwards, editor;* 281 pp., 1990.

Vol. 65: Structure-Function Relationship of Gonadotropins, *D. Bellet and J.-M. Bidart, editors;* 328 pp., 1989.

Vol. 64: Membrane Technology, *R. Verna, editor;* 155 pp., 1989.

Vol. 63: GIFT: From Basics to Clinics, *G.L. Capitanio, R.H. Asch, L. De Cecco and S. Croce, editors;* 454 pp., 1989.

Vol. 62: Unexplained Infertility, *G. Spera and L. Gnessi, editors;* 304 pp., 1989.

Vol. 61: Microbiological, Chemotherapeutical and Immunological Problems in High Risk Patients, *E. Garaci, G. Renzini, F. Filadoro, A. Goldstein and J. Verhoef, editors;* 310 pp., 1989.

Vol. 60: General Surgery: Current Status and Future Trends, *T.E. Starzl and W. Montorsi, editors;* 473 pp., 1989.

Vol. 59: Pathogenesis and Control of Viral Infections, *F. Aiuti, editor;* 328 pp., 1989.

In press.

Serono Symposia Publications from Raven Press
Volume 87

"Redo" Vascular Surgery Renal, Aorto-Iliac and Infrainguinal Areas

Editors

Carlo Spartera, M.D.
Department of Vascular Surgery
University of L'Aquila
L'Aquila, ITALY

Department of Cardiovascular Surgery
Hopital St. Joseph
Marseille, FRANCE

Paolo Fiorani, M.D.
Department of Vascular Surgery
University of Rome
Rome, ITALY

Anthony M. Imparato, M.D.
Department of Vascular Surgery
University of New York
New York, USA

Compiling Editor

Carla Petrassi

Raven Press ■ New York

Raven Press, 1185 Avenue of the Americas, New York, New York 10036

"REDO" VASCULAR SURGERY - RENAL, AORTO-ILIAC AND INFRAINGUINAL AREAS
(Serono Symposia Publications from Raven Press; v. 87)

International Standard Book Number 0-88167-908-9
Library of Congress Catalog Number 91-051157

Printed in Rome, Italy
by Christengraf

Preface

In recent years Vascular Surgery has improved its knowledge in the field of the correction of arterial lesions that are the cause of several disabling diseases. However, these successes obtained in nearly all the areas and regarding an ever-increasing number of cases have brought to light new problems.

In fact, whereas in the past the vascular surgeon was quite satisfied with patient survival and acceptable hemodynamic results, growing technical progress and technological developments from both a diagnostic and instrumental point of view, have stimulated the vascular surgeon to expect better and longer results.

The longer terms of follow-up, though, gave rise ever more frequently to late complications in direct arterial re-constructions necessitating at times an emergency surgical decision. The motivations and aims of re-operations have undergone through the course of time a marked evolution. The first phase was characterized by early re-operations mainly due to technical errors. Subsequently, re-operations had to be effected when alarming symptoms evidenced the failure of the previous operation. The epoch we are now living is that of programed re-operations that have been made possible thanks also to the present diagnostic methods (Ecocolor Doppler, Magnetic Resonance, Digital Subtraction Angiography) that can individuate the failing procedures. On the other hand, the new therapeutic methods of the last decade (Laser, PTA, Stents) raised hopes that a growing number of vascular lesions could be resolved with a minimum of trauma to the patients with results that were comparable to those obtained through surgery.

This was not always true. These methods, which in some cases modified the natural history of some lesions (iliac artery, superficial femoral artery), led themselves to re-operation when the failure of these procedures was evidenced after a brief or long period of time. Consequently, the vascular surgeon has been faced ever more frequently with re-operations whose indications and technical aspects are very different from the original therapeutic procedure.

To define our present knowledge in this field, it was decided to organize an international symposium that could help to clarify the causes of failures, and examine the possibility to effect an early diagnosis of failing procedures in order to avoid - often through a new operation - the development of a pathological situation that could become irreversible and without solution.

This volume contains the papers presented at the international symposium "Redo Vascular Surgery" held in L'Aquila, Italy, June 25-27, 1992, that I was able to organize thanks to the expertise, enthusiasm and collaboration of the members of the scientific committee (A.D. Callow, R. Courbier, P. Fiorani, R.M. Greenhalgh, A.M. Imparato and A.V. Pokrovsky). My profound gratitude goes to them for their assistance in gathering the leading European, North American and Italian experts in re-operations of the renal, aorto-iliac and infrainguinal areas. My staff and I dedicated ourselves totally to the organization of this meeting and we again are grateful to our colleagues for the exceptional scientific quality of the contributions published in this volume by Raven Press.

It was not our presumption that this symposium could solve all the problems that Vascular Surgery has to face today but it is our hope that the debate and discussion on the problems related to this field will have focused attention also to aspects which at times can appear less important, but that, in certain circumstances, can be determinant. In this light, I hope that the symposium "Redo Vascular Surgery - L'Aquila 1992" will be remembered as an important moment for the progress of modern Vascular Surgery.

Carlo Spartera

Acknowledgements

The realization of this volume in such a brief time was made possible only through the hard work of all the speakers who handed in their papers well before the actual conference date. I am grateful to them for their efforts and help towards this goal.

I would like to thank my co-workers for their unfailing contributions towards the scientific, logistic and editorial tasks involved in all the phases of the congress, and in particular, Drs. Carla Petrassi, Giuseppe Morettini, Marco Ventura, Giovanni Marino e Gaetano La Barbera.

A sincere word of thanks goes to Mrs. Marzia Colista for her patience and availability during the past months which were not easy.

A particular acknowledgement must be given to Dr. Sergio Rossetti and his staff at Ares-Serono Symposia for their professional assistance in the difficult task of preparing this book.

Furthermore, I am grateful to the Organizing Secretatiat, CON.OR. International for their guidance and support in all the organizational phases, and in particular, I want to thank Mrs. V. Fares and Mrs. D. Monticelli for their experienced and valuable collaboration.

Lastly, a debt of recognition goes to the spontaneous help and friendly support of the sponsors without which the meeting and the publication of this book would not have been possible. It is my sincere hope that this volume will reap the success for which all of us strived.

Contents

BASIC CONSIDERATIONS

REDO SURGERY IN RENAL AREA

REDO SURGERY IN INFRAINGUINAL AREA

Contributors

G. AGRIFOGLIO, MD
Chief
Institute of Vascular Surgery and
Angiology
University of Milan
Via Commenda, 12
20122 Milan, ITALY

A. ASCOLI MARCHETTI, MD
Department of Vascular Surgery
University of Rome "Tor Vergata"
Ospedale S. Eugenio
Piazzale dell'Umanesimo, 10
00144 Rome, ITALY

G.P. AVRUSCIO, MD
Service of Angiology
Padua Hospital
Padua, ITALY

H. BASSIOUNY, MD
Assistant Professor of Surgery
Department of Surgery
and Pathology
University of Chicago
5841 South Maryland
Avenue MC 5028
Chicago, Illinois 60637, U.S.A.

D. BERGQVIST, MD, PhD
Associate Professor
Department of Surgery
Lund University
Malmo General Hospital
S-214 01 Malmo, SWEDEN

B. BERNARDO, MD
Department of Vascular Surgery
II° School of Medicine
University of Naples
Via S. Pansini, 5
80131 Naples, ITALY

D. BERTINI, MD
Chief
Department of Vascular Surgery
University of Florence
Ospedale Careggi
Viale Morgagni, 55
50134 Florence, ITALY

M. BEZZI, MD
Department of Radiology
University of Rome, "La Sapienza"
Policlinico Umberto I°
00161 Rome , ITALY

G. BIASI, MD
Chief
Department of Vascular Surgery
University of Milan
Bassini Hospital
Via Massimo Gorki, 50
20092 Cinisello Balsamo (MI), ITALY

N. BOM, MD
Thoraxcenter Institute
University Hospital Rotterdam
Dr Molewaterplein 40,
3015 GD Rotterdam, The Netherlands

G. BRACALE, MD
Chief
Department of Vascular Surgery
II° School of Medicine
University of Naples
Via S. Pansini, 5
80131 Naples, ITALY

A. BRANCHEREAU, MD
Professor
Université Aix-Marseille II
Service de Chirurgie Vasculaire
des Hopitaux Sud
Hopital Sainte Marguerite
BP 29 13274 Marseille Cedex 9,
FRANCE

A.D. CALLOW, MD, PhD
Research Professor of Surgery
Division of General Surgery
Washington University School of
Medicine
Box 8109, 4960 Audubon Avenue
St. Louis, Missouri 63110, U.S.A.

D. CHARLESWORTH, DSc,
MD, FRCS
Consultant Vascular Surgeon
University Hospital of South
Manchester
Nell Lane
West Didsbury
Manchester M20 8LR, U.K.

A.W. CLOWES, MD
Professor of Surgery
Department of Surgery, RF-25
University of Washington
Seattle, Washington 98195,
U.S.A.

D. COGNOLATO, MD
Department of Vascular Surgery
University of Padua
V. Giustiniani, 2
35128 Padua, ITALY

M.D. COLBURN, MD
Resident Dept. of General Surgery
UCLA School of Medicine
10833 Le Conte Ave.
Los Angeles, CA 90024, U.S.A.

R. COURBIER, MD
Chief
Department of Cardiovascular Surgery
Hopital St. Joseph
26,Boulevard de Louvain
13285 Marseille Cedex 8, FRANCE

E. CRISPO, MD
Department of Vascular Surgery
University of Rome "Tor Vergata"
Ospedale S. Eugenio
Piazzale dell'Umanesimo, 10
00144 Rome, ITALY

M. D'ADDATO, MD
Chief
Department of Vascular Surgery
University of Bologna
Policlinico S. Orsola
Via Massarenti, 9
40138 Bologna, ITALY

R.H. DEAN, MD
Director
Division of Surgical Sciences
The Bowman Gray
School of Medicine
Wake Forest University
300 South Hawthorne Road,
Winston-Salem, NC 27103,
U.S.A.

G.P. DERIU, MD
Chief
Dept. of Vascular Surgery
University of Padua
Via Giustiniani, 2
35128 Padua, ITALY

E. DI CESARE, MD
Dept. of Radiology
University of L'Aquila
Ospedale S.M. Collemaggio
67100 L'Aquila, ITALY

E.B. DIETHRICH, MD
Dept. of Cardiovascular Surgery
Arizona Heart Institute
Medical Director
2632 North 20th Street
Phoenix, AR 85006, U.S.A.

M. DOMANIN, MD
Institute of Vascular Surgery and
Angiology
University of Milan
Via Commenda, 12
20122 Milan , ITALY

N.A.J.J. DU BOIS, MD
Dept. of Vascular Surgery
University Hospital Rotterdam
Dr Molewaterplein 40,
3015 GD Rotterdam,
The Netherlands

G. J. ECKHOLDT, MD
Alton Ochsner Medical Foundation
New Orleans, Louisiana, USA

H. ESPINOZA, MD
Université Aix-Marseille II
Service de Chirurgie Vasculaire
des Hopitaux Sud
Hopital Sainte Marguerite
BP 29 13274 Marseille Cedex 9,
FRANCE

M. FERDANI, MD
Dept. of Cardiovascular Surgery
Hopital St. Joseph
26, Boulevard de Louvain
13285 Marseille Cedex 8,
FRANCE

O. FILICE, MD
Department of Vascular Surgery
II° School of Medicine
University of Naples
Via S. Pansini, 5
80131 Naples, ITALY

P. FIORANI, MD
Chief
Department of Vascular Surgery
University of Rome "La Sapienza"
Policlinico Umberto I
00161, Rome, ITALY

R.L. GEARY, MD
Vascular Surgery Fellow
Department of Surgery, RF-25
University of Washington
Seattle, Washington 98195, U.S.A.

D. P. GIDDENS, PhD
Department of Aerospace Engineering
Georgian Institute of Technology

G.A. GIORDANO, MD
Department of Vascular Surgery
University of Rome "Tor Vergata"
Ospedale S. Eugenio
Piazzale dell'Umanesimo, 10
00144 Rome, ITALY

S. GLAGOV, MD
Department of Surgery and Pathology
University of Chicago
5841 South Maryland Avenue MC 5028
Chicago, Illinois 60637, U.S.A.

J. GOLDSTONE, MD
Professor and Vice-Chairman
Department of Surgery
Chief, Vascular Surgery
U.C.S.F.
M488, Box 0222
505 Parnassus Avenue
San Francisco, CA 94143-0222,
U.S.A.

R.G. GOSLING, MD
Professor "Emeritous"
United Medical and Dental Schools
St. Thomas Hospital,
London, U.K.

D. GREEN, MD, PhD
Division of Hematology/Oncology
Department of Medicine, Northwestern
University Medical School and the
Rehabilitation Institute,
345 E. Superior Street Room 1407
Chicago, Illinois 60611, U.S.A.

**R.M. GREENHALGH, MA, MD,
MChir, FRCS**
Chief
Department of Surgery
Charing Cross and Westminster
Medical School
University of London
Fulham Palace Road
London W6 8RF, U.K.

W.J. GUSSENHOVEN, MD, PhD
Thoraxcenter and Intercardiology Inst.
University Hospital Rotterdam
Dr Molewaterplein 40,
3015 GD Rotterdam, The Netherlands

K.J. HANSEN, MD
Division of Surgical Sciences
The Bowman Gray
School of Medicine
Wake Forest University
300 South Hawthorne Road,
Winston-Salem, NC 27103, U.S.A.

L.H. HOLLIER, MD, FACS, FACC
Chairman
Department of Surgery
Ochsner Clinic and
Alton Ochsner Medical Foundation
Clinical Professor of Surgery
Louisiana State Univ. Medical Center
and Tulane University Medical Center
1514 Jefferson Highway
New Orleans, LA 70121, U.S.A.

A.M. IMPARATO, MD
Professor of Surgery
Director, Division of Vascular Surgery
New York University
550 First Avenue
New York, NY 10016, U.S.A.

A. IPPOLITI, MD
Department of Vascular Surgery
University of Rome "Tor Vergata"
Ospedale S. Eugenio
Piazzale dell'Umanesimo, 10
00144 Rome, ITALY

J.M. JAUSSERAN, MD
Dept. of Cardiovascular Surgery
Hopital St. Joseph
26, Boulevard de Louvain
13285 Marseille Cedex 8,
FRANCE

C.T. LANCEE, MD
Thoraxcenter Institute
University Hospital Rotterdam
Dr Molewaterplein 40,
3015 GD Rotterdam, The Netherlands

P. LEWIS, MD, FRCS
Department of Vascular Surgery
St. Mary's Hospital
Praed Street
London W2 1NY, U.K.

G. LORENZI, MD
Institute of Vascular Surgery and
Angiology
University of Milan
Via Commenda, 12
20122 Milan , ITALY

F. MACCIONI, MD
Department of Radiology
University of Rome, "La Sapienza"
Policlinico Umberto I°
00161 Rome , ITALY

P.E. MAGNAN, MD
Université Aix-Marseille II
Service de Chirurgie Vasculaire
des Hopitaux Sud
Hopital Sainte Marguerite
BP 29 13274 Marseille Cedex 9,
FRANCE

J.P. MATHIEU, MD
Université Aix-Marseille II
Service de Chirurgie Vasculaire
des Hopitaux Sud
Hopital Sainte Marguerite
BP 29 13274 Marseille Cedex 9,
FRANCE

S. MICHELAGNOLI, MD
Department of Vascular Surgery
University of Florence.
Ospedale Careggi
Viale Morgagni, 55
50134 Florence, ITALY

D. MILITE, MD
Department of Vascular Surgery
University of Padua
Via Giustiniani, 2
Padua, ITALY

P.M. MINGAZZINI, MD
Department of Vascular Surgery
University of Milan
Bassini Hospital
Via Massimo Gorki, 50
20092 Cinisello Balsamo (MI),
ITALY

W.S. MOORE, MD
Professor of Surgery
Chief, Section of Vascular Surgery
UCLA School of Medicine
Center for the Health Sciences
10833 Le Conte Avenue
Los Angeles, CA 90024-1749, U.S.A.

P. MORACCHINI, MD
Université Aix-Marseille II
Service de Chirurgie Vasculaire
des Hopitaux Sud
Hopital Sainte Marguerite
BP 29 13274 Marseille Cedex 9,
FRANCE

A.C. NOVICK, MD
Chairman
Department of Urology
The Cleveland Clinic Foundation
9500 Euclid Avenue
Cleveland, Ohio 44195 5041, U.S.A.

F. ORSI, MD
Department of Radiology
University of Rome, "La Sapienza"
Policlinico Umberto I°
00161 Rome , ITALY

R. PASSARIELLO, MD
Chief
Department of Radiology
University of Rome, "La Sapienza"
Policlinico Umberto I°
00161 Rome, ITALY

B. PERRETTI, MD
Department of Vascular Surgery
II° School of Medicine
University of Naples
Viu S. Pansini, 5
80131 Naples, ITALY

H. PIETERMAN, MD
Dept. of Radiology
University Hospital Rotterdam
Dr Molewaterplein 40,
3015 GD Rotterdam,
The Netherlands

G. R. PISTOLESE, MD
Chief
Department of Vascular Surgery
University of Rome "Tor Vergata"
Ospedale S. Eugenio
Piazzale dell'Umanesimo, 10
00144 Rome, ITALY

A.V. POKROVSKY, MD
Professor
A.V. Vishnevsky Institute of Surgery
27, B. Serpukhovskaya Str.
113811 Moscow, Russia

C. PRATESI, MD
Associate Professor
Department of Vascular Surgery
University of Florence
Ospedale Careggi
Viale Morgagni, 55
50134 Florence, ITALY

T.K. RAMOS, MD
Division of Vascular Surgery
U.C.S.F. San Francisco
California, U.S.A.

P. RICCI, MD
Department of Radiology
University of Rome, "La Sapienza"
Policlinico Umberto I°
00161 Rome , ITALY

S. RONCHEY, MD
Department of Vascular Surgery
University of Rome "Tor Vergata"
Ospedale S. Eugenio
Piazzale dell'Umanesimo, 10
00144 Rome, ITALY

M. ROSSI, MD
Department of Radiology
University of Rome, "La Sapienza"
Policlinico Umberto I°
00161 Rome, ITALY

P. ROSSI, MD
Chief
Department of Radiology
University of Rome,
"La Sapienza"
Policlinico Umberto I°
00161 Rome, ITALY

L.R. SAUVAGE, MD
Director
The Hope Heart Institute
528, 18th Avenue
Seattle, WA 98122- 5798, U.S.A.

G.P. SIGNORINI, MD
Service of Angiology
Padua Hospital
Padua, ITALY

C. SPARTERA, MD
Chief
Dept. of Vascular Surgery
University of L'Aquila
Pineta Signorini
Viale della Croce Rossa
67100 L'Aquila, ITALY

M.G. TAYLOR, MD
Division of Radiological Sciences and
Medicine, Guy's Campus, United
Medical and Dental Schools,
University of London
London, U.K.

S.H.K. THE, MD
Thoraxcenter and Intercardiology Inst.
University Hospital Rotterdam
Dr Molewaterplein 40,
3015 GD Rotterdam,
The Netherlands

F.C. VAN EGMOND, MD
Thoraxcenter Institute
University Hospital Rotterdam
Dr Molewaterplein 40,
3015 GD Rotterdam,
The Netherlands

H. van URK, MD, PhD
Department of Vascular Surgery
University Hospital Rotterdam
Dr. Molewaterplein, 40
3015 GD Rotterdam,
The Netherlands

A. VOSA, MD
Department of Vascular Surgery
II° School of Medicine
University of Naples
Via S. Pansini, 5
80131 Naples, ITALY

F.J. VEITH, MD
Professor of Surgery
Chief of Vascular Surgical Service
Montefiore Medical Center/
Albert Einstein College of Medicine
111 East 210th Street
Bronx, New York NY 10467-2490, U.S.A.

F. VERLATO, MD
Service of Angiology
Padua Hospital
Padua, ITALY

S. WHITE, MD
Department of Surgery and Pathology
University of Chicago
5841 South Maryland.
Avenue MC 5028
Chicago, Illinois 60637, U.S.A.

S.P. WARD, MD
Division of Radiological Sciences and
Medicine, Guy's Campus, United
Medical and Dental Schools,
University of London
London, U.K.

J.H.N. WOLFE, MS, FRCS
Department of Vascular Surgery
St. Mary's Hospital
Praed Street
London W2 1NY, U.K.

C.K. ZARINS, MD
Department of Surgery and Pathology
University of Chicago
5841 South Maryland Avenue MC 5028
Chicago, Illinois 60637, U.S.A.

BASIC CONSIDERATIONS

Basic Considerations

A.D. Callow

Department of Surgery, Washington University
School of Medicine
St. Louis, Missouri, U.S.A.

Reoperation in any anatomical region or organ system is a substantial challenge to the surgeon, to available treatment options, and to the patient's well being.

Reoperation within the vascular system is often more difficult and the outcome often less rewarding than elsewhere. Failure of redo vascular reconstructions may threaten life as well as the target limb or organ and do so more frequently than in other systems such as the musculoskeletal system and the gastrointestinal tract. Unlike primary operations, redo procedures must often be designed at the instant of operation.

Few guidelines for preoperative planning exist. Successful innovation is prized and outcome is difficult to predict. Until approximately a decade ago vascular surgery was in the fast lane of heady success engendered by sometimes dazzling technological innovations following one another in swift succession. Imaginative and creative surgeons, supported by improvements in diagnostic imaging and better medical evaluation and patient management, liberalized their operative indications. Surgical interventions extended into smaller arterial beds and into increasingly complex clinical problems. Vascular surgery was developed on large arteries without much technical analysis and little supporting basic science. These techniques, so successful with large vessels, were applied to vessels a tenth the size of those first subjected to endarterectomy or bypass grafting. The wonder and the exhilaration that followed the initial successes of large artery operations changed to disappointment and disenchantment as small arteries such as the dorsalis pedis and secondary and tertiary branches of the renal artery failed to retain intermediate and long term patency. Reality returned to the clinical scene with the realization that arterial reconstructive procedures were not immortal. Certain generalizations gradually emerged:

1) Duration of patency is
   a) inversely related to the resistance of the bypass channel; thus the longer the channel the shorter the period of patency;
   b) the smaller the lumen of the recipient vessel and the higher the resistance of the recipient arterial bed the shorter the period of patency;
2) The size of the anastomosis is not constant but dwindles over time;
3) The healing response of the "injured" artery is mediated by multiple factors, poorly understood, only partially identified and largely beyond therapeutic control;
4) The smaller the functional lumen of the recipient vessel the more vulnerable continued patency becomes to anastomotic hyperplasia.
5) The nonanatomic bypass reconstruction lack collaterals and thus depends on the continuing patency of the outflow tract to a greater extent than does a normal or "anatomic" vessel of similar length even with occlusive disease, and
6) Small vessel reconstructive procedures are less forgiving than are large vessels subjected to the same technical manipulations of vascular surgery.

The causes of acute failure which occurs within a few hours to days of operation are almost without exception identical in small and large vessel reconstructions. These are usually technical errors such as an improperly placed suture, the inadvertent creation of flap-like material within the lumen, which adds to the turbulence of flow, imperfect coaptation of the semi-rigid graft to the more pliable recipient arterial wall, inadequate anticoagulation or an overlooked thrombus within the graft or the vessel. Completion arteriography can be of great assistance in the detection of these technical imperfections.

The second large cause of acute failure is the improper selection of the patient in terms of the recipient vascular bed. This is the consequence of incomplete arteriography by intent or by error. It can usually be easily corrected by intraoperative distal arteriography.

Late failure of both small and large diameter vessel reconstructions may be due to one or a number of factors. Predominant among these are progressive atherosclerosis in distal vessels and anastomotic hyperplasia. A small reduction of flow in a small vessel exerts a greater hemodynamic effect distally than an equal reduction in a large vessel. Intimal hyperplasia that reduces the stoma of a 2 mm outflow vessel by approximately one third has no clinically detectable influence upon flow in a 10-15 mm reconstruction. It is not surprising therefore that late failure in an aortobifemoral bypass graft may not occur in the majority of patients until years later. Distal tibial grafts by contrast experience a rapid decrease in primary patency after 30 months.

PREVENTION

The incidence of early failure can be reduced by improvement in operating skills and better selection of patients. Late failures are not so readily in-fluenced. These are the result of the inexorable progression of two poorly understood events sometimes operating singly, other times jointly: the exten-sion of the atherosclerotic occlusive lesion and the proliferative cellular response with its inexorable accumulation of extracellular matrix. Those fac-tors considered risks for the development of the atherosclerotic lesion are equally if not more potent for the development of restenosis. Thus, patients undergoing arterial revascularization procedures of any type, whether en-darterectomy, bypass graft, atherectomy, or balloon angioplasty, either as primary or as adjuvant procedures, should be strongly and repetitively coun-selled concerning the hazards of cigarette use, the desirability of controlling hypertension, diabetes mellitus, excess weight, and the alleged beneficial ef-fects of regular exercise.

We have demonstrated in a rabbit model the synergistic effect of hyper-cholesterolemia on the volume extent of postarterial injury hyperplasia. In-timal hyperplasia is a major cause of failure in small diameter arterial reconstructions. Precise mechanisms mediating the cellular response of both intimal hyperplasia and atherosclerosis remain enigmatic. There are several similarities. The players for each lesion include: the smooth muscle cell, the endothelial cell, the lipid laden macrophage, the platelet, various mitogens, cytokines, and the activated T lymphocyte. Mechanistically, both are fueled by inflammatory pathways and driven by autocrine and paracrine systems. Both manifest complications of unchecked cellular proliferation. The endothelial cell and the smooth muscle cell play pivotal roles in the pathogenesis of both.

In an attempt to clarify this confusion New Zealand white rabbits were subjected to a standardized balloon catheter injury and fed a 0.25% cholesterol supplemented diet. These were administered alone or together for from 0 to 12 weeks with the aorta, the carotid and the iliac arteries as the target vessels as detailed in Table 1.

Table 1

I.	No mechanical injury, no cholesterol diet (n=5);
II.	No injury, 6 weeks cholesterol diet (n=5);
III.	No injury, 12 weeks cholesterol diet (n=11);
IV.	12 weeks injury, no cholesterol diet (n=5);
V.	6 weeks injury, 12 weeks cholesterol diet (n=6);
VI.	12 weeks injury, 6 weeks cholesterol diet (n=5);
VII.	12 weeks injury, 12 weeks cholesterol diet (n=5).

Cholesterol supplemented diets were initiated either 6 weeks prior to bal-loon injury, concurrent with injury, or 6 weeks post injury in the above 7 test groups.

Balloon injury alone induced uniform intimal smooth muscle cell proliferation and production of extracellular matrix. Vessels from animals treated with cholesterol alone showed periorificial fatty streaks dominated by foam cells. Combined cholesterol and balloon injury treatment elicited an exuberant intimal lesion characterized by fibrous tissue, smooth muscle cells at the perimeter, and centrally located foam cells. Indexed by intimal thickness or area fraction of lesioned intima, singly administered treatment, that is balloon injury or cholesterol supplementation, rarely resulted in significant lesion development. However, combinations of injury and cholesterol resulted in statistically significant and synergistic lesion enhancement. Marked lesion enhancement occurred in both the carotid and iliac arteries when cholesterol diet and mechanical injury were combined. This synergistic effect was seen regardless of when the cholesterol regimen was initiated, prior to, concurrent with, or following mechanical injury. The lipid lesions were seen only in cholesterol fed animals. Complete endothelial repaving of all denuded vessels, and leukocytes located preferentially over lesioned areas all lend credence to a priming effect of mechanical injury on lesion pathogenesis. The marked lesion increase seen in this combined catheter injury plus cholesterol diet model presents obvious clinical implications. Since hypercholesterolemia and mechanical injury have synergistic effects on intimal hyperplasia, success of vascular procedures may be impaired by co-existenting hypercholesterolemia. The benign nature of cholesterol reduction makes aggressive dietary modification in both the pre- and post-operative period attractive as well as practical and may improve patency of small diameter vascular reconstructions (Fig. 1).

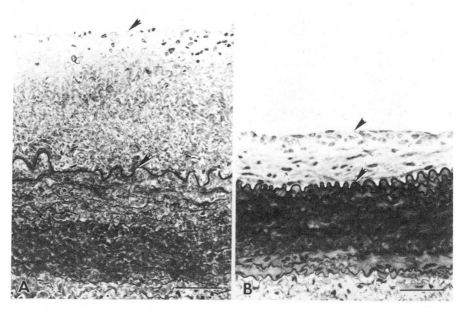

Fig. 1. The combination of injury and cholesterol resulted in statistically significant and synergistic lesion enhancement. * p=<0.05; ** p=<0.01 (Callow, et al, Ann Vasc Surg, in press.)

Additional laboratory evidence which may be of eventual usefulness in the prevention of intimal hyperplasia are our studies on the use of an endothelial cell specific mitogen to accelerate postinjury endothelial restitution. Damage to the endothelium occurs in the performance of any revascularization procedure. Endothelial damage also occurs in atherosclerosis. We postulated that more rapid endothelial repair might attenuate the hyperplastic response following arterial injury. Vascular permeability factor (VPF), a specific endothelial cell mitogen, was administered by intravenous injection to rabbits over a 4 week period following balloon denudation of the carotid artery. Rabbits were randomly divided into two treatment groups and received either recombinant VPF or vehicle. Endothelial cell repaving was significantly enhanced and intimal thickening was significantly less in the VPF treated animals versus the controls. The response of enhanced reendothelialization was clearly manifest as early as two weeks. Intimal thickening as measured by maximum intima-media ratio was significantly less in the VPF treated animals. Thus, it seemed reasonable to conclude that there was a correlation between rapid reendothelialization and reduction of post-injury intimal thickness.

The diagnosis of failed grafts has been immeasurably improved by advances in noninvasive techniques. For the failing peripheral graft, duplex scanning provides the most convenient and least hazardous diagnostic modality. Indeed, some authorities recommend routine noninvasive surveillance of peripheral bypass grafts to detect any changes in flow prior to the occurrence of symptoms and prior to complete thrombosis of the entire graft. Restoration or reconstitution is not only easier but more satisfactory when some flow is still present than after complete thrombosis and retrograde or prograde extension with clot organization and conversion into a fibrous scar. CT scanning is available for intracavitary reconstruction, even for such deeply situated and small vessels as the renal artery. To wait for symptoms to appear may result in loss of the ideal time for angiographic delineation of the problem and prompt therapeutic intervention. Reoperation may also be required for complications that may arise from graft impingement on viscera. These include aorto duodenal or other enteric fistulae and scar tissue entrapment of surrounding structures such as the ureter and other organs. Thus the complications of arterial surgery requiring reoperation may involve investigation of the urinary tract from the kidney to the bladder, of the gastrointestinal tract from stomach to rectum, as well as a search for causes of low grade and delayed onset infection, perigraft seroma, lymph fistula and cutaneous fistulae. Such redo operations may require the utmost ingenuity to remove the fistula, evacuate the hematoma, drain the abscess and preserve adequate distal arterial flow.

In general redo operations are far more frequent than were once anticipated, are technically more demanding, are associated with poorer short and long term revascularization results and often may require concomitant operative intervention on other organ systems than the vascular system alone.

Utilization of non-anatomic, and, at first glance, seemingly unphysiologic routes are frequently needed. Aside from avoidable technical errors, that is the errors of commission, the second single most frequent contribution to a poor result, if not a disaster, is the error of omission - surgical procrastination. When faced with the herald bleed of an aortoenteric fistula, a sudden change in the perfusion status of a lower extremity, or the gradual appearance of swelling in the groin, the site of a previous vascular anastomosis, delay is dangerous. With rare exception, these complications can only progress.

REFERENCES

1. VPF and intimal hyperplasia. Unpublished data.
2. Clowes AW, Gown AM, Hanson SR, et al. Mechanisms of arterial graft failure. I. Role of cellular proliferation in early healing of PTFE prostheses. *Am J Path*, 118:43-54,1985.
3. Clowes AW, Reidy MA, Clowes MM. Mechanisms of stenosis after arterial injury. *Lab Invest*, 49:208-215, 1983.
4. Rutherford RB, Flanigan DP, Gupta SK, et al. Suggested standards for reports dealing with lower extremity ischemia. *J Vasc Surg*, in press.
5. Gooding GAW, Effeney DJ, Goldstone J. The aortofemoral graft: Detection and identification of healing complications by ultrasonography. *Surgery*, 89:91-100, 1981
6. Whittemore AD, Clowes AW, Couch NP, et al. Secondary femoropopliteal reconstruction. *Ann Surg*, 193:35-42, 1981.
7. Ascer E, Veith FJ, Morin L, et al. Components of outflow resistance and their correlation with graft patency in lower extremity arterial reconstructions. *J Vasc Surg*, 1:817-828, 1984.
8. Mark A, Moss AA, Lusby R, et al. CT evaluation of complications of abdominal aortic surgery. *Radiology*, 145:409-414, 1982.
9. Reilly LM, Altman H, Lusby RJ, et al. Late results following surgical management of vascular graft infection. *J Vasc Surg*, 1:36-44, 1984.
10. Reilly LM, Goldstone J, Ehrenfeld WK, et al. Gastrointestinal tract involvement by prosthetic graft infection: The significance of gastrointestinal hemorrhage. *Ann Surg*, 202:1985
11. O'Donnell TF Jr, Scott G, Shepard AD, et al. Improvements in the diagnosis and management of aortoenteric fistula. *Am J Surg*, 149:481-486, 1985.
12. Stevens SL, Hilgarth K, Ryan US, Callow AD. The synergistic effect of hypercholesterolemia and mechanical injury on intimal hyperplasia. *Ann Vasc Surg*, in press.
13. Callow AD. Recurrent stenosis after carotid endarterectomy. *Arch Surg*, 117:1082-1085, 1982.
14. DePalma RG. Atherosclerosis in vascular grafts. *Athero Rev*, 6:147-177, 1979.
15. Echave V, Koornick AR, Haimov M, et al. Intimal hyperplasia as a complication of the use of the polytetrafluorethylene graft for femoral-popliteal bypass. *Surgery*, 86:791-798, 1979.
16. Chervu A, Moore WS. An overview of intimal hyperplasia. *Surg Gyn Obstet*, 171:433-447, 1990.
17. Clowes AW, Reidy MA, Clowes MM. Kinetics of cellular proliferation after arterial injury. I. Smooth muscle growth in the absence of endothelium. *Lab Invest*, 49:327-333, 1983.
18. Ross R. Cellular interactions, growth factors, and atherogenesis. *Atherosclerosis Rev*, 21:53-58, 1990.
19. Holm J, Hansson GK. Cellular and immunologic features of carotid artery disease in man and experimental animal models. *Eur J Vasc Surg*, 4:49-55, 1990.
20. Witztum JL. Current approaches to drug therapy for the hypercholesterolemic patient. *Circulation*, 80:1101-1114, 1989.
21. Sottiurai VS. Biogenesis and etiology of distal anastomotic intimal hyperplasia. *Int Angiol*, 9:359-69, 1990.
22. Fingerle J, Au YPT, Clowes AW, Reidy MA. Intimal lesion formation in rat carotid arteries after endothelial denudation in absence of medial injury. *Arteriosclerosis*, 10:1082-1087, 1990.
23. Campeau LC, Enjalbert M, Lesperance J, et al. The relation of risk factors to the development of atherosclerosis in saphenous-vein bypass grafts and the progression of disease in the native circulation. *N Engl J Med*, 311:1329-1332, 1984.

Thrombogenesis in Relation to Aging

D. Green

*Division of Hematology/Oncology, Department of Medicine,
Northwestern University Medical School and the Rehabilitation Institute,
Chicago, Illinois, U.S.A.*

Many diseases occur with greater frequency in the aged, including atherosclerosis, cancer of the prostate, and degenerative disorders of the brain. A predisposition to thrombosis, especially in those with advanced atherosclerosis, is commonly observed. Is this thrombotic tendency solely to the vascular disease, or are there biochemical changes in the blood that are age-related and contribute to the thrombotic risk? Assuming such changes do occur, could they be due to the effects of atherosclerosis on the delicate vascular endothelium; in other words, are they secondary phenomenons? If there is hypercoagulability of the blood, does this augment atherogenesis? Answers to these questions remain elusive, but a variety of age-related changes in hemostasis have been established and will be described in this report. Wherever possible, these alterations in coagulability will be linked to the pathologic processes of vascular occlusion.

PLATELETS

While platelet number remains constant with aging, platelets in the elderly are more likely to release their granules and spontaneously aggregate. Platelet factor 4 and beta-thromboglobulin, two components of the platelet alpha granules, were found in higher concentrations in the plasma of elderly as compared to young subjects[12,19]. Platelets are activated by shear stress and by exposure to subendothelial connective tissue. Zahavi et al.[19] suggest that contact of platelets with narrowed, atheromatous vessels may be responsible for the activation of the platelets and release of their granular contents.

Spontaneous platelet aggregation is defined as the ability of platelets to aggregate in stirred platelet-rich plasma at 37° C, and has been reported with both normal and increased platelet counts; it may be present even when platelet aggregation induced by standard aggregating agents is not excessive[15]. It has been shown to increase with increasing age[3], hematocrit, and fibrinogen concentration[5]. Patients with this phenomenon often have transient ischemic attacks, strokes and ischemic peripheral vascular disease[15,17].

The mechanism of the increased platelet activation and aggregation with aging has been investigated recently. Phosphoinositides play a critical role in platelet activation; inositol 1,4,5-triphosphate mobilizes calcium ions from the vescicles of the platelet dense tubular system, and 1,2-diacylglycerol, a metabolic product of the phosphoinositide pathway, activates protein kinase C; the latter phosphorylates myosin light chain, which is important in platelet secretion[9]. Bastyr et al.[1] found that phosphoinositide turnover stimulated by thrombin progressively increased with advancing age, and that the incorporation of labelled phosphorus into phosphoinositide metabolites correlated with platelet aggregation and beta thromboglobulin release. They concluded that the enhanced platelet activity found in the aged might be a consequence of increased platelet polyphosphoinositide turnover.

COAGULATION FACTORS

There have been several studies of clotting factors in the elderly[7,10,14]. Hager et al.[7] compared clotting factor concentrations in three groups of subjects: young (n=21, age 29+6); old, healthy (n=32, age 79+7); and old, diseased (n=31, age 77+5). The most striking differences were in the levels of fibrinogen (mg/dl): 246 vs. 367 vs. 578, respectively; the difference between young and old was significant at $p<0.001$.

In addition, factor VII(%) (114 vs. 143 vs. 124) and factor VIII(%) (100 vs. 128 vs. 147) were also significantly different between young and old. Fibrinogen concentrations in the elderly have been shown to fluctuate seasonally, reaching their highest values in the winter months when cardiovascular mortality is highest[14]. The increases in factor VII include both activity and antigen, and the highest activity levels are observed in those with atherosclerotic disease[10]. The relationship between elevated levels of fibrinogen and factor VII, and ischemic heart disease has been documented by the Northwick Park Heart Study, which showed that subjects with increased concentrations of these clotting factors were at highest risk[13]. Hyperfibrinogenemia, perhaps because it is associated with hyperviscosity, was associated with the greatest risk of myocardial infarction. Stroke incidence has also been correlated with raised fibrinogen concentrations[18].

von Willebrand factor is an adhesive glycoprotein that also increases with advancing age. Studies in pigs have shown that von Willebrand factor is required for the development of coronary thrombosis in animals fed an atherogenic diet[4]. The factor is necessary for a carpet of platelets to be laid down on the sub-endothelium. Monoclonal anti-von Willebrand factor antibodies markedly decrease the deposition of platelets and thrombus formation after both superficial and deep vascular injury[4,6]. Whether increased levels of von Willebrand factor are thrombogenic or atherogenic is uncertain.

In summary, clotting factors associated with atherothrombotic disease increase with advancing age, but whether these increases are primary, secondary to atherosclerosis, or promote atherosclerosis and its complications, has not been established.

FIBRINOLYTIC SYSTEM

Prekallikrein and high molecular weight kininogen play an important role in the activation of fibrinolysis. Hager et al.[7] observed a significant increase in both factors in the healthy elderly as compared to young persons. Plasminogen, the precursor of the fibrinolytic enzyme plasmin, and alpha-2 antiplasmin, an inhibitor of fibrinolysis, did not differ between young and old. Taken together, these results suggest that fibrinolytic activity would either be no different, or enhanced, in the elderly. However, Hashimoto et al.[8], who studied subjects up to age 60, found that plasminogen activator activity showed a significant decrease ($p < 0.01$) with aging. This loss of capacity to convert plasminogen to the active enzyme would result in impaired ability to lyse thrombi.

CLOTTING FACTOR INHIBITORS

Proteins C, S, and Antithrombin III

The principal plasma inhibitors of coagulation are proteins C, its cofactor protein S, and antithrombin III. Hager et al.[7] noted no differences in protein C, but antithrombin III levels were significantly lower in the old, both healthy and diseased, as compared with the young. Bauer et al.[2] took this one step further and measured age-associated changes in indices of thrombin generation and protein C activation. During coagulation, factor X becomes activated and cleaves a fragment from prothrombin (fragment F_{1+2}). The levels of this fragment were found to increase as a function of age (up to age 80; only males were examined). This observation suggests a subtle activation of coagulation with aging.

To confirm these results, the investigators also assayed levels of fibrinopeptide A and the activation peptide of protein C, since thrombin generated during coagulation would be expected to cleave peptides from both fibrinogen and protein C. Both these peptides showed significant age-related correlations. The authors concluded that many apparently normal males demonstrate a hypercoagulable state, but that the etiology of this hypercoagulability is speculative. Aging of endothelium with loss of binding sites for antithrombin III would be one possible mechanism, since such binding is important in the activation of antithrombin III.

Anti-Phospholipid Antibodies

Antibodies directed against a variety of natural and synthetic phospholipids are found in higher concentrations in the old than in the young[11]. Some of these phospholipids accelerate coagulation reactions in vitro, and antibodies to such phospholipids have been designated "lupus anticoagulants", although the patients may not meet the clinical criteria for lupus, and do not exhibit a bleeding tendency. On the contrary, about a third of the patients with "lupus anticoagulants" have recurrent arterial or venous thrombosis.

The mechanism for such thrombosis is not clear; inhibition of prostacycline generation, prevention of factor Va inactivation by activated protein C, interference with the release of tissue plasminogen activator, as well as other theories have been proposed. These antiphospholipid autoantibodies constitute another risk factor for thrombosis in the elderly.

ENDOTHELIUM

The endothelium serves a variety of critical functions in the regulation of hemostasis[16]. As mentioned above, it provides specific proteoglycans important in the activation of antithrombin III. It is also a source of tissue plasminogen activator and prostacycline, the latter a vasodilator and potent inhibitor of platelet aggregation. Thrombomodulin, a thrombin receptor required for protein C activation, is an endothelial cell membrane protein. A local vasoconstrictor, endothelin-1, is synthesized by endothelial cells and is a paracrine activator of phospholipase C in these cells. Lastly, endothelium releases endothelial cell relaxing factor-nitric oxide, a strong vasodilator and inhibitor of platelet adhesion and aggregation. The effect of aging on the ability of vascular tissue to synthesize and release these various regulators of hemostasis is still largely unknown.

SUMMARY

With aging, there are increases in the plasma concentrations of fibrinogen, factor VII, factor VIII and von Willebrand factor. Elevated levels of these factors identify a population at high risk for ischemic heart disease and stroke. Furthermore, tissue plasminogen activator activity, a key component of the fibrinolytic system, declines with age. Sensitive methods have shown that in elderly men there is activation of the coagulation system, as defined by raised amounts of prothrombin fragments and protein C activation peptide in the circulation. In addition, there is evidence of platelet activation with aging, with increases in the plasma content of platelet granule contents, hypersensitivity to platelet aggregating agents, and spontaneous platelet aggregation.

Finally, age-related changes in the endothelium may have a major impact on hemostasis. Whether changes in the circulating factors or endothelium are the cause or the result of the vascular occlusive disease observed in the elderly is a provocative question for investigators in this field.

GRANT ACKNOWLEDGEMENT

This work was supported by grant HL-43758-01 from the NHLBI, National Institutes of Health, USA

REFERENCES

1. Bastyr EJ, Kadrofske MM, Vinik AI. Platelet activity and phosphoinositide turnover increase with advancing age. *Am J Med,* 1990; 88: 601-606.
2. Bauer KA, Weiss LM, Sparrow D, Vokonas PS, Rosenberg RD. Aging-associated changes in indices of thrombin generation and protein C activation in humans. *J Clin Invest,* 1987; 80: 1527-1534.
3. Breddin K, Grun H, Krzywanek HJ, Schremmer WP. On the measurement of spontaneous platelet aggregation. *Thromb Haemostas,* 1976; 35: 669-691.
4. Brinkhous KM, Reddick RL, Read MS, Nichols TC, Bellinger DA, Griggs TR. Von Willebrand factor and animal models: contributions to gene therapy, thrombotic thrombocytopenic purpura, and coronary artery thrombosis. *Mayo Clin Proc,* 1991; 66: 733-742.
5. Burgess-Wilson ME, Green S, Heptinstall S, Mitchell JRA. Spontaneous platelet aggregation in whole blood: dependence on age and haematocrit. *Lancet,* 1984; ii: 1213 (letter).
6. Fuster V, Badimon L, Badimon JJ, Ip JH, Chesebro, JH. The porcine model for the understanding of thrombogenesis and atherogenesis. *Mayo Clin Proc,* 991; 66: 818-831.
7. Hager K, Setzer J, Vogl T, Voit J, Platt D. Blood coagulation factors in the elderly. *Arch Gerontol Geriatr,* 1989; 9:277-282.
8. Hashimoto Y, Kobayashi A, Yamazaki N, Sugawara Y, Takada Y, Takada A. Relationship between age and plasma t-PA, PA-inhibitor, and PA activity. *Thromb Res,* 1987; 46: 625-633.
9. Haslam RJ. Signal transduction in platelet activation. In Thrombosis and Haemostasis 1987, edited by Verstraete M, Vermylen J, Lijnen R, Arnout J. Leuven University Press, Leuven, Belgium, 1987, pp 147-174.
10. Kario K, Matsuo T, Nakao K. Factor VII hyperactivity in the elderly. *Thromb Haemostas,* 1991; 65: 25-27.
11. Love PE, Santoro SA. Antiphospholipid antibodies: anti-cardiolipin and the lupus anticoagulant in systemic lupus erythematosus(SLE) and in non-SLE disorders. *Ann Intern,* Med 1990; 112: 682-698.
12. Ludlam CA. Evidence for the platelet specificity of B-thromboglobulin and studies on its plasma concentration in healthy individuals. *Br J Haematol,* 1979; 41: 271-278.
13. Meade TW, Brozovic M, Chakrabarti RR, Haines AP, Imeson JD, Mellows S, Miller GJ, North WRS, Stirling Y, Thompson SG. Haemostatic function and ischaemic heart disease: principal results of the Northwick Park Heart Study. *Lancet,* 1986; ii: 533-537.
14. Stout RW, Crawford V. Seasonal variations in fibrinogen concentrations among elderly people. *Lancet,* 1991; 338: 9-13.
15. Ts'ao Ch, Ali N, Kolb T. Spontaneous platelet aggregation: its characteristics and relation to aggregation by other agents. *Thromb Haemostas,* 1978; 39: 379-385.

16. Vane JR, Anggard EE, Botting RM. Regulatory functions of the vascular endothelium. *N Engl J Med,* 1990; 323: 27-36.
17. Vreeken J, van Aken WG. Spontaneous aggregation of blood platelets as a cause of idiopathic thrombosis and recurrent painful toes and fingers. *Lancet,* 1971; ii: 1394-7.
18. Wilhelmsen L, Svardsudd K, Korsan-Bengtsen K, Larsson B, Welin L, Tibblin G. Fibrinogen as a risk factor for stroke and myocardial infarction. *N Engl J Med,* 1984; 311: 501-505.
19. Zahavi J, Jones NAG, Leyton J, Dubiel M, Kakkar VV. Enhanced in vivo platelet "release reaction" in old healthy individuals. *Thromb Res,* 1980; 17: 329-336.

Hemodynamic Factors in Anastomotic Intimal Hyperplasia

H.S. Bassiouny, C.K. Zarins,
S. Glagov, S. White and D.P. Giddens *

Department of Surgery and Pathology , University of Chicago
Chicago, Illinois, U.S.A.
* *Department of Aerospace Engineering, Georgian Institute of Technology*

INTRODUCTION

Anastomotic intimal hyperplasia, a nonatherosclerotic form of intimal thickening is a major cause of arterial stenosis, occurring typically at the distal end to side anastomosis of bypass grafts[1-3]. The pathobiologic mechanisms underlying the early development of this lesion and it's progression to an occlusive lesion is the focus of considerable basic and clinical research. Two major hypothesis are under investigation. The first is the "response to injury" hypothesis which emphasizes the roles of endothelial injury, platelet adherence and activation, and elaboration of smooth muscle cell mitogenic factors[4-6]. This concept has evolved from innumerable animal experiments in which balloon catheter injury of the intima is induced[7-10] Pharmacologic agents to minimize this process at vascular anastomosis have nonetheless been unsuccessful.[11-12] The second hypothesis implicates biomechanical forces. The de novo anastomotic geometry and implanted graft engender major alterations in flow velocities, near wall flow patterns, wall shear, tensile stress compliance mismatch and tissue vibration[13-15]. These forces may stimulate smooth muscle proliferation through mechanisms that are, to a limited extent, understood. In vitro, endothelial cells respond to changes in shear stress by alteration in morphology and cytoskeletal structure,[16-17] prostacyclin, mitogen secretion, tissue plasminogen activator transcription and potassium channel activation[20-23]. Smooth muscle cells submitted to increased cyclical stretch responds by increasing collagen production[34].

It is our contention that all anastomotic thickening is not the same; different types exist, and the underlying mechanism regulating each type may vary. We have conducted invivo animal experiments and concordant elaborate model flow studies to characterize the location and magnitude of anastomotic intimal thickening in end to side autogenous vein and PTPE anastomosis, and qualitatively correlated these histopathologic findings with the hemodynamic patterns characterized in the flow models.

INVIVO STUDIES

Previous experiments in our laboratory have demonstrated the reproductibility of anastomotic intimal thickening in a canine model. The lesion consists of proliferating smooth muscle cells in an abundant stroma with scanty matrix fibers (Fig. 1). This particular form of intimal thickening resembles another form of intimal proliferation, intimal fibrocellular hypertrophy; an orderly layered thickening of the intima, similar to, but not identical to arterial wall medial architecture. This type of intimal thickening appears to represent an adjustment or adaptive response to maintain the structural in-

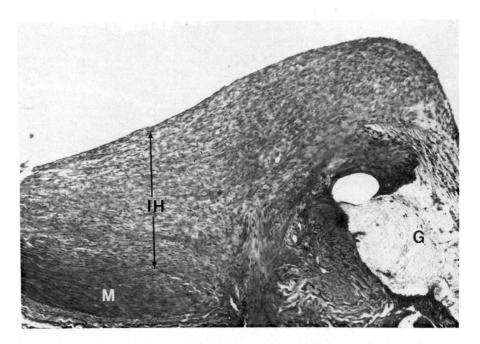

Fig. 1. Typical intimal hyperplastic reaction (IH) above the media (M) at an and to side PTFE anastomosis. Typically IH is composed of proliferating smooth muscle cell in abundant stroma with scanty matrix fibers.

tegrity of the artery wall at bends, geometric transitions, and in regions of altered flow[24-29].

To investigate the precise location and magnitude of anastomotic intimal thickening, iliofemoral bypasses were implanted using autogenous reverse saphenous vein on one side and thin walled PTFE grafts on the contralateral side in a canine model. Both external iliac arteries were ligated to simulate an arterial occlusion and produce an inflow outflow pressure gradient. Distal anastomotic geometry was standardized with a hood length to vessel diameter ratio of 4:1 and a maximum hood width of 6 mm's at the center of the anastomosis. The outflow conditions were standardized such that all distal end to side anastomosis were constructed beyond the deep femoral artery in a superficial femoral artery segment devoid of side branches. Housing and handling of animals were in compliance with "Principles of Laboratory Animal Care" and "Guide for the Care and Use of Laboratory Animals" (NIH publication #80-23, revised 1985).

Blood flow was measured in the common iliac artery proximal to the bypass grafts and in the proximal and distal outflow limbs of the distal end to side anastomosis and systemic blood pressure was measured with an indwelling 21 gauge brachial arterial cannula. The invivo hemodynamic data were recorded simultaneously on a four channel FM tape recorder. Mean systemic blood pressure was 93 ± 9.5 mmHg (range 75 to 110). Mean blood flow in the PTFE grafts was 192 ± 32 mls/min and in the vein grafts was 160 ± 68 mls/min. At the distal anastomosis, mean flow through the proximal outflow limb of PTFE bypass was 34 ± 26 mls/min and of vein bypass 59 ± 32 mls/min. Mean flow through the distal outflow limb of PTFE grafts was 149 ± 74 mls/min and 121 ± 82 mls/min. There were no significant differences between inflow or outflow volumetric flow rates in PTFE and vein grafts. The in vivo distal to proximal outflow division ratio was 75:25. Peak Reynold numbers for these conditions was 650 based on graft diameters and assuming an kinematic viscosity of blood, v, to be 0.035 cm^2/sec. The average Reynolds number for the entire cycle was 260, and the frequency, f, of the waveforms was 2 Hz, the Womersley parameter was 3.8. Postoperatively, all animals received 125 mg. of aspirin daily to reduce platelet aggregation and promote graft patency. After 8 weeks, the animals were sacrificed. The distal aorta, iliac arteries, bypass grafts and distal anastomoses were pressure perfusion fixed with 3% glutaraldehyde at 100 mmHg. The distal anastomosis including the graft hood, suture line and proximal and distal outflow tracts were harvested en bloc and sectioned in the sagittal and transverse planes (20-24 samples/specimen). The samples were embedded in paraffin and adjacent 5 mm sections were stained with hematoxylin and eosin, and the Gomori-trichrome-aldehyde fuchsin procedure for connective-tissue differentiation. Regions of anastomotic intimal thickening were identified using light microscopy and their location in relation to anastomotic junction (sinus, toe, heel) and host artery (floor, proximal, distal outflow tracts) mapped. Intimal thickness was measured using a Zeiss oculomicrometer.

Topography of Intimal Thickening

Histologic sections from the anastomoses revealed 2 separate and distinct regions of anastomotic intimal thickening; one at the suture line and the other on the floor of the artery. Suture line intimal thickening was observed in all PTFE and vein anastomoses and developed at the graft/vessel wall junction; in the sinus, at the toe and the heel of the anastomoses (Fig. 2). Arterial floor intimal thickening was noted in 84% of the anastomoses. The arterial lesion was located in the midplane opposite the distal portion of the graft hood and was relatively closer to the distal than the proximal outflow tract. Intimal thickening was not identified in the proximal or distal outflow arterial segments.

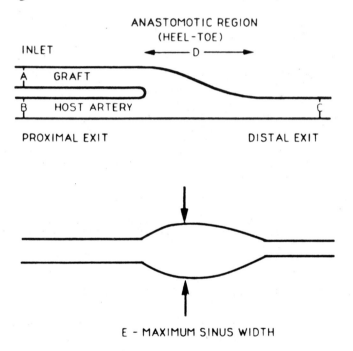

Fig. 2. An illustration of a sagittal section of the end to side anastomosis depicting sites of localization of intimal thickening at the suture line and artery floor.

Histopathologic and Quantitative Morphometry

Intimal thickening consisted of proliferating cells, predominantly smooth muscle and myfibroblasts within a loose connective tissue matrix above the intimal elastic lamina. The overlying endothelium was intact with no evidence of immediate surface thrombosis or organization of previous thrombi. Along the lateral walls of the anastomoses, at the suture line, a hyperplastic tissue pannus consisting of a structured layer of subintimal cells migrated from the artery onto graft surface. This covered the triangulation deformity at the anastomotic junction in the sinus region resulting in a more circular lumen configuration (Fig. 3). In the heel and toe regions suture line intimal thickening projected slight into the lumen. Suture line intimal thickness was significantly greater in PTFE anastomoses than in vein anastomoses. The magnitude of arterial floor intimal thickness was not different between PTFE and vein grafts.

Topography of Anastomotic Intimal Thickening (IT)

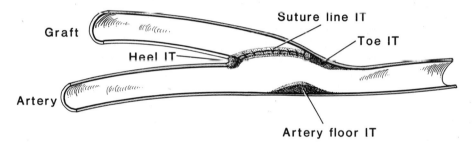

Fig. 3. Anastomotic measurements used in flow model construction. The major geometric features of the anastomosis were replicated including the slope of the hood and the anastomotic sinus.

MODEL FLOW VISUALIZATION STUDIES

The flow patterns in regions of anastomotic intimal thickening were characterized in upscaled (7.5 times) transparent sylgard models constructed with the identical in vivo end to side anastomotic geometry and dimensions (Fig. 4). The invivo pulsatile flow conditions; Reynolds number, outflow division, (80 distal: 20 proximal) and pulsatile waveforms, were simulated in the model with a computer controlled Teel pump. The flow system is represented in Fig. 5. Neutrally buoyant 200 micron amberlite particles were infused into the flow system and particle trajectroy in the pulsatile flow field was visualized using 15 m w He-Ne laser sheet of light in the horizontal planc of the model. Particle path lines were photographed on at six selected times during the pulse cycle using and exposure time of 0.5 secs. Three dimensional particle movement was also determined in the vertical plane under incandescent lighting using a video camera.

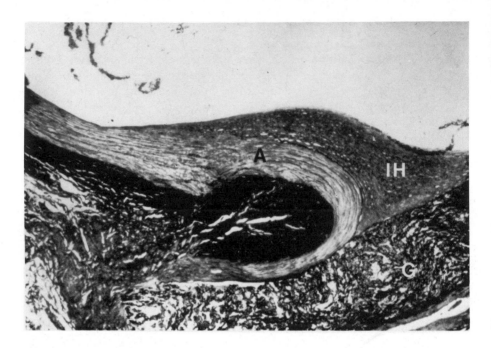

Fig. 4. Suture line intimal thickening in the anastomotic sinus (transverse section). A pannus of proliferating smooth muscle cells (IH) extendes from the artery (A) to the graft surface (GH), thus covering the triangular deformity at the anastomotic junction (Hematoxylin and eosin; original magnification x40).

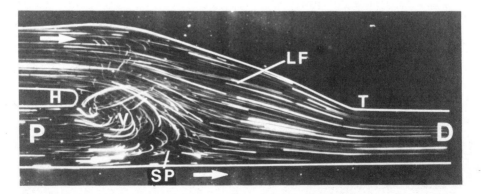

Fig. 5. Model flow visualization studies. Neutrally buoyant particles are illuminated in the pulsatile flow field using He-Ne laser sheet of late. Early in the acceleration phase of laminar flow (LF) is observed along the hood of graft. A starting vortex (V) develops at the heel near the proximal outflow tract. Flow reattaches on the arterial floor along the stagnation point (SP).

End to side graft anastomosis to the arteriotomy produced lumen cross sectional enlargement and an adverse pressure gradient. As a result of this geometric transition, distinct secondary flow patterns developed in the anastomosis and varied during the different phases of the pulse cycle. Regions of relatively high and low particle velocities were indicative of high and low shear.

During the acceleration phase in early systole, flow is laminar with skewing of particles toward the hood of the anastomoses (Fig. 5). On the arterial floor a stagnation point which oscillated in the proximal/distal direction was identified. Streamlines falling lateral to the midplane exhibited a circumferential velocity component toward the sinus region, with particles becoming entwined into the separation region along the side walls. Particles traversing near the midplane assumed a laminar trajectory to the proximal or distal outflow tracts. The location of the stagnation point oscillated in direction and shear throughout the pulse cycle, moving distally during the acceleration phase of systole and in a reverse direction proximally during the deceleration phase (Figs. 6,7).

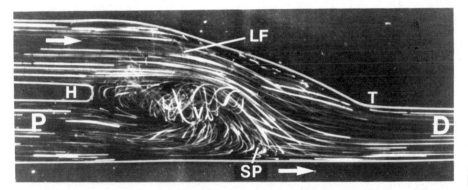

Fig. 6. In mid systole, the vortex structure rolls into the sinus region. The stagnation point (SP) has moved distally during the acceleration phase of systole.

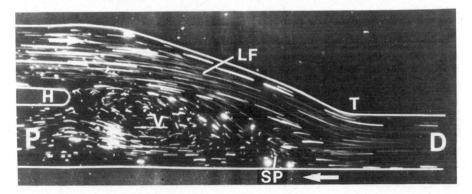

Fig. 7. During diastole, the stagnation point (SP) moves in the reverse direction towards the proximal outflow tract.

In the region of the suture line and lateral wall, (anastomotic sinus), secondary flow patterns were observed. Early in each cycle, flow separated from the heel of the anastomosis where vortex formation started and rolled into the sinus region (Fig. 5). Flow separation also occurred along the lateral sinus walls where particle residence time was prolonged with delayed clearing and accumulation of the particles.

In a different set of experiments, increasing the anastomotic hood length ratio to 8:1, outflow division ratio and Re number had a demonstrable effect on the flow field. A flow separation region occurred along the distal section of the hood with tendency of the stagnation point to move distally with increasing proximal outflow ratio and Re number (Fig. 8).

Qualitative correlation between the histopathologic findings observed in the invivo anastomoses and the flow visualization studies indicate that: 1) Intimal thickness was absent along the graft hood where flow was laminar and high shear, short particle residence time prevailed, 2) Arterial floor intimal thickening developed in the region where the stagnation point oscillated during the pulse cycle and shear was low. Flow patterns consistent with separation, relatively low shear and long particle residence time also formed along the heel and lateral wall of the anastomotic sinus where suture line intimal thickness was present. Model flow studies designed to measure rear wall velocity gradients using laser doppler anemometry methods are ongoing. Early results indicate exceedingly low shear stress levels in the stagnation point region (-2 to + 5 dynes/cm^2) and shear stress levels over 40 dynes/cm^2 along the anastomotic hood.

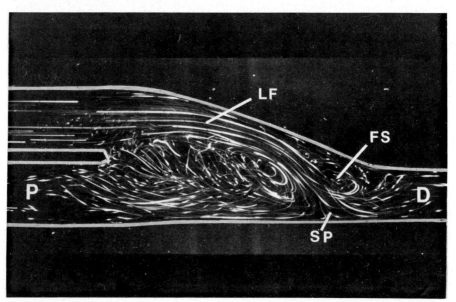

Fig. 8. During the descending phase of systole increasing flow division to 50:50 resulted in flow separation (FS) along the toe of the anastomosis.

DISCUSSION

The quest for elucidating the precise etiology of anastomotic intimal hyperplasia has driven investigators in the field of vascular research to utilize a plethora of animal models, injurious agents and counteragent such as cytotoxic, immunosuppressive drugs, thermal injury, growth factor antibodies. It should be emphasized that intimal smooth muscle proliferative response observed in these studies is a normal feature of vascular healing in response to mechanical injury. As such it is usually self limited and not a runaway response. These models of intimal thickening should not be misconstrued as a models of intimal hyperplasia which produces anastomotic stenosis and graft failure in humans. Occlusive intimal hyperplasia is characteristically poorly organized, consists of nonoriented smooth muscle cells in a uniform ground substance with few collagen or elastin fibers. This tissue reaction maintains an intact endothelium with no evidence of platelet aggregation on medial injury. The important question is, why does, adaptive intimal thickening progress to an uncontrolled occlusive lesion resulting in anastomotic stenosis, low flow and eventual graft thrombosis. To resolve this query, we have sought initially to establish an animal model that closely resembles the human clinical setting, to characterize the different types of anastomotic intimal thickening and define the associated hemodynamic alterations[30].

Intimal thickening, in this model developed at two distinct and separate sites, at the suture line and along the floor of the artery opposite the anastomotic hood. Suture line intimal thickening appears to represent vascular hoaling and remodelling in response to mechanical injury or compliance mismatch. The prominence of the lesion with prosthetic grafts in this study, may be a consequence of the greater cyclic deformations associated with the marked difference in the mechanical properties between PTFE and native artery as compared with vein wall and native artery.

Considerable attention has been focused on compliance mismatch as a significant determinant of graft patency and intimal hyperplasia[14, 31-33]. It is suggested that differences in the mechanical properties of graft and artery may promote anastomotic intimal thickening. Regions of hypercompliance have also been demonstrated in end to end isocomplaint arterial anastomoses suggesting that the mere existence of a suture line can produce this biomechanical perturbation. Although hypercompliance may result in increased smooth muscle cyclical stretch and collagen synthesis[34], in vivo experimental evidence supporting this tenet is lacking. Conversely, reduction of arterial wall motion has been shown to reduce arterial wall metabolism, biosynthesis of matrix components and atherosclerotic lesion formation[35]. Further studies correlating peranastomotic strain and compliance measurements with intimal thickening are underway to clarify the role of compliance mismatch.

Although surgical trauma and endothelial injury have been shown to induce smooth muscle cell proliferation and subsequent intimal thickening, the role of acute vascular injury has been questioned by a number of investigators and conflicting reports exist on the efficacy of antiplatelet agents in promoting graft patency and limiting intimal hyperplasia[12,36,37]. Clowes and others have demonstrated that the smooth muscle proliferative response to acute injury is short lived and eventually regresses[38].

Model flow visualization[30,39] studies revealed complex secondary flow patterns in the vicinity of the suture line. The adverse pressure gradient created by the relatively large anastomotic sinus resulted in flow separation along the lateral walls, at the anastomotic heel where helical formations developed and rolled into the sinus region during the acceleration phase of systole. These secondary flow patterns may interact with other biomechanical and humoral factors to modulate suture line intimal thickening. The process may be self-limiting and abate once the local intimal thickening has remodelled the surface irregularities which result in the secondary flow patterns.

Arterial intimal thickening at the floor of the anastomosis was identified in all but one PTFE and one vein anastomosis. This change developed where flow entering the anastomosis reattached along the arterial floor and oscillated in direction during the pulsatile cycle. The reattachment zone or stagnation point appeared similar to the three dimensional separation region observed along the outer wall in the sinus of the human internal carotid artery. In other studies by White et al[40], this stagnation point moved distally if proximal outflow increased from 0 to 50% or the hood length doubled. Additionally, significant changes in the secondary flow patterns along the lateral sinus and heel of the anastomosis were observed. Hence the anastomotic flow field is greatly influenced by the anastomotic geometry and outflow divisions. Ojha[41] and others[13] studied steady and pulsatile flow fields in an end to side arterial anastomosis model and noted that low axial wall shear stress was present at the reattachment point on the artery floor, the toe of the anastomosis and the proximal region of the host artery. The hemodynamic patterns elucidated in our study are similar to their findings.

It is well recognized that arteries adapt to chronic changes in flow or pressure by alterations in dimension, configuration or wall composition[42-44]. These adaptations appear to be self limiting and cease when ideal hemodynamic conditions are established at the endothelial surface. Increased flow velocity results in artery enlargement until lumen radius results in restitution of normal baseline wall shear levels[45,46]. Conversely, a reduction in flow velocity may result in lumen narrowing to achieve the same goal[47]. In both human and experimental vessels, intimal thickening is a common response to lowered or oscillatory shear. Moreover, the degree of intimal thickening is inversely related to wall shear stress levels[48]. Inflow, outflow resistance and geometric configurations such as end to side anastomoses create adverse local hemodynamic conditions that may incite an intimal proliferative response.

The topography and morphologic features of anastomotic intimal thickening observed suggest an adaptive or remodelling response to the imposed biomechanical and flow conditions. If baseline conditions are achieved, intimal proliferation would be expected to cease. However, with persistence of abnormal configurations and low flow velocities, the stimulus of intimal proliferation may continue and progressive intimal hyperplasia would occur leading eventually to lumen stenosis and graft occlusion.

In conclusion, we have identified two different types of anastomotic intimal thickening and the conditions underlying their initiation. Suture line intimal thickening may be related to compliance mismatch, and focal geometric deformations which result in complex secondary flow patterns. Arterial floor intimal thickening remote from the sture line develops in regions of flow reattachment and low and oscillating shear. These findings corroborate with observations in the clinical setting where occlusive intimal occurs predominantly on the floor of the host vessel and extending to the outflow tracts. Specific investigations of microanatomy, smooth muscle kinetics and molecular events which initiate and perpetuate the smooth muscle proliferative response with varying hemodynamic conditions will help identify those factors responsible for progression of anastomotic intimal thickening to an occlusive stenosis.

REFERENCES

1. Imparato AM, Bracco A, Kim GE, Zeff R. Intimal and neointimal fibrous proliferation causing failure of arterial reconstruction. *Surgery,* 1972; 72:1007-17
2. Echave V., Koornick A., Haimov M., and Jacobson J. Intimal hyperplasia as a complication of the use of the polytetrafluoroethylene graft for femoral-popliteal bypass. *Surgery,* 86(6):791-798, 1979.
3. Garratt K.N., Edwards W.D., Kaufmann U.P., Vlietstra R.E., Holmes D.R. Jr.: Differential histopathology of primary atherosclerotic and restenotic lesions in coronary arteries and saphenous vein bypass grafts: Analysis of tissue obtained from 73 patients by directional atherectomy. *J Am Coll Cardiol,* 1991; 17:442-448.
4. M.A. Golden, Y.P.T. Au, R.D. Kenagy and A.W. Clowes: Growth factor gene expression by intimal cells in healing polytetrafluoroethylene grafts. *J Vasc Surg,* 4, 580-585 (1990).
5. Baumgartner HR, Hadenschild C. Adhesion of platelets to subendothelium. *Ann NY Acad Sci,* 1972; 201:22-36.
6. Barrett TB, Benditt EP. Sis (platelet-derived growth factor B chain) gene transcript levels are elevated in human atherosclerotic lesions compared to normal artery. *Proc Natl Acad Sci USA,* 1987;84:1099-1103.
7. Clowes AW, Reidy MA, Clowes MM: Kinetics of cellular proliferation after arterial injury. I. Smooth muscle growth in the absence of endothelium. *Lab Invest,* 1983;49:327-333.
8. Kohler TR, Jawien A, Clowes AW: Effect of shear on intimal hyperplasia following arterial injury in rats (abstract). *Circulation,* 1990:82(suppl III):III-400.
9. Clowes AW, Schwartz SM: Significant of quiescent smooth muscle migration in the injured rat carotid artery. *Circ Res,* 1985;56:139-145.
10. Clowes A W, Clowes M.M., Reidy M.A.: Kinetics of cellular proliferation after arterial injury. III Endothelial and smooth muscle growth in chronically denuded vessels. *Lab Invest,* 1986;54:295-303.
11. Clowes AW, Karnovsky MJ: Failure of certain antiplatelet drugs to affect myointimal thickening following arterial endothelial injury in the rat. *Lab Invest,* 36(4):452-464, 1977.
12. McCready R, Price M, Kryscio R, Hyde G, Mattingly S, Griffen W Jr.: Failure of antiplatelet therapy with ibuprofen (Motrin) to prevent neointimal fibrous hyperplasia. *J Vasc Surg,* 2(1):205-13, 1985.

13. LoGerfo FW, Soncrant T, Teel T, Dwey F Jr. Boundary layer separation in models of side to end arterial anastomoses. *Arch Surg,* 1979; 1141:1369-73.
14. W.M. Abbott, J. Megerman, J. Hasson, G. L'Italien and D.F. Warnock: Effect of compliance mismatch on vascular graft patency. *J Vasc Surg,* 2, 376-382 (1981).
15. M. Fillinger, E. Reinitz, and R. Schwartz: Graft geometry and venous intimal-medial hyperplasia in arteriovenous loop grafts. *Am J Surg,* 11, 556-566 (1990).
16. Dewey CF, Bussolari SR, Gimbrone MA, Davies PF: The dynamic response of vascular endothelial cells to fluid shear stress. *J Biomech Eng,* 1981:103:177-185.
17. Eskin SG, Ives CL, McIntire LV, Navarro LT: Response of cultured endothelial cells to steady flow. *Microvasc Res,* 1984; 28:87-94.
18. Franke RP, Grafe M, Schnittler H, Seiffge D, Mittermayer C: Induction of human vascular endothelial stress fibres by fluid shear stress. *Nature,* 1984;307:648-649.
19. Kim DW, Gottlieb AI, Langille BI: In vivo modulation of endothelial F-actin micorfilaments by experimental alterations in shear stress. *Arteriosclerosis,* 1989;9:439-445.
20. Frangos JA, Eskin SG, McIntire LV, Ives CL: Flow effects on prostacyclin production by cultured human endothelial cells. *Science,* 1985;227:1477-1479.
21. Davies PF, Dewey CF, Bussolari SR, Gordon EJ, Gimbrone MA: Influence of hemodynamic forces on vascular endothelial function: In vitro studies of shear stress and pinocytosis in bovine aortic cells. *J Clin Invest,* 1984;73:1121-1129.
22. Olesen SP, Clapham DE, Davies PF: Hemodynamic shear stress activates a K current in vascular endothelial cells. *Nature,* 1988;331:168-170
23. Diamond SL, Sharefkin JB, Dieffenbach C, Frasier-Scott K, McIntire LV, Eskin SG: Tissue plasminogen activator messenger RNA levels increase in cultured endothelial cells exposed to laminar shear stress. *J Cell Physiol,* 1990;143:364-371.
24. S. Glagov, D.P. Giddens, H. Bassioouny, S. White and C.K. Zarins: Hemodynamic effects and tissue reactions at graft to vein anastamoses for vascular access. In: Vascular Access for Hemodialysis-II B.G. Sommer and M.L. Henry (Eds.), 3-20, W.L. Gore and Associates and Precept Press (1991).
25. Zarins CK, Giddens D, Bharadvaj BK, et al. Carotid bifurcation atherosclerosis: Quanititative correlation of plaque localization with flow velocity profiles and wall shear stress. *Circ Res,* 53:502-514, 1983.
26. Ku DN, Giddens DP, Zarins CK, and Glagov S. Pulsatile flow and atherosclerosis in the human carotid bifurcation: Positive correlation between plaque location and low and oscillation shear stress. *Arteriosclerosis,* 5:293-302, 1985.
27. Glagov S. and Zarins C.K.: What are the determinants of plaque instability and its consequences. *J Vasc Surg,* 9,389-390;1989.
28. Glagov S. and Zarins C.K., Giddens D.P. and Ku D.N.: Hemodynamics and atherosclerosis: insights and perspectives gained from studies of human arteries. *Arch Path Lab Med,* 112,1018-1031; 1988.
29. Glagov S., Zarins C.K., Giddens D.P.: Hemodynamic and tissue reactive factors during human atherogenesis. *Giorn It Cardiol,* 20,1070-1074;1990
30. Bassiouny, H.S., White, S., Glagov, S., Choi, E., Giddens, D.P., Zarins, C.K., Anastomotic Intimal Hyperplasia: Mechanical Injury of Flow Induced, *J Vasc Surg,* (In Press) 1991.
31. Hasson J, Megerman J, Abbott WM: Increased compliance near vascular anastomoses. *J. Vasc Surg,* 2(3): 419-423, 1985.
32. Megerman J, Abbott WM: Compliance in vascular grafts. In Vascular Grafting, Wright C (ed.). John Wright - PSB, Boston, pp 344-64, 1983.
33. Walden R, L'Italien GJ, Megerman J, Abbott WM: Matched elastic properties and successful arterial grafting. *Arch Surg,* 115:1166-9, 1980.
34. Lelung DYM, Glagov S, and Mathews MB. Cyclic stretching stimulates synthesis of matrix components by arterial smooth muscle cells in vitro. *Science,* 191:475, 1976.
35. Lyon R. Runyon-Haas A, Davis H, et al. Protection from atherosclerotic lesion formation by reduction of artery wall motion. *J Vasc Surg,* 5(1):59-67, 1987.
36. Kohler TR, Kaufman JL, Kacoyanis GP, et al. Effect of aspirin and dipytridamole on the patency of femoral artery bypass grafts. *Surgery,* 1984;95:462-66.
37. Radic ZS, O'Malley MK, Mikat EM, et al. The role of aspirin and dipyridamole on vascular DNA synthesis and intimal hyperplasia following deendothelialization. *J Surg Res,* 1986;41:8491.
38. Clowes A.W. Pathobiology of arterial healing. In: Strandness, DE Jr., Didisheim P, Clowes AW, Watson JT, eds. Vascular Diseases: Current Research and Clinical Applications. Orlando, FL: Grace and Stratton: 1987: 351-62.

39. White SS. Visualization of flow phenomena in a vascular graft model. MS Thesis, Georgia Institute of Technology, Atlanta; 1989.
40. White, S.S., Zarins, C.K., Bassiouny, H.S., Loth, F., Glagov, S., Giddens, D.P. Hemodynamic patterns in a model of endo to side vascular graft anastomoses: Effect of pulsatility, flow division and Reynolds number. (In press) 1991.
41. Ojha M, PhD, Ethier CR, PhD, Johnston KW, MD, FRCS (C), and Cobbold RSC, PhD: Steady and pulsatile flow fields in an end-to-side arterial anastomosis model. *J. Vasc Surg*, (12):747-753, 1990.
42. Kamiya A and Togawa T. Adaptive regulation of wall shear stress to flow change in the canine carotid artery. *Am J. Physiol* 239:H14-H21, 1980.
43. Zarins CK, Zatina MA, Giddens DP, Ku DN and Glagov S. Shear stress regulation of artery lumen diameter in experimental atherogenesis. *J Vasc Surg*, 5:413-420, 1987.
44. Lelung DYM, Glagov Sand Mathews MB. Elastin and collagen accumulation in rabbit ascending aorta and pulmonary trunk during postnatal growth: Correlation of cellular synthetic response with medial tension. *Circ Res*, 41:316-323, 1977.
45. Masuda H. Bassiouny, H. Glagov S., and Zarins, CK. Artery wall restructuring in response to increased flow. *Surg Forum*, 40:285286, 1989.
46. Is intimal hyperplasia an adaptive response or a pathologic process? observations on the nature of nonatherosclerotic intimal thickening. S. Glagov and CK Zarins. Special Communications, *I Vasc Surg*, 10:5, 571-573, 1989.
47. Languille BL and O'Donnell F. Reductions in arterial diameter produced by chronic decreases in blood flow are endothelium-dependent. *Science*, 231:405407, 1986.
48. Bassiouny, Lieber BB, Giddens DP, Xu CP, Glagov S and Zarins CK. Quantitative inverse correlation of wall shear stress with experimental intimal thickening. *Surg Forum*, 39:328-330, 1988.

Intimal Hyperplasia as a Cause of Graft Failure After Vascular Reconstruction

R.L. Geary and A.W. Clowes

Department of Surgery, University of Washington
School of Medicine
Seattle, Washington, U.S.A.

INTRODUCTION

Vascular surgery has grown rapidly in the past 50 years in large part due to the development of techniques for long segment arterial bypass grafting with autologous vein and synthetic materials[63,73,82]. Arterial grafting remains largely a palliative procedure and both autologous and synthetic grafts fail at a significant rate. For example, at least one half of infrainguinal vein bypasses fail within 5 years of implantation[87,100,101].

Early graft thrombosis is often related to technical problems in vein graft procurement, preparation or implantation[40,74,98]. Improper selection of patients with inadequate arterial inflow or runoff and multiple level disease can contribute to graft failures[2,98,101]. Late graft failure on the other hand is often due to intimal hyperplasia or progression of underlying atherosclerosis[51,57].

Intimal hyperplasia accounts for a significant number of graft failures in the period 6 to 24 months after implantation[11,98,101]. Failure rates (10-30%) vary with graft materials and location of implantation. In autologous vein grafts significant intimal thickening occurs chiefly at anastomoses and in areas damaged by vascular clamps, temporary ligatures and at valvulotomy sites. Fibrotic stenoses of vein valves also contribute. A similar pattern of anastomotic thickening is seen in synthetic conduits as ingrowth of cellular elements from adjacent arteries accumulate at anastomoses.

This review will address our current understanding of the pathologic processes and mediators underlying intimal hyperplasia in both autologous and synthetic arterial conduits. Since vascular injury is an important stimulus for intimal hyperplasia we will review first what is known about the arterial response to endothelial cell (EC) denudation before discussing the factors involved in graft healing. Evidence from animal models will be considered and potential interventions aimed at controlling intimal hyperplasia will be explored.

ARTERIAL INJURY AND REPAIR

In the rat, injury to the carotid artery by balloon catheter denudation results in predictable intimal thickening and lesions similar to those in humans[22,23]. The endothelium is scraped off and the media is damaged by the passage of the distended balloon catheter. Approximately 20% of the smooth muscle cells (SMCs) are killed. Immediately, platelets adhere to the exposed media forming a carpet of thrombus. To the extent that the platelet granules are released vectorially into the media, the underlying SMCs are exposed to a number of factors including the potent EC and SMC mitogens such as platelet derived growth factor (PDGF), transforming growth factor ß (TGFß), and an epidermal growth factor-like protein (EGF)[89,90]. These agents may contribute to the initial SMC proliferative response. The nonocclusive platelet thrombus is transient and replaced by the regenerating EC monolayer.

Within hours of injury a cohort of the remaining medial SMC population begins to proliferate. With tritiated-thymidine labeling techniques it can be shown that approximately 20-30% of remaining SMCs begin synthesizing DNA at 24 hours (S-phase)[25,76]. The labeling index is maximal at 33 hours following injury, and proliferation continues for a number of days. Approximately 4 days following injury SMCs can be seen migrating across the internal elastic lamina into the intima underneath the platelet layer[25]. This population of migrating SMCs is comprised not only of proliferating SMCs but also a cohort of non-dividing SMCs (approximately 50%). This can be demonstrated using continuous tritiated-thymidine labeling, a technique that allows all dividing cells to be identified by autoradiography and distinguished from nondividing cells. The significance of the non-dividing cohort is not yet understood.

Once in the intima SMCs proliferate further and secrete matrix proteins. While SMCs accumulate in the intima, ECs are migrating from adjacent areas to reform a luminal monolayer overlying the remodeling intima. As the endothelium becomes confluent in previously denuded areas the underlying SMCs resume a quiescent state. ECs have a limited ability to regenerate a luminal surface, and the central portion of the carotid remains devoid of endothelium indefinitely[88]. Within 4 weeks SMCs will normalize their proliferative rate even in areas where EC coverage is incomplete. In these exposed areas luminal SMCs take on an altered morphology and, like endothelium, form a smooth non-thrombogenic luminal surface[15,17].

The overall SMC proliferative process in the intima is augmented by the deposition of matrix consisting of elastin, collagen and proteoglycans. A steady state is reached after approximately 3 months and at this point the matrix accounts for 80% of intimal area[23].

INTIMAL THICKENING IN VEIN GRAFTS

Intimal hyperplasia has long been recognized in both synthetic and autologous conduits placed into the arterial circulation. Carrel and Guthrie were the first investigators to describe the thickening of the vein graft wall after implantation and the accumulation of connective tissue in both media and intima[4,5]. Areas adjacent to anastomoses developed a smooth white "scar like appearance" and the process was termed "arterialization". Initially this was felt to be a normal adaptation of vein to the stress of arterial hemodynamics. It is now recognized that, at times, this healing process is poorly regulated and can produce atherosclerotic lesions which can cause luminal encroachment and graft thrombosis.

Subsequent investigators have noted that the initial response of arterialized vein grafts is characterized microscopically by EC denudation, particularly near anastomoses, in part due to intraoperative handling[40]. Denuded areas become carpeted acutely with platelet thrombi and leukocytes. The underlying media contains regions of hemorrhage, swelling and SMC necrosis[74]. The injury can be limited with meticulous technique in dissecting, clamping, valvulotomy and by avoiding over distension of vein grafts. The contribution of these factors to acute graft failure is undeniable but long-term consequences are less clear.

In man the intimal hyperplastic response is difficult to characterize as grafts are unavailable for serial pathologic examination. The fragmentary evidence available has been largely corroborated by animal studies.

The etiology of intimal hyperplasia has as its underpinnings proliferation of medial SMCs and their migration into the intima of arteries, vein grafts, and the perianastomotic regions of synthetic grafts. This normal repair process is necessary for anastomotic healing and restoration of a nonthrombogenic luminal surface. It often continues beyond what is required for graft healing and results in luminal encroachment.

In a rabbit vein graft model, there is patchy loss of endothelium throughout the graft because of surgical trauma. Platelets adhere where endothelium is missing and form a monolayer. Re-endothelialization of jugular vein grafted into the carotid circulation is complete within 2 weeks of implantation at which point platelets and leukocytes are again excluded from the graft luminal surface[59,106].

Intimal thickening begins very early and is characterized by SMC replication, migration and extracellular matrix deposition. The SMC proliferation is maximal at one week and returns to baseline levels in one month. When this period of SMC proliferation ends the intima continues to thicken for up to 12 weeks from further extracellular matrix production[105].

The structure of grafts at later times is similar to grafts at 12 weeks but degenerative changes take place[59]. One year after implantation, these grafts have developed increased endothelial permeability, red blood cell deposition in the graft wall as well as subendothelial fibrin deposits, and associated foam cells in the intima. These changes are not unlike early atherosclerotic lesions in human vessels and may be precursors to degenerative lesions such as those seen in human vein grafts[3,28,68].

Hypercholesterolemia and changes in blood flow alter proliferative responses of healing vein grafts. Using the jugular vein graft model discussed above, Zwolak et al. have shown that rabbits fed high cholesterol diets (serum levels 200 to 600 mg/dl) develop increased graft intimal thickening when looked at 3 and 6 months after implantation[106].

Immunohistochemical analysis showed that the thickening was caused largely by lipid laden macrophages (foam cells) accumulating within the intima. SMC and EC proliferation were not significantly different than in normo-cholesterolemic controls. Hemodynamic factors have also been shown to modify the intimal thickening response in vein grafts[30,105].

In the rabbit vein graft model it appears that wall thickness and luminal area adjust in response to wall tangential stress[105]. Dobrin et al. have correlated intimal thickening in canine vein grafts with low blood flow (shear stress) and medial thickening with radial deformation of the vein graft wall (pulse and pressure changes)[30,31].

INTIMAL THICKENING IN SYNTHETIC GRAFTS

The development of synthetic vascular grafts, particularly Dacron and expanded polytetraflouroethylene (PTFE), is a milestone in the history of vascular surgery. These prostheses are invaluable in large vessel reconstructions. In small vessel reconstructions synthetic grafts provide an alternative when autogenous vein is not available but have proven to be less durable. Despite their relative inertness these grafts develop lesions similar in composition and equally as detrimental as those described above in vein grafts[100,101]. The magnitude of this problem is underscored by the high failure rates of these grafts in infrainguinal locations. For example, Veith et al., in a randomized trial of PTFE vs. saphenous vein femoropopliteal grafts, reported 5 year primary patency rates in PTFE of 38% compared to 68% in vein grafts[100]. This can be contrasted with 85-95% patency of synthetic grafts in the aortofemoral location.

Intimal hyperplasia in PTFE grafts in man is limited to the few centimeters adjacent to anastomoses. Smooth, white, fibrotic lesions develop at the anastomoses soon after implantation while the center portion of the graft is left unhealed and thrombogenic even years after grafting. The SMCs in these lesions probably come from two sources: ingrowth from adjacent arterial cut edges and from invading capillaries in the graft interstices.

A non-human primate model of PTFE graft healing has been established in our laboratory[18,20,21,42]. In conventional low-porosity grafts (30 micrometer internodal distance) anastomotic thickening begins as SMCs migrate inward beneath an advancing EC layer[20]. The SMCs proliferate only in areas covered by EC. This form of intimal hyperplasia differs from intimal thickening in injured arteries where SMCs underlying regenerated endothelium become quiescent. The endothelial ingrowth stops 2 to 3 centimeters from the anastomosis leaving grafts incompletely healed when followed up to one year. Anastomotic thickening increases as SMCs continue to divide and deposit extracellular matrix. The resulting lesions resemble those in injured arteries and vein grafts.

When the porosity of PTFE grafts in this model is increased (60 micrometer internodal distance) the healing process goes to completion[21]. Capillaries from surrounding granulation tissue traverse the graft matrix providing multiple sources for ECs and SMCs. By two weeks a confluent endothelium is established under which SMC proliferation and matrix production continue. Intimal thickening stops only after three months.

MEDIATORS OF SMOOTH MUSCLE CELL PROLIFERATION

The intimal thickening responses in different conditions of vascular repair are quite similar. The common features in each are SMC proliferation, migration and matrix deposition. It is tempting then to propose potential interventions that might retard intimal thickening under all circumstances. In order to due so we must first understand how SMC growth is regulated. Factors thought to be important include blood borne elements (platelets and leukocytes), hemodynamic factors (compliance mismatch, flow separation, shear-stress, and wall tension) and growth factors or inhibitors released from blood cells or from vessel wall cells themselves.

The "response-to-injury hypothesis" proposed by Ross and Glomset in 1976 was based on three main observations: 1) platelet adherence and degranulation in injured vessels precede SMC proliferation; 2) induced thrombocytopenia attenuates the intimal thickening response; and 3) platelets contain a number of potent SMC mitogens[38,89,90]. This hypothesis subsequently stimulated a great number of investigators to examine the role of platelets and antiplatelet agents both *in vitro* and *in vivo* . These drugs prevent platelet aggregation but have little effect on platelet adherence and to date have failed to impact the intimal thickening process in clinical trials[9,10].

In a rat model of induced thrombocytopenia, levels of adherent platelets can be reduced to 5% of control animals by administering antiplatelet antibodies[37]. After vessel injury SMC proliferation in the thrombocytopenic group is no different than in controls. These observations support the conclusion that platelets are unnecessary for the first wave of medial SMC proliferation. Subsequent intimal thickening is reduced in the thrombocytopenic animals so that while proliferation remains high migration of SMCs from the media to the intima may be inhibited.

The hypothesis that platelet factors are important for SMC migration while having little effect on SMC proliferation is further supported by recent studies. PDGF, a growth factor for SMCs *in vitro*, is found in abundance in platelets and released when they degranulate. Jawien et al. infused PDGF into rats following carotid balloon injury and found little change in SMC proliferation while SMC migration increased dramatically[54]. At two weeks the intimal area in injured arteries of treated animals increased twenty-fold compared with untreated controls. Ferns et al. reported that antibodies to PDGF when infused following vessel injury reduced the intimal thickening response by 40% largely by inhibiting SMC migration; antibody treatment did not affect proliferation[35]. Taken together, the evidence suggests that PDGF is important for stimulating the migration of SMCs from the media to the intima following injury.

PDGF is present not only in platelets but also in SMCs and ECs, and PDGF derived from cells could act locally on the cells themselves (autocrine) or on their neighbors (paracrine) within the vessel wall. This is intriguing when we consider that platelets are likely to have only a brief role in stimulating SMCs since EC regeneration excludes platelets from the vessel wall soon after injury.

Another growth factor of importance is basic fibroblast growth factor (bFGF)[70]. Unlike PDGF which appears to primarily affect SMC migration bFGF seems to affect the initial SMC proliferative response. This protein is found in vascular SMCs and ECs, is released by injured cells, and is mitogenic for SMCs *in vitro*[70]. Interest in this molecule has been stimulated by the observation that medial SMC proliferation is proportionate to the extent of the initial injury[36]. Recently investigators have provided evidence that bFGF, released from the vessel wall by balloon injury, stimulates proliferation of adjacent medial SMCs. Infused bFGF stimulates intimal thickening, and antibodies against bFGF inhibit SMC proliferation after balloon injury[72]. Additionally, bFGF is mitogenic for ECs and stimulates them to cover denuded segments of artery that would be to extensive for spontaneous EC repair[71]. These observations coupled with those of PDGF above suggest a role for bFGF in stimulating the first wave of SMC proliferation and for PDGF in stimulating migration of both proliferating and quiescent SMCs into the intima where these and other factors stimulate further proliferation and matrix deposition.

Other growth factors might play a role in the injury response. Lymphocytes are present in injury-induced intimal thickening and human atheroma and growing evidence exists for a role for lymphokines in cell proliferation[48,69]. For instance, it has been noted that a significant number of SMCs in atheroma express class II major histocompatibility antigens, possibly in response to interferon, which has been shown to inhibit vascular SMC proliferation *in vivo* and *in vitro*[47].

Hemodynamic factors are an important influence on vascular structure[56,62,66,103,104]. Vascular cells are constantly reacting to changes in blood flow (shear stress), pressure (wall tension), and turbulence (flow separation). Clinical studies have identified low blood flow and low shear as risk factors for intimal thickening and graft thrombosis in infrainguinal bypass grafts[2]. How hemodynamic forces translate into changes in vessel structure is unknown. Shear forces are likely to act through ECs as they are of low magnitude and not transmitted throughout the vessel wall. Vessel diameter is regulated by blood flow and shear. In response to an increase in blood flow vessels dilate[56].

This observation has been interpreted to mean that vessels attempt to maintain physiological levels of shear stress at the luminal surface by changing vessel diameter. Langille and O'Donnell showed that compensatory vasoconstriction in response to reduced blood flow is endothelium-dependent[66]. They reported that removing the endothelium from carotid arteries abolished a 21% decrease in luminal caliber observed in control arteries subjected to low flow. Wall tension (pressure) is transmitted to all layers of the vessel wall and teleologic evidence supports the premise that wall thickness increases in response to wall tension by adding lamellar units as tension increases[103]. This is dramatically illustrated by the observation on the pulmonary artery and aorta of newborns during growth and development. At birth the vessels are the same thickness. As the neonatal circulation matures aortic pressure far exceeds pulmonary pressure and the aorta becomes many times thicker. Mediators of this phenomenon may also be active within diseased vessels. Hypertension enhances the thickening response to vascular injury[12,95]. The renin-angiotensin system, involved in blood pressure homeostasis, may also play an important role in the development of intimal hyperplasia[32,46,67,99]. Powell and colleagues have inhibited intimal hyperplasia in the rat carotid injury model with both angiotensin converting enzyme (ACE) inhibitors and the angiotensin receptor inhibitor DuP 753 [81,84-86]. The inhibitory effects of these agents can be reversed in part be administering exogenous angiotensin[27].

Kohler and Kraiss have studied the effects of blood flow (shear) in the baboon PTFE model in our laboratory. These experiments were conducted using two different models. In the first model, blood flow was increased through aorto-iliac grafts by a small fistula in the mid thigh[60]. Intimal thickening was decreased in the grafts with increased blood flow. In some animals, the fistula was ligated and normal flow restored at two months.

This maneuver produced a five-fold increase in intimal thickening. In the second model, variations of shear within a physiologic range were created by diverting aortic flow into a single aorto-aortic graft which in turn emptied into two identical aorto-iliac grafts distally[61]. The intimal thickening was significantly less in the proximal, high flow graft compared to the distal, normal flow grafts. These data support the hypothesis that blood flow may regulate wall structure as well as vessel diameter.

As the EC surface is restored following arterial injury the underlying SMCs become quiescent. It may be that the endothelium is preventing blood-borne agents from reaching the underlying intima or that the ECs themselves release inhibitors of SMC proliferation. A potential inhibitor is heparan sulphate. The related molecule heparin inhibits SMC growth and migration in animal models of injury as well as in tissue culture[14,19,49,50,75]. ECs and SMCs synthesize and secrete heparan sulphate[6,7,39]. In addition to its inhibitory effects on SMCs heparin also alters the composition of extracellular matrix and may in this way interfere with SMC movement[96,97].

The response in clinical situations is likely controlled in part by all of the above mechanisms. Growth factors and inhibitors from both the vessel wall and blood borne elements, leukocytes, cytokines, and hemodynamic forces all interact in the balance of cell growth and suppression.

PREVENTION AND TREATMENT OF INTIMAL HYPERPLASIA

The recognition of the importance of intimal hyperplasia has prompted several pharmacological trials. The data from these trials will be discussed in brief below. First, it is important to point out that graft patency rates are largely determined by the type of graft employed and that only postoperative surveillance with early intervention into failing grafts has significantly impacted patency rates[1,2,26,101]. Bandyk et al. have recomended screening to identify patent but compromised grafts before they fail. Using noninvasive hemodynamic testing and angiography they were able to identify 85 primary and 18 recurrent lesions in 396 infrainguinal bypass grafts before they failed. Following surgery or endovascular intervention a 5 year cumulative graft patency rate of 85% was achieved[1]. In contrast, Whittemore et al. have reported poor graft salvage following vein graft thrombosis[101]. Once thrombosed, thrombectomy and vein patching of underlying graft stenoses resulted in five year patency rates of only 19%. On the other hand, grafts repaired prior to thrombosis had an 86% five year patency. These observations underscore the importance of detecting and repairing lesions prior to graft failure.

As mentioned above, anti-platelet agents have been studied extensively and have proven of limited benefit in prolonging graft patency[9,10]. These agents likely affect acute graft thrombosis rather than late stenosis. A randomized multicenter trial was recently reported. It compared aspirin plus dipyridamole to placebo in maintaining patency of femoropopliteal vein grafts[77]. There was no difference in graft patency between the two treatment groups but the authors noted a reduction in stroke and myocardial infarction in patients receiving aspirin plus dipyridamole. Aspirin has been shown to improve both synthetic infrainguinal[58] and coronary bypass graft[41,43] patency if given perioperatively, but has not helped to prevent post-coronary angioplasty restenosis[34,65,94].

The ACE inhibitors are another group of agents currently being tried in man for prevention of intimal hyperplasia. These agents have proven safe in clinical use as antihypertensives. Familiarity with these agents as well as the animal studies commented on above has prompted clinical trials in the USA and Europe to assess their efficacy in reducing restenosis after coronary angioplasty. In the rat, the ACE inhibitor cilazapril blocks the proliferative response to balloon injury as does the angiotensin II receptor antagonist DuP 753[46,81,84-86]. In the rat carotid injury model we have recently reported that a short course of heparin and cilazapril together decrease SMC proliferation and intimal thickening[16]. The affect of the two drugs together was more than either agent alone, resulting in 80% reduction of intimal area in the treatment group.

Another drug that may help to reduce graft intimal hyperplasia is heparin. Our laboratory and others have shown that heparin inhibits SMC and EC growth *in vitro*. In animal models heparin decreases intimal thickening following injury by decreasing SMC proliferation[13,14,50,76] and migration[75] and by altering the pericellular matrix composition[96,97]. It also promotes EC regrowth in denuded vessels. In the rat, a short course of heparin following injury (7 days) is as effective as longer periods of treatment (28 days)[14]. These data from animal models justify a trial of heparin in man following vascular grafting. Trials are hampered by the procoagulant properties of heparin. To date, trials in man of appropriate dosage and timing of heparin therapy are lacking.

Nonanticoagulant fractions of heparin are available and have been shown in animals to inhibit intimal thickening[24,25]. As these agents become available for trials in man improved graft patency rates may be achieved. It is likely that only a short course of heparin would be needed.

Other agents that have been employed in an attempt to prevent intimal hyperplasia include the fish oils, calcium channel blockers[33], and immunosuppressive agents[8,55]. Fish oils reduce intimal thickening in animal models and have been shown to decrease platelet adhesion and PDGF production[34,44]. Trials in preventing intimal hyperplasia following angioplasty and vein grafting have unfortunately produced inconclusive results[64,78,91]. Steroids[8] and immunosuppressive agents decrease intimal hyperplasia in animal grafts but human studies have not been performed as these agents have a number of adverse affects. Calcium channel blockers, another group of drugs that have favorable affects in animal models of intimal hyperplasia[52,93], have had little impact on the human situation[53,92].

A novel approach to inhibit intimal thickening after vascular injury has recently been proposed[79,83,102]. Gene therapy techniques have been developed by which transfected vascular cells are placed into the arterial system where they release introduced gene products. Ideally, cells seeded with a gene for an inhibitory protein would be introduced into grafts at the time of implantation. Inhibitors could then act locally, within the graft and adjacent arteries, to inhibit intimal thickening[29,80]. Further work is needed before introducing transfected cells into man but the approach is appealing.

SUMMARY

We have presented clinical evidence that intimal hyperplasia is a significant problem in vascular grafting. Data from animal experiments and clinical studies invoke similar mechanisms of repair and intimal thickening in grafts and injured arteries. Events common to each are SMC proliferation, migration and the production of pericellular matrix. Factors controlling the proliferative response include mitogens and inhibitors. Although new methods to prevent intimal hyperplasia are under study, currently the only effective method of decreasing graft failure from intimal hyperplasia is an aggressive surveillance program. Identification of grafts that are failing but patent allows more effective intervention and improved longterm patency rates.

REFERENCES

1. Bandyk, D.F., T. M. Bergamini, J. B. Towne, D. D. Schmitt, and G. R. Seabrook. 1991. Durability of   vein graft revision: The outcome of secondary procedures. *J. Vasc. Surg.* 13:200-210.
2. Bandyk, D.F., D. D. Schmitt, G. R. Seabrook, M. B. Adams, and J. B. Towne. 1989. Monitoring functional patency of in situ saphenous vein bypasses: The impact of a surveillance protocol and elective revision. *J. Vasc. Surg.* 9:286-296.
3. Bourassa, M.G., L. D. Fisher, L. Campeau, M. J. Gillespie, M. McConney, and J. Lesperance. 1985. Long-term fate of bypass grafts: the coronary artery surgery study (CASS) and Montreal Heart Institute experiences. *Circulation,* 72:V-71-V-78.
4. Carrel, A. and C. C. Guthrie. 1906. Results of the biterminal transplantation of veins. *Am. J Med. Sci.* 132:415-422.
5. Carrel, A. and C. C. Guthrie. 1906. Uniterminal and biterminal venous transplantations. *Surg. Gynecol. Obstet.* 2:266-286.
6. Castellot, J.J.,Jr., M. L. Addonizio, R. Rosenberg, and M. J. Karnovsky. 1981. Cultured endothelial ells produce a heparin-like inhibitor of smooth muscle cell growth. *J. Cell Biol.,* 90:372-379.
7. Castellot, J.J.,Jr., L. V. Favreau, M. J. Karnovsky, and R. D. Rosenberg. 1982. Inhibition of vascular smooth muscle cell growth by endothelial cell-derived heparin. Possible role of a platelet endoglycosidase. *J. Biol. Chem.,* 257:11256-11260.
8. Chervu, A., W. S. Moore, W. J. Quinones-Baldrich, and T. Henderson. 1989. Efficacy of corticosteroids in suppression of intimal hyperplasia. *J Vasc. Surg.* 10:129-134.
9. Clagett, G.P., E. Genton, and E. W. Salzman. 1989. Antithrombotic therapy in peripheral vascular disease. *Chest,* 95:128S-139S.
10. Clowes, A.W. 1986. The role of aspirin in enhancing arterial graft patency. *J. Vasc. Surg.* 3:381-385.
11. Clowes, A.W. 1989. Pathologic intimal hyperplasia as a response to vascular injury and reconstruction, p. 266-275. In R. B. Rutherford (ed.), Vascular Surgery. W.B.Saunders Company, Philadelphia.
12. Clowes, A.W. and M. M. Clowes. 1980. Influence of chronic hypertension on injured and uninjured arteries in spontaneously hypertensive rats. *Lab. Invest.* 6:535-541.
13. Clowes, A.W. and M. M. Clowes. 1985. Kinetics of cellular proliferation after arterial injury. II. Inhibition of smooth muscle growth by heparin. *Lab. Invest.,* 52:611-616.
14. Clowes, A.W. and M. M. Clowes. 1986. Kinetics of cellular proliferation after arterial injury. IV. Heparin inhibits rat smooth muscle mitogenesis and migration. *Circ. Res.,* 58:839-845.
15. Clowes, A.W., M. M. Clowes, and M. A. Reidy. 1986. Kinetics of cellular proliferation after arterial   injury. III.Endothelial and smooth muscle growth in chronically denuded vessels. *Lab. Invest.* 54:295-303.

16. Clowes, A.W., M. M. Clowes, S. C. Vergel, R. K. M. Müller, J. S. Powell, F. Hefti, and H. R. Baumgartner. 1991. Heparin and cilazapril together inhibit injury-induced intimal hyperplasia. *Hypertension* 18 Suppl.:II65-II69.
17. Clowes, A.W., R. E. Collazzo, and M. J. Karnovsky. 1978. A morphologic and permeability study of luminal smooth muscle cells after arterial injury in the rat. *Lab. Invest.* 39:141-150.
18. Clowes, A.W., A. M. Gown, S. R. Hanson, and M. A. Reidy. 1985. Mechanisms of arterial graft failure. I. Role of cellular proliferation in early healing of PTFE prostheses. *Am. J Pathol.*, 118:43-54.
19. Clowes, A.W. and M. J. Karnovsky. 1977. Suppression by heparin of smooth muscle cell proliferation in injured arteries. *Nature,* 265:625-626.
20. Clowes, A.W., T. R. Kirkman, and M. M. Clowes. 1986. Mechanisms of arterial graft failure. II. Chronic endothelial and smooth muscle cell proliferation in healing polytetrafluoroethylene prostheses. *J Vasc. Surg.,* 3:877-884
21. Clowes, A.W., T. R. Kirkman, and M. A. Reidy. 1986. Mechanisms of arterial graft healing. Rapid transmural capillary ingrowth provides a source of intimal endothelium and smooth muscle in porous PTFE prostheses. *Am. J Pathol.,* 123:220-230.
22. Clowes, A.W., M. A. Reidy, and M. M. Clowes. 1983. Kinetics of cellular proliferation after arterial injury.I.Smooth muscle growth in the absence of endothelium. *Lab. Invest.,* 49:327-333.
23. Clowes, A.W., M. A. Reidy, and M. M. Clowes. 1983. Mechanisms of stenosis after arterial injury. *Lab. Invest.,* 49:208-215.
24. Clowes, A.W., R. D. Rosenberg, and M. M. Clowes. 1983. Regulation of arterial smooth muscle cell proliferation by heparin in vivo. *Surgical. Forum.,* 34:357-360.
25. Clowes, A.W. and S. M. Schwartz. 1985. Significance of quiescent smooth muscle migration in the injured rat carotid artery. *Circ. Res.,* 56:139-145.
26. Cohen, J.R., J. A. Mannick, N. P. Couch, and A. D. Whittemore. 1986. Recognition and management of impending vein-graft failure. Importance for long-term patency. *Arch. Surg.,* 121:758-759.
27. Daemen, M.J.A.P., D. M. Lombardi, F. T. Bosman, and S. M. Schwartz. 1991. Angiotensin II induces smooth muscle cell proliferation in the normal and injured rat arterial wall. *Circ. Res.,* 68:450-456.
28. DePalma, R.G. 1979. Atherosclerosis in vascular grafts. *Atherosclerosis. Reviews.* 6:146-177.
29. Dichek, D.A., R. F. Neville, J. A. Zwiebel, S. M. Freeman, M. B. Leon, and W. F. Anderson. 1989. Seeding of intravascular stents with genetically engineered endothelial cells. *Circulation,* 80:1347-1353.
30. Dobrin, P.B., F. N. Littooy, and E. D. Endean. 1989. Mechanical factors predisposing to intimal hyperplasia and medial thickening in autogenous vein grafts. *Surgery.* 105:393-400.
31. Dobrin, P.B., F. N. Littooy, J. Golan, B. Blakeman, and J. Fareed. 1988. Mechanical and histologic changes in canine vein grafts. *J. Surg. Res.* 44:259-265.
32. Dzau, V.J., G. H. Gibbons, and R. E. Pratt. 1991. Molecular mechanisms of vascular renin-angiotensin system in myointimal hyperplasia. *Hypertension* 18 Suppl.:II100-II105.
33. El-Sanadiki, M.N., K. S. Cross, J. J. Murray, R. W. Schuman, E. Mikat, R. L. McCann, and P-O. Hagen. 1990. Reduction of intimal hyperplasia and enhanced reactivity of experimental vein bypass grafts with verapamil treatment. *Ann. Surg.* 212:87-96.
34. Fanelli, C. and R. Aronoff. 1990. Restenosis following coronary angioplasty. *Am. Heart J.* 119:357-368.
35. Ferns, G.A.A., E. W. Raines, K. H. Sprugel, A. S. Motani, M. A. Reidy, and R. Ross. 1991. Inhibition of neointimal smooth muscle accumulation after angioplasty by an antibody to PDGF. *Science,* 253:1129-1132.
36. Fingerle, J., Y. P. T. Au, A. W. Clowes, and M. A. Reidy. 1990. Intimal lesion formation in rat carotid arteries after endothelial denudation in absence of medial injury. *Arteriosclerosis,* 10:1082-1087.
37. Fingerle, J., R. Johnson, A. W. Clowes, M. W. Majesky, and M. A. Reidy. 1989. Role of platelets in smooth muscle cell proliferation and migration after vascular injury in rat carotid artery. *Proc. Natl. Acad. Sci. USA* 86:8412-8416.
38. Friedman, R.J., M. B. Stemerman, B. Wenz, S. Moore, J. Gauldie, M. Gent, M. L. Tiell, and T. H. Spaet. 1977. The effect of thrombocytopenia on experimental atherosclerotic lesion formation in rabbits. Smooth muscle cell proliferation and re-endothelialization. *J. Clin. Invest.,* 60:1191-1201.

39. Fritze, L.M.S., C. F. Reilly, and R. D. Rosenberg. 1985. An antiproliferative heparan sulfate species produced by postconfluent smooth muscle cells. *J. Cell Biol.* 100:1041-1049.
40. Fuchs, J.C., J. S. Mitchener,3d., and P. O. Hagen. 1978. Postoperative changes in autologous vein grafts. *Ann. Surg.,* 188:1-15.
41. Fuster, V. and J. J. Chesebro. 1985. Aortocoronary artery vein-graft disease: experimental and clinical-approach for the understanding of the role of platelets and platelet inhibitors. *Circulation,* 72:V-65-V-70.
42. Golden, M.A., S. R. Hanson, T. R. Kirkman, P. A. Schneider, and A. W. Clowes. 1990. Healing of polytetrafluoroethylene arterial grafts is influenced by graft porosity. *J. Vasc. Surg.,* 11:838-845.
43. Goldman, S., J. Copeland, T. Moritz, W. Henderson, K. Zadina, T. Ovitt, J. Doherty, R. Read, E. Chesler, Y. Sako, L. Lancaster, R. Emery, G. VRK. Sharma, M. Josa, I. Pacold, A. Montoya, D. Parikh, G. Sethi, J. Holt, J. Kirklin, R. Shabetai, W. Moores, J. Aldridge, Z. Masud, H. DeMots, S. Floten, C. Haakenson, and L. A. Harker. 1988. Improvement in early saphenous vein graft patency after coronary artery bypass surgery with antiplatelet therapy: results of a Veterans Administration Cooperative Study. *Circulation,* 77:1324-1332.
44. Goodnight, S.H., M. Fisher, G. A. Fitzgerald, and P. H. Levine. 1989. Assessment of the therapeutic use of dietary fish oil in atherosclerotic vascular disease and thrombosis. *Chest,* 95:19S-25S.
45. Guyton, J.R., R. D. Rosenberg, A. W. Clowes, and M. J. Karnovsky. 1980. Inhibition of rat arterial smooth muscle cell proliferation by heparin. I. In vivo studies with anticoagulant and non-anticoagulant heparin. *Circ. Res.,* 46:625-634.
46. Hanson, S.R., J. S. Powell, T. Dodson, A. Lumsden, A. B. Kelly, J. S. Anderson, A. W. Clowes, and L. A. Harker. 1991. Effects of angiotensin converting enzyme inhibition with cilazapril in injured arteries and vascular grafts in baboons. *Hypertension* (in press).
47. Hansson, G.K., L. Jonasson, J. Holm, M. M. Clowes, and A. W. Clowes. 1988. Gamma interferon regulates vascular smooth muscle proliferation and Ia espression in vitro and in vivo. *Circ. Res.,* 63:712-719.
48. Hansson, G.K., L. Jonasson, P. S. Seifert, and S. Stemme. 1989. Immune mechanisms in atherosclerosis. *Arteriosclerosis* 9:567-578.
49. Hirsch, G.M. and M. J. Karnovsky. 1991. Inhibition of vein graft intimal proliferative lesions in the rat by heparin. *Am. J. Pathol.,* 139:581-587.
50. Hoover, R.L., R. Rosenberg, W. Haering, and M. J. Karnovsky. 1980. Inhibition of rat arterial smooth muscle cell proliferation by heparin. II. In vitro studies. *Circ. Res.,* 47:578-583.
51. Imparato, A.M., A. Bracco, G. E. Kim, and R. Zeff. 1972. Intimal and neointimal fibrous proliferation causing failure of arterial reconstructions. *Surgery.* 72:1007-1017.
52. Jackson, C.L., R. C. Bush, and D. E. Bowyer. 1988. Inhibitory effect of calcium antagonists on balloon catheter-induced arterial smooth muscle cell proliferation and lesion size. *Atherosclerosis,* 69:115-122.
53. Jackson, C.L., R. C. Bush, and D. E. Bowyer. 1989. Mechanism of antiatherogenic action of calcium antagonists. *Atherosclerosis* 80:17-26.
54. Jawien, A., D. F. Bowen-Pope, V. Lindner, S. M. Schwartz, and A. W. Clowes. 1992. Platelet-derived growth factor promotes smooth muscle migration and intimal thickening in a rat model of balloon angioplasty. *J. Clin. Invest.* (in press).
55. Jonasson, L., J. Holm, and G. K. Hansson. 1988. Cyclosporin A inhibits smooth muscle proliferation in the vascular response to injury. *Proc. Natl. Acad. Sci.* USA 85:2303-2306.
56. Kamiya, A. and T. Togawa. 1980. Adaptive regulation of wall shear stress to flow change in the canine   carotid artery. *Am. J Physiol.* 239:14-21.
57. Karayannacos, P.E., J. R. Hostetler, and M. G. Bond. 1978. Late failure in vein grafts, mediating factors in subendothelial fibromuscular hyperplasia. *Ann. Surg.* 187:183-188.
58. Kohler, T.R., J. L. Kaufman, G. Kacoyanis, A. W. Clowes, M. C. Donaldson, E. Kelly, J. Skillman, N.   P. Couch, A. D. Whittemore, J. A. Mannick, and al. 1984. Effect of aspirin and dipyridamole on the patency of lower extremity bypass grafts. *Surgery.* 96:462-466.
59. Kohler, T.R., T. R. Kirkman, D. Gordon, and A. W. Clowes. 1990. Mechanism of long-term degeneration of arterialized vein grafts. *Am. J. Surg.,* 160:257-261.
60. Kohler, T.R., T. R. Kirkman, L. W. Kraiss, B. K. Zierler, and A. W. Clowes. 1991. Increased blood flow inhibits neointimal hyperplasia in endothelialized vascular grafts. *Circ. Res.* (in press).
61. Kraiss, L.W., T. R. Kirkman, T. R. Kohler, B. Zierler, and A. W. Clowes. 1991. Shear stress regulates   smooth   muscle   proliferation   and   neointimal   thickening   in   porous

polytetrafluoroethylene grafts. *Arteriosclerosis and Thrombosis,* 11:1844-1852.
62. Ku, D.N., D. P. Giddens, C. Zarins, and S. Glagov. 1985. Pulsatile flow and atherosclerosis in the human carotid bifurcation: Posative correlation between plaque location and low and oscillating shear stress. *Arteriosclerosis,.* 5:293-302.
63. Kunlin, J. 1949. Le traitement de l'arterie par la greffe veineuse longue. *Arch Mal Coeur,* 42:371-372.
64. Landymore, R.W., M. S. Manku, M. Tan, M. A. MacAulay, and B. Sheridan. 1989. Effects of low-dose marine oils on intimal hyperplasia in autologous vein grafts. J. Thorac. Cardiovasc. *Surg.* 98:788-791.
65. Lange, R.A., E. D. Flores, and L. D. Hillis. 1991. Restenosis after coronary balloon angioplasty. *Annu. Rev. Med.,* 42:127-132.
66. Langille, B.L. and F. O'Donnell. 1986. Reductions in arterial diameter produced by chronic decreases in blood flow are endothelium-dependent. *Science,* 231:405-407.
67. Larrue, J., J. Demond-Henri, and D. Daret. 1989. Renin-angiotensin system in cultured human arterial smooth muscle cells. *J. Cardiovasc. Pharmacol. 14 Suppl.,* 4:S43-S45.
68. Lawric, G.M., J. T. Lie, G. C. Morris, and H. L. Beazley. 1976. Vein graft patency and intimal proliferation after aortocoronary bypass, Early and long-term angiopathologic correlations. *Am. J Cardiol.,* 38:856-862.
69. Libby, P. and G. K. Hansson. 1991. Involvement of the immune system in human atherogenesis: Current knowledge and unanswered questions. *Lab. Invest.,* 64:5-15.
70. Lindner, V., D. A. Lappi, A. Baird, R. A. Majack, and M. A. Reidy. 1991. Role of basic fibroblast growth factor in vascular lesion formation. *Circ. Res.,* 68:106-113.
71. Lindner, V., R. A. Majack, and M. A. Reidy. 1990. Basic fibroblast growth factor stimulates endothelial regrowth and proliferation in denuded arteries. *J. Clin. Invest.,* 85:2004-2008.
72. Lindner, V. and M. A. Reidy. 1991. Proliferation of smooth muscle cells after vascular injury is inhibited by an antibody against basic fibroblast growth factor. *Proc. Natl. Acad. Sci, USA,* 88:3739-3743.
73. Linton, R.R. 1955. Some practical considerations in surgery of blood vessel grafts. *Surgery,* 38:817-835.
74. LoGerfo, F.W., W. C. Quist, N. L. Cantelmo, and C. C. Haudenschild. 1983. Integrity of vein grafts as a function of initial intimal and medial preservation. *Circulation,* 68:II-117-II-124.
75. Majack, R.A. and A. W. Clowes. 1984. Inhibition of vascular smooth muscle cell migration by heparin-like glycosaminoglycans. *J Cell. Physiol.,* 118:253-256.
76. Majesky, M.W., S. M. Schwartz, M. M. Clowes, and A. W. Clowes. 1987. Heparin regulates smooth muscle S phase entry in the injured rat carotid artery. *Circ. Res.,* 61:296-300.
77. McCollum, C., C. Alexander, N. Dip, G. Kenchington, P. J. Franks, and R. Greenhalgh. 1991. Antiplatelet drugs in femoropopliteal vein bypasses: A multicenter trial. *J. Vasc. Surg.,* 13:150-162.
78. Milner, M.R., R. A. Gallino, A. Leffingwell, A. D. Pichard, S. Brooks-Robinson, J. Rosenberg, T. Little, and Jr. Lindsay,J.. 1989. Usefulness of fish oil supplements in preventing clinical evidence of restenosis after percutaneous transluminal coronary angioplasty. *Am. J. Cardiol.,* 64:294-299.
79. Nabel, E.G., G. Plautz, F. M. Boyce, J. C. Stanley, and G. J. Nabel. 1989. Recombinant gene expression in vivo within endothelial cells of the arterial wall. *Science,* 244:1342-1344.
80. Nabel, E.G., G. Plautz, and G. J. Nabel. 1990. Site specific gene expression in vivo by direct gene transfer into the arterial wall. *Science,* 249:1285-1288.
81. Osterrieder, W., R. K. M. Müller, J. S. Powell, J. -P. Clozel, F. Hefti, and H. R. Baumgartner. 1991. Role of angiotensin II in injury-induced neointima formation in rats. *Hypertension* 18 Suppl.:II60-II64.
82. Oudot, J. 1951. Un deuxieme cas de greffe de la bifurcation aortique pour thrombose de la fourche aortique. *Mem Acad Chir,* 77:644-645.
83. Plautz, G., E. G. Nabel, and G. J. Nabel. 1991. Introduction of vascular smooth muscle cells expressing recombinant genes in vivo. *Circulation,* 83:578-583.
84. Powell, J.S., J. P. Clozel, R. K. M Muller, H. Kuhn, F. Hefti, M. Hosang, and H. R. Baumgartner. 1989. Inhibitors of angiotensin-converting enzyme prevent myointimal proliferation after vascular injury. *Science,* 245:186-188.
85. Powell, J.S., R. K. M. Muller, and H. R. Baumgartner. 1991. Suppression of the vascular response to injury: The role of angiotensin-converting enzyme inhibitors. *J. Am. Coll. Cardiol.* 17 Suppl. B:137B-142B.

86. Powell, J.S., R. K. M. Müller, M. Rouge, H. Kuhn, F. Hefti, and H. R. Baumgartner. 1990. The proliferative response to vascular injury is suppressed by angiotensin-converting enzyme inhibition. *J. Cardiovasc. Pharmacol. 16 Suppl.* 4:S42-S49

87. Reichle, F.A., K. P. Rankin, R. R. Tyson, A. J. Finestone, and C. Shuman. 1979. Long-term results of 474 arterial reconstructions for severely ischemic limbs: A fourteen year follow-up. *Surgery* 85:93-100.

88. Reidy, M.A., A. W. Clowes, and S. M. Schwartz. 1983. Endothelial regeneration. V. Inhibition of endothelial regrowth in arteries of rat and rabbit. *Lab. Invest.,* 49:569-575.

89. Ross, R., J. Glomset, B. Kariya, and L. Harker. 1974. A platelet-dependent serum factor that stimulates the proliferation of arterial smooth muscle cells in vitro. *Proc. Natl. Acad. Sci. USA,* 71:1207-1210.

90. Ross, R. and J. A. Glomset. 1976. The pathogenesis of atherosclerosis. *N. Engl. J Med.,* 295:369-377; 420-425.

91. Sarris, G.E., J. I. Fann, M. H. Sokoloff, D. L. Smith, M. Loveday, J. C. Kosek, R. J. Stephens, A. D. Cooper, K. May, A. L. Willis, and D. C. Miller. 1989. Mechanisms responsible for inhibition of vein-graft arteriosclerosis by fish oil. *Circulation* 80 Suppl.:I109-I123.

92. Schlant, R.C. and S. B. King,III. 1989. Usefulness of calcium entry blockers during and after percutaneous transluminal coronary artery angioplasty. *Circulation* 80 Suppl.:IV88-IV92.

93. Schmitz, G., J. Hankovitz, and E. M. Kovacs. 1991. Cellular processes in atherogenesis: Potential targets of Ca^{2+} channel blockers. *Atherosclerosis* ,88:109-132.

94. Schwartz, L., J. Lesperance, M. G. Bourassa, C. Eastwood, F. Kazim, M. Arafah, and L. Ganassin. 1990. The role of antiplatelet agents in modifying the extent of restenosis following percutaneous transluminal coronary angioplasty. *Am. Heart J.,* 119:232-236.

95. Schwartz, S.M. and M. A. Reidy. 1987. Common mechanisms of proliferation of smooth muscle in atherosclerosis and hypertension. *Hum. Pathol.,* 18:240-247.

96. Snow, A.D., R. P. Bolender, T. N. Wight, and A. W. Clowes. 1990. Heparin modulates the composition of the extracellular matrix domain surrounding arterial smooth muscle cells. *Am. J. Pathol.,* 137:313-330.

97. Snow, A.D., S. Lara, J. Fingerle, S. Certeza, and T. N. Wight. 1988. The effect of heparin on intimal extracellular matrix components after arterial injury. *FASEB J,* 2:810.

98. Szilagyi, D.E., J. P. Elliott, J. H. Hageman, R. F. Smith, and Dall'olmo. 1973. Biologic fate of autogenous vein implants as arterial substitutes. *Ann. Surg.,* 178:232-245.

99. Tang, S.-S., L. Stevenson, and V. J. Dzau. 1990. Endothelial renin-angiotensin pathway: Adrenergic regulation of angiotensin secretion. *Circ. Res.,* 66:103-108.

100. Veith, F.J., S. K. Gupta, E. Ascer, S. White-Flores, R. H. Samson, L. A. Scher, J. B. Towne, V. M. Bernhard, P. Bonier, W. R. Flinn, P. Astelford, J. S. T. Yao, and J. J. Bergan. 1986. Six-year prospective multicenter randomized comparison of autologous saphenous vein and expanded polytetrafluoroethylene grafts in infrainguinal arterial reconstructions. *J. Vasc. Surg.,* 3:104-114.

101. Whittemore, A.D., A. W. Clowes, N. P. Couch, and J. A. Mannick. 1981. Secondary femoropopliteal reconstruction. *Ann. Surg.* 193:35-42.

102. Wilson, J.M., L. K. Birinyi, R. N. Salomon, P. Libby, A. D. Callow, and R. C. Mulligan. 1989. Implantation of vascular grafts lined with genetically modified endothelial cells. *Science,* 244:1344-1346.

103. Wolinsky, H. and S. Glagov. 1967. A lamellar unit of aortic medial structure and function in mammals. *Circ. Res.,* 20:99-111.

104. Zarins, C.K., M. A. Zatina, D. P. Giddens, D. N. Ku, and S. Glagov. 1987. Shear stress regulation of artery lumen diameter in experimental atherogenesis. *J. Vasc. Surg.,* 5:413-420.

105. Zwolak, R.M., M. C. Adams, and A. W. Clowes. 1987. Kinetics of vein graft hyperplasia: association with tangential stress. *J. Vasc. Surg.,* 5:126-136.

106. Zwolak, R.M., T. R. Kirkman, and A. W. Clowes. 1989. Atherosclerosis in rabbit vein grafts. *Arteriosclerosis,* 9:374-379.

Factors Determining The Success or Failure of a Composite Knitted Dacron Biosynthetic Prosthesis

L.R. Sauvage

*The Hope Heart Institute, The Providence Medical Center and
The Department of Surgery, University of Washington
Seattle, Washington, U.S.A.*

Dr. Spartera originally asked me to speak on prosthesis factors that could be related to failure of arterial grafts. I have found this a very difficult subject to handle because I have had broad experience only with the knitted Dacron prosthesis that must be rendered impervious by preclotting prior to implantation. The knitted graft received from the manufacturer is a porous fiber framework that evolves through the proper preclotting process into a highly-sophisticated, complete biosynthetic prosthesis in which every Dacron fiber is coated and every interstice closed by a matrix of the patient's own vascular protein, fibrin. Fibrin is a tough, elastic, negatively-charged protein that was designed by nature to cover denuded flow surfaces and to form the pabulum for healing. The blood inside and the tissues outside thus interface with an autogenous protein material that has the attributes of flow surface passivity and outer wall healability. The Dacron fiber framework of the bioprosthesis functions as a lattice for the deposition of a fibrin matrix during preclotting, provides the strength necessary for indefinite dimensional stability after implantation, and serves as a trellis to assist cellular ingrowth from the perigraft tissues.

I have had extensive experience using this composite biosynthetic prosthesis in the abdominal, femorofemoral, axillofemoral, and above-knee femoropopliteal locations. The success rates my partners and I have achieved follow the sequence mentioned because the size of the vessels and their flow rates progressively decrease in this order. Against this background I will discuss the factors that have been important in achieving the results we have obtained since 1978 using a warp-knit, external-velour, knitted Dacron prosthesis. These results are shown in Figure 1.

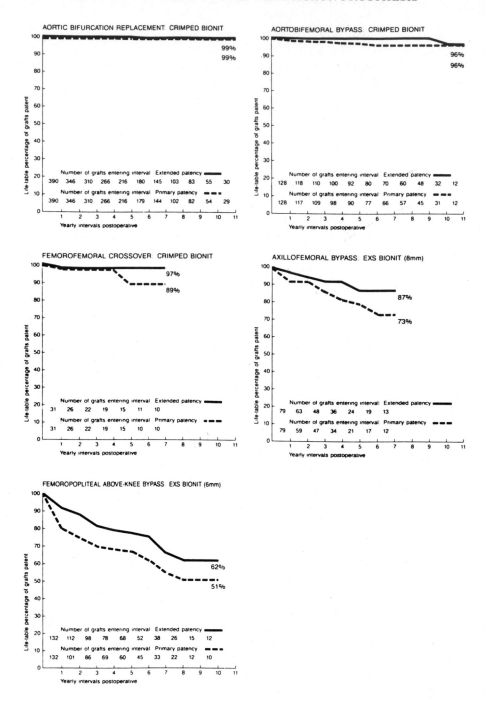

Fig. 1. Extended and primary patencies obtained with warp-knit, external-velour knitted Dacron prostheses.

We shall consider in sequence: blood/graft flow-surface interactions, formation of the fibrin matrix of the biosynthetic graft by preclotting, importance of performing precise anastomoses that are correct in every detail, influence of the quality of the perigraft bed on graft healing, and the value of long-term surveillance of patients in whom arterial prostheses have been implanted. Each of these considerations has an important influence on whether the graft functions long term or fails in the early, middle, or late period.

BLOOD/GRAFT FLOW-SURFACE INTERACTIONS

Prosthesis patency is determined by the interaction between the blood and the flow surface. The blood's reactivity to the flow surface of the graft is largely determined by the degree of platelet aggregability and the concentration of prothrombin and fibrinogen. The thrombogenicity of the flow surface is largely determined by its capacity to activate the platelets. If the platelets do not become activated, thrombosis does not occur. This lack of activation may be due to a high resistance of the platelets to be activated, to a significant lack of activating capacity by the surface, or to any combination of these characteristics that fails to reach the activation threshold. The capacity of the flow surface to activate platelets is determined by its physical, electrical, and chemical characteristics. The ability of a flow surface to activate platelets is enhanced by irregularities that produce turbulence, eddies, and stasis, by a positive charge, and by the presence of chemicals such as ADP, collagen, thrombin, thromboxane A_2 and many others.

We are testing the hypothesis that a high concentration of hyperaggregable platelets combined with a high concentration of fibrinogen (over 400 mg/dl) are the most important prothrombotic factors enabling the blood to be activated into a thrombotic reaction on the flow surface of the prosthesis. The velocity of blood across the flow surface determines whether there is time for a thrombotic reaction to occur. This velocity varies with the concentration and activity of the prothrombotic factors of the blood and with the capacity of the flow surface to activate platelets. If the surface has little capacity to activate platelets, the flow can become very slow before there is time for the platelets to adhere to the surface, be activated, attract and activate other platelets, and catalyze the conversion of fibrinogen to fibrin. The flow velocity which allows thrombosis to begin may be termed the thrombotic threshold velocity (Fig. 2)[3]. This velocity is a definable characteristic of the flow surface which in theory remains constant so long as the prothrombotic factors of the blood also remain constant.

In 1986 we demonstrated that 4-mm Dacron grafts work well in the carotid arteries of mongrel dogs which were pre-selected on the basis of a low platelet aggregatory potential. The same graft would fail in other dogs with a high aggregatory potential[2]. However, the platelet aggregatory potential was not of consequence to the uniform success of 8-mm grafts of this

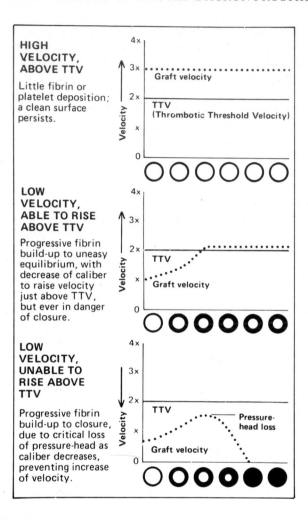

Fig. 2. Relationship between fibrin buildup and blood flow velocity through graft. *From* Sauvage, L.R. (1984) Opportunities and responsibilities in the use of arterial grafts. In Surgery Annual, Volume 16, edited by Nyhus, L., pp 91-117, Appleton-Century-Crofts, Norwalk, Connecticut.

same type when implanted in the large-caliber, high-flow descending thoracic aorta. In recent years we have instituted the testing of our patients' blood in the same way we test that of our dogs and believe the information gained is of much value. We no longer implant synthetic grafts in the above- or below-knee femoropopliteal position in patients whose platelet aggregatory potentials cannot be controlled to low levels. The closures that we have observed in the past in these areas occurred primarily in the first year. We now believe that these early closures were in patients in whom the hematologic environment was unfavorable. We are currently doing both retrospective and prospective studies to challenge this hypothesis. In order to do these studies we have had to develop a credible method for measuring the platelet aggregation of our patients. In view of the obvious importance of this information, it is unfortunate that it can be obtained in so few hospitals.

The comparatively poor results observed with the knitted Dacron grafts in the above-knee femoropopliteal location (Fig. 1) could likely have been changed to a more favorable long-term result if the grafts had been implanted only in patients whose platelet aggregatory potentials were either naturally low or had been rendered low by antiplatelet agents. In my current practice, a patient whose platelets cannot be controlled by aspirin or a medication we have developed called "Citramine" will not receive a synthetic graft. Such a patient will receive a good saphenous vein graft if one is present. Because of occasional closure of apparently good saphenous grafts even in above-knee locations, I also give antiplatelet agents to these patients.

There is a time to commit the patient's best resources, the saphenous veins, and, in my opinion, that applies even to the above-knee femoropopliteal location if the hematologic factors are unfavorable (high aggregator platelets that cannot be modified and/or high fibrinogen). There is no question that a good saphenous graft is preferable to any synthetic prosthesis for unfavorable anatomic locations such as the below-knee popliteal or tibial runoff areas. The greater saphenous vein can be used in these areas with little concern about preserving them for potential use in the heart, because in my cardiac practice I have routinely used the internal thoracic arteries since 1984 for extensive revascularization of the entire heart with excellent success[4].

If a good vein is not available for use below the knee I would avoid operation unless the patient had severe rest pain or threatened limb loss. Under these circumstances I would only use a synthetic graft if the aggregatory potential of the platelets could be reduced to a low level.

FORMATION OF THE FIBRIN MATRIX OF THE BIOSYNTHETIC GRAFT BY PRECLOTTING

As mentioned earlier, the knitted Dacron prosthesis that is received from the manufacturer is an incomplete graft that must be converted into an impervious biosynthetic composite which presents an autogenous protein matrix largely composed of fibrin to the tissues externally and to the blood internally (Fig. 3). The manufacturer makes the fiber framework which most surgeons mistakenly regard as the "complete graft". They do not fully appreciate the importance of their role in forming the fibrin matrix of the completed graft. The quality of this matrix determines the biologic quality of the biosynthetic prosthesis that the patient will receive. It has been a bitter dis-

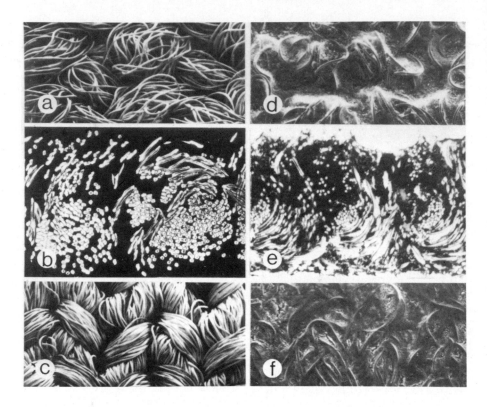

Fig. 3. LEFT: Microstructure of a knitted, warp-knit external velour Dacron prosthesis as received from the manufacturer. a. Outer surface, SEM; b. Longitudinal section, LM; c. Flow surface, SEM. RIGHT: Completed biosynthetic prosthesis after preclot. d. Outer surface, SEM; e. Longitudinal section, LM; f. Flow surface, SEM. Original magnification x50 for all SEM's. Left panel *from* Mathisen, S.R., et al., (1986) The influence of denier and porosity on performance of a warp-knit Dacron arterial prosthesis. Ann. Surg., 203:382-389. Right panel *from* Sauvage, L.R. (1984) Opportunities and responsibilities in the use of arterial grafts. In Surgery Annual, Volume 16, edited by Nyhus, L., pp 92-117, Appleton-Century-Crofts, Norwalk, Connecticut.

appointment to me that so few surgeons have recognized the importance of their vital role in constructing the definitive form of this biosynthetic prosthesis. The surgeon is responsible for the matrix phase of graft construction in which fibrinogen is catalyzed into fibrin by the enzymatic action of thrombin, the most powerful procoagulant. There is a paradox here: fibrinogen cannot be converted to fibrin without the action of thrombin, and the continued presence of thrombin makes the surface exceedingly thrombogenic. Although necessary during the reaction, thrombin's presence after the reaction has been completed is most undesirable. The inactivation of the thrombin is most conveniently achieved by repeatedly inflating the preclotted graft with heparinized blood. Heparin works by the intense activation of the antithrombin III in the blood: the activated antithrombin III forms a complex with thrombin to render it inactive.

The technique of preclotting that I use is shown in Figure 4. Two pans of heparinized blood are always used for femorofemoral, axillofemoral, or femoropopliteal bypass grafts. Often, the blood in the first pan will slowly form a soft clot after having been used to repeatedly inflate the graft, indicating that there still is residual thrombin on the surface and in the substance of the fibrin matrix of the graft, whereas the blood in the second pan remains totally fluid, indicating that all thrombin has been complexed and, in addition, that there is residual heparin-activated antithrombin III on the surface and in the substance of the fibrin matrix of the now-completed biosynthetic prosthesis. The presence of this antithrombin III gives the graft a measure of true antithrombogenicity. I have always had a sense of pride in preclotting a graft in a careful and accurate manner and believe that the final product is well worth the 15 minutes required to produce it.

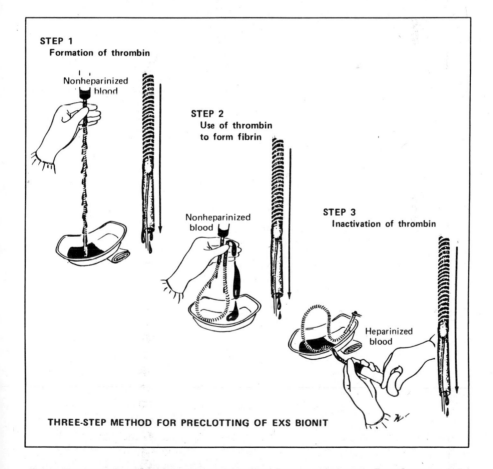

Fig. 4. Essence of preclotting technique for knitted Dacron prostheses. *From* Sauvage, L.R., (1991) Cardio-vascular grafts and synthetic materials. Adv. Card. Surg., 1:199-222

IMPORTANCE OF PERFORMING PRECISE ANASTOMOSES THAT ARE CORRECT IN EVERY DETAIL

Joining a prosthesis to a host artery must be done accurately and securely. There are both short- and long-term consequences of doing vascular anastomoses in an improper manner. The most obvious short-term consequence is occlusive thrombosis. The junction between the endothelial surface of the host artery and the dethrombinated fibrin surface of the prosthesis should be beautifully smooth without any part of the edge of the prosthesis projecting into the blood stream. This is readily accomplishable if sufficient care is taken. Optical magnification is of great help in obtaining this objective. I use 4x loupes and would be lost without them. It is helpful to keep the obvious in mind: if there are irregularities in the suture line, or if adventitial strands are pulled inward to the flow surface with the sutures, platelets will adhere, activate and lead to thrombotic problems at the anastomosis.

I use an interrupted everting mattress technique for joining grafts to the abdominal aorta when circumstances and time allow (Fig. 5a), and for end-to-end anastomosis to the iliacs I use a simple interrupted suture method that accomplishes the same purpose by going through a double layer of the prosthesis (Fig. 5b). Major size discrepancy between the graft limb and a

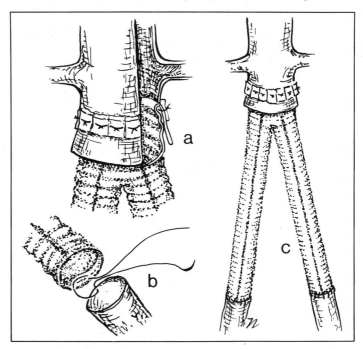

Fig. 5. a. Intussuscepting, interrupted everting mattress anastomosis to abdominal aorta. b. Interrupted simple suture anastomosis assuring smooth junction of prosthesis to iliacs. c. Completed implantation.

larger common iliac can be accommodated if the interrupted sutures are placed at right angles to the wall of each structure, in essence compensating for the disproportion in an equal manner beginning with the second stitch and continuing with all subsequent ones.

The integrity of the anastomosis of a synthetic to the host artery depends forever on the suture line. The scar-tissue union that occurs between the prosthesis and the host artery is not able to withstand the constant pounding of the arterial pressure over long periods of time. This means that the suture one employs must have sufficient strength to remain intact indefinitely, and have a sufficient hold on the arterial wall so that it will not cut out over time.

If there is excessive axial tension on the anastomosis because the graft is too short, the anastomosis will have undue tension on it and over time the sutures may cut through the wall leading to the development of a false aneurysm (Fig. 6). Also, if the opening in the artery is made larger than the opening in the prosthesis, excessive suture-line tension develops which may cause the sutures to cut through the wall with possible false aneurysm.

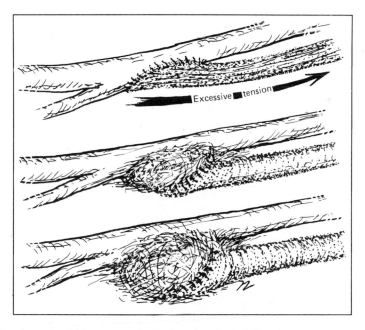

Fig. 6. Development of false aneurysm due to excessive axial tension.

A key point I have learned over my years in practice is that sutures should always be placed at right angles to the wall whether the structure being su-tured is skin, fascia, prosthesis, or arterial wall. This right-angled placement to the wall of a circular anastomosis is difficult if there is significant disproportion between the ends being joined except at the 6, 9, 12, and 3 o'clock positions. In those locations I can pass the needle through both walls in one motion and achieve right-angle orientation for both sides. Elsewhere, I must pass the needle through each wall separately in order to achieve this right-angle relationship. It is helpful to envision a long anastomosis as composed of a half circle at each end, connected by an intervening straight line. For the straight line portion of the anastomosis, the right-angle relationship is conveniently achieved by passing the needle through both walls with one motion.

For an interrupted everting mattress anastomosis of a prosthesis to the abdominal aorta I use 3-0 or 4-0 Tycron. If I employ a continuous suture I use a 3-0 or 4-0 Prolene. For the interrupted suture anastomosis to the iliacs, I use 4-0 Tycron. For the anastomosis of the nonconforming supported end of an EXS Dacron graft to the common femoral I also use interrupted 4-0 Tycron. However, I use continuous 5-0 Prolene for anastomosis of a prosthesis to the above- or below-knee popliteal and continuous 6-0 Prolene for anastomosis to the tibial runoff vessels.

INFLUENCE OF THE QUALITY OF THE PERIGRAFT BED ON GRAFT HEALING

Most surgeons exercise great skill in the performance of the anastomosis of the prosthesis to the host artery. Few surgeons have anywhere near the same concern to form the quality of the perigraft bed which surrounds the

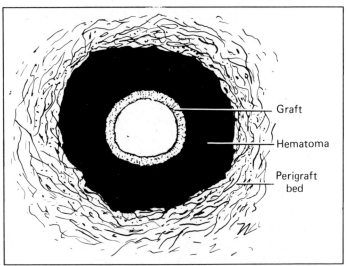

Fig. 7. Prevention of tissue ingrowth into outer wall due to hematoma between prosthesis and perigraft bed.

prosthesis. This lack of concern is unfortunate because the only way the body of the graft can be healed is by contact of perigraft tissues with its outer wall. If a hematoma occurs around the graft the tissues are prevented from reaching the prosthesis (Fig. 7). Under these circumstances, the reproductive capacity of the areolar tissues in the perigraft bed becomes exhausted by the magnitude of the effort to organize the hematoma before ingrowth into the outer wall of the prosthesis can occur. Also, so long as there is space around the prosthesis, the graft is at risk for the delayed development of perigraft infection.

Over the years I have come to regard the perigraft bed of a prosthesis much as a gardener regards the soil into which he plants a special bush or plant. If the conditions are right for patency and healing, the prosthesis will remain patent and the perigraft tissues will grow into the outer wall and incorporate it as a part of its own. The Biblical statement "as you sow, so shall you reap" is also applicable to what we as surgeons do with prostheses.

THE VALUE OF LONG-TERM SURVEILLANCE OF PATIENTS IN WHOM ARTERIAL PROSTHESES HAVE BEEN IMPLANTED

In my years of practice, I have never discharged a patient with an arterial prosthesis from continuing followup. I always ask the patient to come back at 6- to 12-month intervals if everything is going well, or at shorter intervals if I have some concern. If the patients choose not to come back, that is their responsibility, but it is my responsibility to invite them to return at stated intervals. This is important because patients with arterial grafts may develop signs of impending trouble in subtle ways that can be detected at times when they can still be corrected readily. False aneurysms may develop and should be repaired if they are large or increasing in size. Lower extremity graft stenosis can be ascertained by changes in the ankle-brachial index and by the development of murmurs along the course of the graft. The development of murmurs worries me and signals the need for close observation because they result from the turbulence of blood going through stenotic areas. If a graft closes, I will reopen or replace it if the patient's general condition and extremity status both indicate that this should be done. To prevent reocclusion the thrombotic reactivity of the blood to the flow surface must be reduced, often necessitating the use of both Coumadin and antiplatelet agents.

Early in our experience we saw quite a few grafts develop fiber breakdown with perigraft false aneurysm formation. We observed this with grafts produced by all the major manufacturers[1]. Because it has been reasonably established that such fiber breakdown was due to degradation of the Dacron, induced by excessive attempts with chemicals and/or heat treatment to reduce the porosity of the wall; such harsh processes are no longer used and the danger of post-implant fiber breakdown is now largely a thing of the past for all grafts produced by current manufacturers.

As a closing note, I wish to say that during my years in the practice of cardiovascular surgery, I have come to appreciate the factor of judgment at least as much as technical skill. Skill without direction is dangerous and so is the reverse. Both attributes are essential if excellent results are to be consistently obtained with any type of arterial prosthesis.

REFERENCES

1. Berger, K., Sauvage, L.R., (1981) Late fiber deterioration in Dacron arterial grafts. *Ann. Surg.*, 193:477-491.
2. Kaplan S., Marcoe, K.F., Sauvage, L.R., Zammit, M., Wu, H.-D., Mathisen, S.R., Walker, M.W., (1986) The effect of predetermined thrombotic potential of the recipient on small-caliber graft performance. *J. Vasc. Surg.*, 3:311-321.
3. Sauvage, L.R., Walker, M.W., Berger, K., Robel, S.B., Lischko, M.M., Yates, S.G., Logan, G.A., (1979) Current arterial prostheses: Experimental evaluation by implantation in the carotid and circumflex coronary arteries of the dog. *Arch. Surg.*, 114:687-691.
4. Sauvage, L.R., Wu, H.-D., Kowalsky, T.E., Davis, C.C., Smith, J.C., Rittenhouse, E.A., Hall, D.G., Mansfield, P.B., Mathisen, S.R., Usui, Y., Goff, S.G., (1986) Healing basis and surgical techniques for complete revascularization of the left ventricle using only the internal mammary arteries. *Ann. Thorac. Surg.*, 42:449-465.

Pharmacological Prevention of Graft Occlusion - A Review

D. Bergqvist

Department of Surgery, Lund University,
Malmo General Hospital
Malmo, Sweden

Although it may be interesting to discuss pharmacological prevention of graft occlusion after every type of peripheral arterial reconstruction, this review will restrict itself to deal with femorocrural reconstruction. This is the type of surgery where graft patency should be better and where pharmacological methods might be of some value.

This is also the type of surgery where there have been a number of studies which can be analyzed and hopefully form the basis for some practical conclusions. It is in a way remarkable how resistant peripheral vascular surgeons have been to perform adequate studies on this topic, which is in contrast to coronary bypass surgeons[9,28]. The purpose of this review is to determine the efficacy of pharmacological therapy in preventing graft occlusion after femorocrural bypass surgery. Before doing so some background data will be given on factors of importance for graft occlusion and the natural history of grafts inserted from the groin and distally.

NATURAL COURSE AND CAUSES OF GRAFT OCCLUSION

Graft occlusion is a multifactorial and complex process. During the temporal course after insertion of a graft, there are several factors which may cause failure, and their relative importance changes over time. The situation is somewhat simplified in Table 1, but it is evident that all factors can not easily be counteracted by pharmacological modalities, and when the temporal endpoint in a study is set is therefore important as the various factors overlap. The part which is possible to influence pharmacologically is moreover in most cases small and hidden among other causes and thus studies on pharmacological prophylaxis have to be fairly large concerning the population sample. Several other factors are of importance but will not be further discussed in this paper: anatomic location of the reconstruction, joint crossing, peripheral resistance, type of reconstruction, adjunctive surgical procedures such as vein collars and AV fistulae, graft material, indication for surgery, presence of diabetes, and skill of the vascular surgeon. Another very potent factor is smoking habits, and a few comments may be relevant. Smoking influences in a negative way a number of factors which are of importance both for graft occlusion and progression of the atherosclerotic disease[36]. It is now quite clear that continued smoking after femorocrural bypass surgery has a great influence on graft patency[44,50]. This fact becomes especially evident when objective criteria are used to define ongoing smoking such as determination of isothiocyanate[41]. It may be relevant to notice that differences in patency between high and low isothiocyanate patients are at least of the order of magnitude, which is discussed when pharmacological interventions are considered.

Table 1 - Temporal classification of graft occlusion

Time in relation to surgery	Interval from operation	Cause of occlusion
1 Intraop or immediately postop	Hours to a few days	Technical errors Poor run-in Poor run-off High blood viscosity Light thrombogenicity
2 Postop	Days to a few weeks	Graft thrombogenicity High blood viscosity
3 Postop	Weeks to a few months	Graft thrombogenicity Vein graft stricture Pseudointimal hyperpl. Graft blood viscosity
4 Postop	Months to years	Pseudointimal hyperpl. High blood viscosity Arteriosclerosis

Concerning pathophysiology of graft occlusion, early in the form of thrombosis and late in the form of pseudointimal hyperplasia, much is known[11,15,16] but still more knowledge must be obtained before the "perfect" pharmacological investigation can be designed and performed. Many studies have been focused on the role of fibrinogen and platelets, few on leucocytes, the role of which in the blood surface interaction is unknown, but important to evaluate. Their role in ischemic diseases has been increasingly discussed[21].

DESIGN OF CLINICAL STUDIES

The main requirements that should be fulfilled in a trial of pharmacological prophylaxis against graft occlusion are summarized in Table 2. Only few, if any studies, fulfill all these criteria. The number of studies and reports on femorocrural bypass surgery is large, but only rarely do they report on pharmacological principles, neither perioperatively nor in the long-term perspective[3]. As can be suspected from the introductory remarks on graft occlusion as a multifactorial process, the results between studies are extremely variable. Therefore a minimal criterion, where pharmacological intervention is concerned, is that the studies are properly randomized and only such studies will be further discussed in this review. The studies have been identified through Medline and in bibliographies of the identified articles. Abstracts have not been included in the analysis.

Table 2 - Which requirements should be fulfilled in studies on prophy-laxis against arterial graft occlusion?

1 - The pathophysiological background should be considered.

2 - The trial design should take into account the natural history of arterial graft occlusion.

3 - Doses and administration intervals must be adequate.

4 - It must be prospective and randomized and, if at all possible, double-blind.

5 - The patients must be well characterized.

6 - The endpoints must be well defined in character as well as time of occurrence.

7 - Inclusion and exclusion criteria must be defined.

8 - Drug compliance must be checked.

9 - Adequate group sizes must be calculated from the potential effect of the substances.

10 - Adverse effects must be recorded.

11 - The representativity of the study sample must be known.

PERIOPERATIVE PROPHYLAXIS

The two main pharmacological principles are heparin and dextran. Heparin is used as an anticoagulant and may be given as a bolus dose - if necessary repeated - intravenously or used in the saline flush solution. The scientific documentation of the effect is largely lacking, but the majority of vascular surgeons use it, and historically it may be said that the use of heparin was one of the main prerequisites for the development and expansion of vascular and cardiac surgery. Those surgeons using heparin have different attitudes towards reversing the effect by protamine, probably because of fear for complications and adverse effects of protamine[38]. However, in a recent study in carotid surgery it was suggested that bleeding complications were significantly diminished if mandatory reversal of the heparin effect was used[48]. Doses of heparin vary from 500 IU per 100 ml in the rinsing solution to 150 IU per kg body weight prior to arterial cross clamping. Some authors recommend continuing heparin for several days[2]. There is a lack of consensus on what is the optimal way of using heparin. Because of great interindividual differences in heparin kinetics it has been suggested to closely monitor the heparin effect during peripheral vascular surgery[40].

In recent years low molecular weight heparin fragments are rapidly replacing heparin for prophylaxis against postoperative venous thromboembolism, the documentation being solid[5]. The efficacy of low molecular weight heparin to prevent early post-reconstructive arterial occlusion is, however, not known. There are a few pilot patients reported[6] and there is definitely a need for systematic research in this field. In this context the antimitogenic activity of heparin is of great interest and this function may be traced to fairly well defined fragments of the heparin molecular[14]. Theoretically it is possible that heparin would counteract early thrombosis as well as later pseudointima.

Some surgeons, especially in Scandinavia, use dextran instead of heparin. Dextran has several effects which makes it rational to use in reconstructive vascular surgery[4] (Table 3). It is usually given as a rapid infusion of 500 ml intraoperatively and then in different amounts during the first postoperative days. Also in this field there is a large lack of properly conducted studies. Waibel showed dextran infused intraoperatively to give a significantly higher three-day patency than no treatment in patients undergoing femoropopliteal reconstruction with poor run-off[49]. Rutherford et al. made a randomized, multicenter trial on the effect of dextran 40 given in addition to a single dose of 100 IU of heparin per kg body weight iv intraoperatively in patients undergoing difficult lower extremity bypass. The overall one-week occlusion rate was significantly lower in the dextran group. By one month the protective effect was partially lost[43]. The combination of dextran and heparin is theoretically interesting but has not been evaluated in a systematic way. This would seem important in a time when volume expansion with blood products is decreasingly used and there is a need for alternative plasma expanders. Experimentally this combination does not influence haemostasis in a negative way[30].

LONGTERM POSTOPERATIVE PROPHYLAXIS

Principally, there are two main types of pharmacological substances, which are of interest in the long-term postoperative course: oral anticoagulants and some type of platelet function inhibitors. At least concerning platelet inhibition there are animal experiments pointing towards an effect, but the data are conflicting[26] (Deen & Sundt 1982, Kon et al. 1984, Gershlick et al. 1984, Lane et al. 1986). It is, however, difficult to draw clinical conclusions based on the animal experiments. An experimental model simulating the human situation with very long-term follow-up in a circulation where the arteriosclerotic process is progressively deteriorating does not exist. There are also human experimental investigations where labelled platelets have been used to study effects of graft implantation and platelet inhibition. Data are not consistent, some studies pointing to an effect[24,46] (Pumphrey et al. 1983), others not (Davies et al. 1982).

In Table 4 the randomized studies on long-term pharmacological prophylaxis are summarized. As can be seen there are several differences between them and some of the studies have a fairly small population sample, creating a possibility for statistical errors. Only three of the studies report the biostatistical basis for the investigation[2,39,47].

Table 3 - Effects of dextran which may be of importance as an anti-thrombotic agent

---

* Volume expansion and hemodilation, decreasing blood viscosity and improving microvascular flow

* Red cell disaggregation

* Influence on haemostasis
  inhibition of platelets
  increased lysability of thrombi
  altered function of factor VIII R:Ag

* Coating of vessel wall and blood cells with a dextran film

The studies are in fact too heterogenous to make statistical analysis on pooled data or meta-analysis meaningful. Two of the studies deal with endarterectomy[7,10] and in three of the remaining a proportion of patients undergoing endarterectomy have been included[2,20,37] and this technical detail may have implications on the results. The study by Harjola et al. has included a great mixture of arterial reconstructions and moreover the follow-up time is only 10 days[27]. Although having used acetylsalicylic acid and dipyridamole it should be regarded more as a study of the immediate postoperative period and data on long-term patency are lacking. A safe conclusion from the study by Swedenborg et al. seems to be that dipyridamole alone is without effect[47]. Whether it potentiates acetylsalicylic acid is still unknown, and the study by Harjola et al. does not have the strict design required to answer that problem[27].

In almost all clinical trials dipyridamole adds little to the antithrombotic effects of acetylsalicylic acid[1,22,45]. That the combination is ineffective when using vein graft to the popliteal artery also seems evident[31]. The British study[31] does not, however, exclude an effect in bypasses distal to the popliteal artery and using non-autologous graft material. Although small in size some studies have indicated that platelet inhibition does increase synthetic graft patency provided that the drug is given before surgery[13,19,23,25], in all acetylsalicylic acid having been combined with dipyridamole. In patients undergoing aorto-coronary bypass surgery there is also indication that antiplatelet therapy started before surgery has an effect[12,28]. Data on oral anticoagulants are contradictory concerning graft patency but consistent in reporting an increased risk for serious bleeding complications[34,2].

One interesting and importing factor is the increased survival seen in patients both on oral anticoagulants[33] and on acetylsalisylic acid[29,35,39]. This is in accordance with other studies summarized in Antiplatelet Trialists' Collaboration[1]. This positive effect may have implications on future studies on how new antiplatelet substances influence graft patency when patients already have background medication with acetylsalicylic acid or ticlopidine to increase survival rate. One negative effect with acetylsalicylic acid, at least in doses above 1g per day, is gastrointestinal problems, also haemorrhagic.

Therefore it is important to keep the dose low, and there are data indicating an equal effect between low (oral 300 mg) and high (oral c:a 1 g) daily versus a diminished frequency of side effects[1,12]. On the other hand, there is still an "aspirin dilemma"[18] in that we do not know which doses and dose intervals that really are optimal. Although very low doses seem theoretically attractive, at least in a recent study after carotid endarterectomy, there was no effect[8].

CONCLUDING REMARKS

The problem of graft occlusion is very complex, the pathologic process being multifactorial. This makes the design of studies diffic ult and they often need to include quite a numbers of patients, which is infected in the low number of adequately performed studies.

Perioperatively heparin or dextran is used by most vascular surgeons but the documentation of an affect is scarce. Oral anticoagulants in the long term peroperative does not seem to influence the graft patency but it increases survival. The frequency of bleeding complications increases with time. In all types of femorocrural reconstruction, which is more complicated than a single vein graft to the popliteal artery, data seem to support antiplatelet prophylaxis for at least 6 months provided it is started preoperatively or at the day of surgery. To quit smoking is, however, probably more effective to improve graft patency than the pharmacological metho ds used today.

Table 4

Author	No of patients	Start of prophy-laxis	Follow up Time	Methodology	Control	ASA	ASA-dip	OA	Ticl	Sulf	Comment	Sign
Arfvidsson et al.[2] (mix)	55,61	1-20	12-36m	C			74-42		75-46		Heparin 5-7d	NS
Bollinger, Brunner [7](TEA)	40,41,39	7d	24m	C,O,AI (A)		84	76	58			ASA 1g 1d	S(ASA)
Castelli et al.[1c](TEA)	23,23	postop	6m	C, Doppler	44				87			S
Clyne et al.[13]	70,78	-48h	12m	C,AI(A)	65		84				ASA 300mg 1d	S
Comberg et al.[17]	27,27	14d	6m	AI,I,O	-					-		NS
Donaldson et al.[19]	38,25	-1	12m	C,Doppler,isot	59		85					S
Ehresman et al.[20](mix)	213,215	2d	12m	C,O(A)	77	91					ASA 1,5g 1d	NS
Goldman, Mc Collum [23]	31,22	-48h	12m	C,Doppler(A)	36		67				ASA 0,9g	S
Green et al.[25]	17,16,16	-48h	12m	C(A)	50	100	100				ASA 325mgx3	S
Harjola et al.[27]	86,92, 93,93	1-2d	10d	C	86	94	100				Dip 94	S
Kester[31]	38,35	?	12m	C	60		85					S
Kohler et al.[32]	44,44	1d	24m	C,AI(A)	67		57				ASA 325mgx3	NS
Kretschmer et al.[35]	59,60	2w	5y	?	71						Survival better	NS
Kretschmer et al.[34]	37,34	2w	18m	C,AI	67			81				S
Lassila et al.[37](mix)	72,72	7d	3m	C,AI(A)	48	72		82			ASA 250mg 1d	NS
McCollum et al.[39]	263,286	-48d	12-36m	C,Dupl,A,AI	72-60		78-61				Survival better	NS
Raithel et al.[42]	59,59	day of op	12m	C,AI(A)		74					Trental 75	NS
Swedenborg et al.[47]	203,209	-1	12m	C,AI(A)							Placebo vs dip	NS
Waibel[49]	62,64	3-7d	6m	C	90			95				NS

C = clinical, O = oscillometry, AI = anklebrachial index, A = angiography, P = plethysmography, ASA = acetylsalicylic acid, dip = dipyridamol, OA = oral anticoagulation, ticl = ticlopidine, sulf = sulfinpyrazon

REFERENCES

1. Antiplatelet trialists' collaboration, (1988) Secondary prevention of vascular disease by prolonged antiplatelet treatment. *Br Med J,* 296:320-331.
2. Arfvidsson, B., Lundgren, F., Drott, C., Scherst n, T., and Lundholm, K., (1990) Influence of coumarin treatment on patency and limb salvage after peripheral arterial reconstructive surgery. *Am J Surg,,* 159:556-560.
3. Bergqvist, D. (1989) Pharmacological intervention to increase patency after peripheral arterial reconstruction - the problem. In: Pharmacological intervention to increase patency after arterial reconstructions, edited by Bergqvist, D., Lindblad, B., pp 11-18 .
4. Bergqvist, D., Bergentz, S-E., (1983) The role of dextran in severe ischemic extremity disease and arterial reconstructive surgery. A review. *VASA,* 12:213-218.
5. Bergqvist, D., Lindblad, B., and Mtzsch, T. (1992) Glycosaminoglycans in prophylaxis against venous thromboembolism. In: Heparin and Related Polysaccharides, edited by Lindahl, U., Lane, D. Plenum Press. In press.
6. Benedetti-Valentini, F., Irace, L., Gattuso, R., Ciossa, F., Aracu, A., Intrieri, F., Marini, P., Massa, R., and Gossetti, B., (1988) Arterial repair of the lower limbs: prevention of prosthetic grafts occlusion by LMW-heparin. *Inter Angio,* 7 (Suppl. 3):29-32.
7. Bollinger, A. and Brunner, U., (1985) Antiplatelet drugs improve the patency rates after femoro-popliteal endarterectomy. *VASA,* 14:272-279.
8. Boysen, G., S rensen, P., Juhler, M., Andersen, A.R., Boas, J., Olsen, J.S., and Joensen, P., (1988) Danish very-low-dose after carotid endarterectomy trial. *Stroke,* 19:1211-1215.
9. Buring, J.E. and Hennekens, C.H., (1990) Antiplatelet therapy to prevent coronary artery bypass graft occlusion. *Circulation,* 82:1046-1048.
10. Castelli, P., Basellini, A., Agus, G.B., Ippolito, E., Pogliani, E.M., Colombi, M., Gianese, F., and Scatigna,M., (1986) Thrombosis prevention with ticlopidine after femoropopliteal thromboendarterectomy. *Int Surg,* 71:252-255.
11. Chervu, A. and Moore, W.S., (1990) An overview of intimal hyperplasia. *Surg Gynecol Obstet,* 171:433-447.
12. Clagett, G.P., (1990) Antithrombotic drugs and vascular surgery. *Perspect Vasc Surg,* 3:79-102.
13. Clyne, C.A.C., Archer, T.J., Atuhaire, L.K., Chant, A.D.B., and Webster, J.H.H., (1987) Random control trial of a short course of aspirin and dipyridamole (Persantin) for femorodistal grafts. *Br J Surg,* 74:246-248.
14. Clowes, A. and Clowes, M., (1985) Kinetics of cellular proliferation after arterial injury. II. Inhibition of smooth muscle growth by heparin. *Lab Invest,* 52:611-616.
15. Clowes, A.W. and Reidy, M.A., (1991) Prevention of stenosis after vascular reconstruction: Pharmacologic control of intimal hyperplasia - a review. *J Vasc Surg,* 13:885-891.
16. Clowes, A.W., Clowes, M.M., Fingerle, J., and Reidy, M.A., (1989) Regulation of smooth muscle cell growth in injured artery. *J Cardiovasc Pharmacol* 14 (Suppl. 6): S12-S15.
17. Comberg, H.-U., Janssen, E.J., Diehm, C., Zimmermann, R., Harenberg, J., Walter, E., Oster, P., Allenberg, J., Horsch, A.K., and M rl, H., (1983) Sulfinpyrazon (AnturanR) versus Placebo nach operativer Rekonstruktion der Oberschenkeletage bei arterieller Verschlusskrankheit. *VASA,* 12:172- 178.
18. De Gaetano, G., Cerletti, C., and Bertele, V., (1982) Pharmacology of antiplatelet drugs and clinical trials on thrombosis prevention: a difficult link. *Lancet,* 2:974-977.
19. Donaldson, D.R., Salter, M.C.P., Kester, R.C., Rajah, S.M., Hall, T.J., Streeharan, N., and Crow, M.J., (1985) The influence of platelet inhibition on the patency of femoro-popliteal dacron bypass grafts. *Vasc Surg,* 19:224-230.
20. Ehresmann, U., Alemany, J., Loew, D., (1977) Prophylaxe von Rezidivverschl ssen nach Revaskularisationseingriffen mit Acetylsalicyls ure. Ergebnisse einer doppeltblinden Langzeitstudie. *Med Welt,* 28:1157-1162.
21. Ernst, E., Hammerschmidt, D.E., Bagge, U., Matrai, A., and Dormandy, J.A., (1987) Leukocytes and the risk of ischemic diseases. *JAMA,* 257:2318-2324.
22. Fitzgerald, G.A., (1987) Dipyridamole. *N Engl J Med,* 316:1247-1257.
23. Goldman, M. and McCollum, C., (1984) A prospective randomized study to examine the effect of aspirin plus dipyridamole on the patency of prosthetic femoro-popliteal grafts. *Vasc Surg,* 18:218-221.
24. Goldman, M., Hall, D., Dykes, J., Hawker, R.J., and McCollum, C.N., (1983) Does 111indium-platelet deposition predict patency in prosthetic arterial grafts? *Br J Surg,* 70:635-638.

25. Green, R.M., Roedersheimer, L.R., and DeWeese, J.A., (1982) Effects of aspirin and dipyridamole on expanded polytetrafluoroethylene graft patency. *Surgery,* 92:1016-1026.
26. Hagen, P.O., Wang, Z.G., and Mikat, E.M., (1982) Antiplatelet therapy reduces aortic intimal hyperplasia distal to small-diameter vascular prostheses (PTFE) in nonhuman primates. *Ann Surg,* 195:328-339.
27. Harjola, P.-T., Meurala, H., and Frick, M.H., (1981) Prevention of early reocclusion by Dipyridamole and ASA in arterial reconstructive surgery. *J Cardiovasc Surg,* 22:141-144.
28. Henderson, W.G., Goldman, S., Copeland, J.G., Moritz, T.E., and Harker, L.A., (1989) Antiplatelet or anticoagulant therapy after coronary artery bypass surgery. A meta-analysis of clinical trials. *Am Coll Phys,* 111:743-750.
29. Hennekens, C.H., Buring, J.B., Sandercock, P., Collins, R., and Peto, R., (1989) Aspirin and other antiplatelet agents in the secondary and primary prevention of cardiovascular disease. *Circulation,* 80:749-756.
30. Holst, J., Lindblad, B., M tzsch, T., and Bergqvist, D., (1992) Effect on primary haemostasis of prophylactic regimens of low molecular weight heparin, unfractionated heparin, dextran and their combinations, an animal experimental study. *Thromb Res.* In press.
31. Kester, R.C., (1984) The thrombogenicity of dacron arterial grafts and its modification by platelet inhibitory drugs. *Ann Royal Coll Surg,* 66:241-246.
32. Kohler, T.R., Kaufman, J.L., Kacoyanis, G., Clowes, A., Donaldson, M.C., Kelly, E., Skillman, J., Couch, N.P., Whittemore, A.D., Man nick, J.A., and Salzman, E.W., (1984) Effect of aspirin and dipyridamole on the patency of lower extremity bypass grafts. *Surgery,* 96:462-466.
33. Kretschmer, G., Wenzl, E., Schemper, M., Polterauer, P., Ehringer, H., Marcost, L., and Minar, E., (1988) Influence of postoperative anticoagulant treatment on patient survival after femoropopliteal vein bypass surgery. *The Lancet,* I:797-799.
34. Kretschmer, G., Wenzl, E., Wagner, O., Polterauer, P., Ehringer, H., Minar, E., and Schemper, M., (1986) Influence of anticoagulant treatment in preventing graft occlusion following saphenous vein bypass for femoropopliteal occlusive dis ease. *Br J Surg,* 73:689-692.
35. Kretschmer, G., Pretschner, T., Prager, M., Wenze, E., Polterauer, P., Schemper, M., Ehringer, H., and Minar, E., (1990) Antiplatelet treatment prolongs survival after carotid bifurcation endarterectomy. Analysis of a clinical series followed by a contr olled trial. *Ann Surg,* 211:317-322.
36. Lassila, R. and Lepntalo, M., (1988) Cigarette smoking and the outcome after lower limb arterial surgery. *Acta Chir Scand,* 154:635-640.
37. Lassila, R., Lepntalo, M., and Lindfors, O., (1991) The effect of acetylsalicylic acid on the outcome after lower limb arterial surgery with special reference to cigarette smoking. *World J Surg,* 15:378-382.
38. Lindblad, B., (1989) Protamine sulphate: A review of its effects: Hypersensitivity and toxicity. *Eur J Vasc Surg,* 3:195-201.
39. McCollum, C., Alexander, C., Kenchington, G., and Greenhalgh, R., (1991) Antiplatelet drugs in femoropopliteal vein bypasses: a multicenter trial. *J Vasc Surg,* 13:150-162.
40. Porte, R.J., de Jong, E., Knot, E.A.R., de Maat, M.P.M., Terpstra, O.T., van Urk, H., and Groenland, T.H.N., (1987) Monitoring heparin and haemostasis during reconstruction of the abdominal aorta. *Eur J Vasc Surg,* 1:397-402.
41. Powell, J. (1991) The patients' contribution to graft patency. In: The maintenance of arterial reconstruction, edited by Greenhalgh, R.M., Hollier, L.H., pp 87-93. W.B. Saunders Company Ltd, Lond on.
42. Raithel, D., Kasprzak, P., and Noppeney, Th., (1986) Rezidivprophylaxe nach femoropoplitealer Rekonstruktion mit PTFE-Prothesen. *Med Welt,* 37:664-667.
43. Rutherford, R., Jones, D.N., Bergentz, S-E., Bergqvist, D., Karmody, A.M., Dardik, H., Moore, W.S., Goldstone, J., Flinn, W.R., Comerota, A.J., Fry, W.J., and Shah, D.M., (1984) The efficacy of dextran 40 in preventing early postoperative thrombosis following difficult lower extremity bypass. *J Vasc Surg,* 1:765-773.
44. Rutherford, R., Jones, D., Bergentz, S-E., Bergqvist, D., Comerota, A., Dardik, H., Flinn, W., Fry, W., McIntyre, K., Moore, W., Sha h, D., and Yano, T., (1988) Factors affecting the patency of infrainguinal bypass. *J Vasc Surg,* 8:236-246.
45. Sanz, G., Pajar n, A., Alegria, E., Coello, I., Dardona, M., Fournier, J.A., Gmez-Recio, M., Ruano, J., Hidalgo, R., Medina, A., Oller, G., Colman, T., Malpartida, F., Bosch, X., and the Grupo Espanol para el S eguimiento del Injerto Coronario (GESIC), 1990 Prevention of early aortocoronary bypass occlusion by low-dose aspirin and dipyridamole. *Circulation,* 82:765-773.
46. Stratton, J.R. and Ritchie, J.L., (1986) Reduction of indium-111 platelet deposition on Dacron vascular grafts in humans by aspirin plus dipyridamole. *Circulation,* 73:325-330.

47. Swedenborg*, J., Brodin, U., Almgren, B., Bj rkman, H., Eriksson, I., Forsberg, J.O., Isaksson, L., Jernby, P., Konrad, P., Larzon, T., Lundqvist, B., Molde, ., Nordstr m, S., Plate, G., Spangen, L., Stenberg, B., and Tro ng, T., Stockholm* and Swedish femoropopliteal trial group, (1989) Influence of dipyridamole and prognostic factors on the patency of femoropopliteal grafts. In: Pharmacological intervention to increase patency after arterial reconstructions, edited by Bergqvist, D., Lindblad, B., pp 86-92 . ICM AB, Malm .
48. Treiman, R., Cossman, D., Foran, R., Levin, P., Cohen, L., and Wagner, W., (1990) The influence of neutralizing heparin after carotid endarterectomy on postoperative stroke and wound hematoma. *J Vasc Surg*, 12:440-4 46.
49. Waibel, P., (1976) Antikoagulation in der Gef sschirurgie. *VASA,* 5:107-110.
50. Wiseman, S., Kenchington, G., Dain, R., Marshall, C.E., McCollum, C.N., Greenhalgh, R.M., and Powell, J.T. Influence of smoking and plasma factors on patency of femoropopliteal vein grafts. *Br Med J,* 299:643-646.

REDO SURGERY IN RENAL AREA

Reoperations Done For Renal Lesions

A.V. Pokrovsky

*The Vishnevsky Institute of Surgery, Academy of Medical Sciences,
Moscow, Russia*

A rate of renal operations is directly related to the treatment of two diseases: symptomatic (renovascular) hypertension and chronic renal failure (as a result of renal artery pathology and of parenchymatous lesions).

Certain achievements in drug therapy of these lesions couldn't influence an increasing number of patients requiring surgical treatment. In its turn it resulted in increased number of reoperations done on renal arteries. We must distinguish three groups of patients, which are to be discussed (Table1).

Table 1 - Redo surgery in renal area

Groups of patients:
a) after renal artery dilatation
b) after reconstructive procedures on renal arteries
c) after kidney transplantation

The first group, in which reoperations may be necessary, these are patients, in whom transcuteneous dilatation of renal arteries has been done.

The second group: patients, in whom various reconstructive operations on renal arteries have been done.

The third group: patients, in whom kidney transplantation has been done.

I'll begin from general regulations, which, to my opinion, define a rate of reoperations.

In the first turn it certainly depends on surgeon's experience, since it is he, who mainly defines proper indications for operation and helps to choose an optimal technique of primary intervention.

Let's discuss the first group of patients in whom renal dilatation is done. Following a description of Gruntzig et al. of the first experience with renal dilatation many thousands of similar interventions have been done in the world. J.C. Stanley[15] wrote, that of 624 renal dilatations complications have been noted in 11%. A.L. Baert et al.[1] having analyzed experience of 10 authors gives a figure of 11%. It has been repeatedly confirmed, that experience defines much. Thus, Martin L. et al.[10] showed, that a per cent of complications in the second group of patients with renal dilatation lowered from 20% to 13% and a number of patients requiring surgical treatment - from 5% to 2% (Table 2).

Table 2 - Renal artery dilatation

	First 100 patients	Consecutive 100 patients
Patients requiring operation: for thrombosis, dissection, perforation, rupture of an artery	5%	2%

L. Martin et al., 1986

One of the scientific committees[13] concluded, that a number of urgent operations required after renal dilatation was 1%.

Such simple measures as nitroglycerine, heparin injection into the renal artery, hydratation of a patient have contributed to reduced number of complications. Success of dilatation is in many respects related to proper indications[1] (Table 3).

Table 3 - Renal artery dilatation (Experience with 250 dilatations)

Aetiology and localization		Per cent of failures
Atherosclerosis:	a) ostium	71%
	b) at length	5.5%
Fibromuscular dysplasia		13%

In 72% it was a failure: unattained dilatation.   A.L. Baert et al., 1990

Diagnosis of complications developed during renal dilatation is quite simple, since control angiography is mandatory. Only in several cases arterial damage can cause delayed thrombosis and occlusion. In such patients it is wise to use noninvasive methods, duplex scanning or transcranial Doppler examination of blood flow to verify a status of the renal artery. These data may be quite convincing for a diagnosis of renal occlusion. DSA with a small contrast medium dose is related to low risk of the development of renal failure and therefore it can be widely used for a diagnosis of early postdilatation complications.

While making a decision of operative intervention choice of the most convenient and optimal approach is an essential problem. Standard median laparotomy can be used. However in obese patients a wound turns to be deep and exposure of distal renal arteries is not always good.

J. Stanley[15] advocates supraumbilical transverse laparotomy with an approach to the right renal artery offered by Kocher and to the left renal artery through the left lateral canal. This method limits an approach to the aorta.

From our viewpoint thoracolumbotomy with a retroperitoneal posterior approach to retract the kidney together with fatty tissue anteriorly and a lateral and posterior approach to the aorta is the best method used in renal reconstruction. This method has been widely used since 1968 and in this country by all vascular surgeons. This approach provides easy mobilization of the renal artery at full length including its branches and a wide approach to aorta allows to perform any type of reconstructive procedure. It is worth to emphasize, that this approach is tolerated much easy than laparotomy.

When we speak about operation after renal dilatation, then taking into consideration arterial wall trauma it is always necessary to resect an artery and to be sure of a normal intima status in the distal artery.

Therefore even in case of simple perforation of the arterial wall by a guide arterial suture shouldn't be done.

Taking it into consideration mobilization of the renal artery must begin with its mobilization in the middle segment, arterial ostium may be not mobilized. If the first arterial segment is involved and arterial wall changes are moderate, then, from our viewpoint, an optimal variant of reconstruction is to resect the artery and implant it caudally into the aorta. Such a variant is especially indicated for children with fibrodysplasia, if the process doesn't involve arterial branches.

Operation of implantation of the renal artery into a new ostium becomes much easier due to good kidney mobility. Thoracophrenolumbotomy contributes to it.

Aortotomy length may be twice as long as an arterial diameter. It is reasonable to tailor a window in the aortic wall. Before renal arterial ligation 5.000 unites of heparin is intravenously injected.

To make implantation easier it is wise to place prolene 4-0 or 5-0 sutures at some distance and then to tighten them. It is possible to place two continuous sutures at certain distance and then to tighten them. These details make operation much easier.

If the second renal artery segment is involved very closely to them arterial resection and subsequent autovein or graft replacement is an optimal variant.

Here, this anastomosis is constructed in an oblique direction with prolene 6-0 after preliminary and longitudinal dissection of the arterial wall. Several authors use autoartery (internal iliac artery).

We adhere to the principal position of using a distal end-to-end anastomosis with the renal artery. Probably a necessary number of operations done after dilatation will be increased due to certain broadening of indications, of trials of recanalization of totally occluded renal arteries in particular.

Such a type of anastomosis can be, when necessary, extended to the renal arterial branches.

In several patients it is possible to use interarterial anastomosis, of splenorenal anastomosis in particular. In children and in patients with very small renal artery it is wise to use several knotted sutures. It must be emphasized, that in 25% of children with fibromuscular dysplasia dilatation is impossible and in 60% nephrectomy is performed.

Nevertheless, it must be emphasized, that all these operations caused minimal mortality.

However, operation may be necessary in the late period after renal artery dilatation. A rate of restenoses and occlusion is closely related to aetiology of the process and is in many respects not changed during desaggregate therapy continued for 6 months.

According to early data of the USA Committee[13] one year after dilatation recurrence is noted in more than 50% of the atherosclerotic patients. Baert A.L. et al.[1] described restenosis already in 8% of the patients, which was undoubtedly related to the refined indications and improved technique of dilatation. Eighty per cent of restenoses develop within first year after dilatation.

For early diagnosis of renal restenoses not only clinical signs (recurrent hypertension), but also repeated ultrasonic and angiographic examinations are important. We must mention such specific complications of dilatation as cholesterol embolism. In case of massive embolism we ought to do nephrectomy.

Among specific features of surgical intervention done in the late period after dilatation we must mention kidney function and size. In case of a markedly reduced kidney size (less 8 cm in length) nephrectomy must be discussed, which must be intracapsullary done.

Choice of a reconstructive procedure is the same, as have been previously discussed. Vary rarely kidney autotransplantation or in vivo operation are discussed. At operation periarterial fibrosis is seen and it is wise to begin with distal renal artery.

The main group of repeated interventions includes operations done after renal artery reconstructions. They can be divided into two groups: those, which have been done in the early postoperative period (within 30 days) and those ones, which have been in the late postoperative period.

Prevention of possible early complications and hence repeated operations is first of all, related to the proper choice of a type of reconstruction and meticulous operative technique. In its turn, it is closely related to the width, depth and convince of an approach, though most authors use median laparotomy[5], and several authors[15,12,18] prefer supraumbilical laparotomy.

We continue advocating and insisting, that thoracolumbotomy with a posterior approach to the vessels and aorta is the most adequate approach of kidney revascularization. Neither intestinum, nor inferior caval vein or renal veins prevent a retroperitoneal approach. Any segment of artery can be reconstructed: from aorta up to its branches.

This approach is low traumatic and easily tolerated by elderly patients.

Indications for reoperations to be done in early period after renal arterial reconstruction are: bleeding, thrombosis, graft rupture.

A rate of all failures relative to lesion aetiology found in the literature is presented by R.H. Dean[6] (Table 4). According to A. Novick[12] a rate of thrombosis or stenosis after renal arterial reconstruction is less 5%. J. Stanley, L. Messina[16] showed that early thrombosis of the autovein graft was seen in 2% of patients with fibromuscular dysplasia.

Table 4 - Early results of operations done for RVH

	Number	Improved	Failed
Atherosclerosis:			
focal	1.173	82%	18%
diffuse	506	72%	28%
Fibromuscular dysplasia	847	90%	10%

R.H. Dean, 1991

Bleeding is extremely rarely seen and its cause is quite clear. Graft rupture is also quite rarely seen and it is related to use of gonadal vein.

Causes of thrombosis are very diverse. They are related to a type of renal reconstruction. Probably, a lower number of similar complications is caused by a method of implantation of the renal artery into the new aortic ostium, since here only one anastomosis is constructed and for simplicity it can be first constructed at a distance and its size can be increased at the expense both of a an aortic "window" and of wall incision in the proper renal artery.

In case of autovein replacement we would like to emphasize several principal regulations, which must be sticked to: first, distal anastomosis to the artery must be always of an end-to-end type with long oblique anastomosis, preferable interruption of continuous suture with knotted suture to avoid a "purse" effect, before anastomosis completion its patency may be tested.

During construction of proximal anastomosis to the aorta it is necessary to avoid placing a too deep suture at the site of anastomosis "heel". For renal artery replacement it is impossible to use a vein with the diameter less 3 mm or a graft with the diameter less 5 mm.

However, an inadequate length and kinkings or bendings are the most common errors of graft use. All these defects must be immediately corrected at the initial operation.

During endarterectomy main danger is related to "blind" intima detachment or a plaque left in the distal renal artery. Therefore, it is extremely important to provide a visual control of the distal arterial lumen. A standard method of transaortic endarterectomy from the transverse aortic incision extended to the renal artery provides it, but requires additional patch insertion. Transaortic endarterectomy from longitudinal aortotomy approached anteriorly doesn't provide a visual control just as endarterectomy with transverse aortic transsection.

That is why in case of atherosclerotic renal artery lesion we believe it to be optimal to use transaortic endarterectomy from thoracolumbotomy approach.

Mobilization of the whole renal artery and its involment into the aortic lumen allows to provide a visual control of the internal arterial surface up to its branching off. It must be, probably, mentioned one more cause of thrombosis: trauma of the distal arterial portion with vascular clamps or tapes during their traction.

Duplex scanning of the renal artery offered by the same authors[18] for a visual intraoperative control of quality of renal arterial reconstruction deserves close attention. Here, we may see intima detachment and residual plaques and registration of peak blood flow velocity and turbulence helps to reveal anastomosis or artery stenosis.

The authors examined 37 patients in 25 of whom there were postendarterectomy defects. To say the truth, 75% of those defects were small seen as a small portion of residual intima or thrombocyte aggregates and had insignificant hemodynamic effect. However, in 9 patients there were large defects and they were reoperated.

In doubtful cases intraoperative duplex scanning is very useful and informative and it must be more widely used.

Postoperative diagnosis and confirmation of renal thrombosis is very difficult problem. Thrombosis may develop within several days. In several patients it can be suspected because of rapidly returned hypertension or absent hypotensive effect. However, this sign is not always reliable just as a renal function; oliguria may be absent and urographic and reno- and scintigraphic data may be noninformative bearing in mind collateral renal circulation.

Of all noninvasive methods duplex scanning and examination of renal artery blood flow by means of transcranial Doppler deserves close attention. In doubtful cases control angiography must be immediately performed. Digital angiography minimizes possible complications on a part of the kidneys.

Sustained patency of the distal vascular bed in the kidney even 1-2 weeks after reconstruction is very important specific feature of renal artery thrombosis. This is a base for principal decision of feasibility of repeated reconstruction of the renal artery for its revascularization.

Here it must be taken into account, that even a control angiogram not always reveals true distal renal artery patency. Nevertheless in case of the sustained kidney size it is wise to try repeated revascularization.

Among methods of repeated reconstruction done for vascular thrombosis autovein replacement is preferable, but if there is no good venous graft, then PTFE graft is preferably used. In extremely rare cases we can speak about kidney autotransplantation or about in vivo reconstruction. For anastomosis it is wise to use prolen 6-0 or even 7-0.

Late reoperations done after kidney revascularization. First of all, it must be emphasized, that necessity to do reoperations in the late period after reconstructive renal artery procedure is related, mainly, to aetiology of the process. For example, according to the data of the Moscow Surgical Center (Knjasev M.D.)[2], which has gained experience with 774 operations done in the patients with vasorenal hypertension, recurrent hypertension is most rarely seen in the patients with fibromuscular dysplasia, twice as often in the patients with atherosclerosis and most commonly seen in the patients with nonspecific aorto arteritis (Takayasu's disease), if inflammation can't be resided. The same tendency is seen by other authors.

Excellent late results were seen in Houston[17]: normal arterial pressure was noted in 85% of the patients, it was not changed in only 2%, in the patients with FMD normal AP was noted in 90%, with atherosclerosis in 80%.

Ten-year survival was 80%, 15 year survival 75% and AP was normal in them. Probably, such results were related to a very strict selection of the patients.

Table 5 - Late results of operations done for RVH (120 patients)

Patent	95%
Restenosis	8%
Occlusion	5%
Dilatation	2.7%
False aneurysm	2.7%

36 angiographies, in 90% bypass graft.   P. Fiorani et al., 1989

P. Fiorani et al.[7] showed, that among 120 patients 15-year survival was 85%, ten-year survival was 68%, here postoperative hypotensive was of the most significance.

According to the data of these authors a rate of late complications seen after revascularization (mainly after bypass grafting with a graft) was: 5% of occlusions, 8% of restenoses (Table 5). It is interesting to note, that restenosis is found 14 months in average after operation. R. Dean and P. Meacham[4] in the publication in 1986 wrote about 10% of late reoperations.

Dean R.[5] mentioned 5% of late restenoses and 2% of late occlusions 1 to 23 years after operation (Table 6). J. Stanley[16] wrote, that stenosis of the autovein transplant used for aorto-renal replacement occurred in 8% of the patients with FMD.

Table 6 - Late results (1 to 23 years after surgical treatment of RVH)

Status	Number of grafts	Per cent
No change	174	88%
Aneurysm dilatation*	7	3.5%
Stenosis	10	5.0%
Occlusion	4	2.0%
False aneurysm	3	1.5%
TOTAL	198	

* autovein and autoartery   R. Dean, 1989

A less rate of restenoses 2.1% seen after renal bypass grafting done for atherosclerosis was written by A. Novick[11]. The terms of restenosis onset varied from 6 months to 5 years.

A total number of thromboses and stenoses seen in atherosclerosis was 4.3% among 254 operations. Among 120 patients with FMD restenosis developed in only 1 patient in 5 years. Attention must be paid to the fact, that in one third of the patients extracorporeal reconstruction of the branches and kidney autotransplantation have been performed, though, bypass grafting was the type of surgical intervention. Even in case of standard bypass grafting reconstruction has involved renal arterial branches in one fourth part of the patients. It has resulted in a small number of complications seen in the late postoperative period.

According to the compiled literature data a rate of repeated operations is 3% in total[6] (Table 7).

Certainly, a number of reoperations done in the late post-revascularization period depends on aetiology, choice of a reconstructive method and surgical thoroughness. Among cases of late reoperations we must mention fibrous changes in autovein valve cusps, subendothelian fibrous proliferation, anastomosis stenosis resulting from subintimal layer proliferation.

Table 7 - Late results of surgical treatment of RVH

Graft patency	91-95%	
Reoperation rate	3%	1.038 patients
Redilatation success	35%	

R.H. Dean, 1991

Indications for late reoperations are anastomosis stenosis, then arterial thrombosis and development of true and false aneurysms.

Development of hemodynamically marked stenosis as well as thrombosis occurrence are most often clinically seen as uncorrectable stable high hypertension, sometimes pressure is suddenly jumped, but most often two first postoperative years are critical. Among noninvasive diagnostic methods only duplex scanning and characteristics of renal blood flow are useful. However, repeated angiography is the main diagnostic method.

Among reconstructive methods renal artery resection and subsequent autovein or graft replacement of wide end-to-end anastomosis with knotted sutures is still most widely used. It is wise to start renal artery mobilization with a portion located outside an anastomosis site and renal vein must be very carefully detached.

In the presence of atherosclerosis it doesn't involve, as a rule, a new distal segment and stenosis develops at the anastomosis site or it may be related to the process progress in the proper aorta. Sometimes, stenosis may be related to the development of intimal or mural fibrosis, in rare cases the anastomosis stenosis may be eliminated by means of an inserted patch.

If a patient has moderate distal anastomosis stenosis then dilatation may be tried.

In case of proximal anastomosis stenosis between the graft and aorta it is wise to perform laparotomy and repeated placement of anastomosis in the new aortic area or at the expense of a graft addition. In case of severe aortic lesion we are forced to discuss a variant of combined aortic and renal reconstruction. In rare cases one of the variant of intraarterial anastomoses may be performed.

In the patients with nonspecific aorto-arteritis a most part of failures is related with further aortic lesion, that is why among 118 operated patients combined procedures have been done in most of them (Pokrovsky A.V.). Thus, in 65 of them both renal arteries have been simultaneously reconstructed and in 56 patients of this group simultaneous reconstruction of the proper aorta has been done. Even in case of revascularization of one kidney done in 53 patients 26 have undergone aortic reconstruction (Table 8).

Table 8

Type of operation	Number
Transaortic endarterectomy	49
Bypass grafting	11
Resection and implantation	29
Miscellaneous	29
TOTAL	108

Late complications: thrombosis + stenosis in 8 patients   A.V. Pokrovsky

In several patients with aortitis and aortic wall involvement a synthetic graft has been inserted at reoperation and then renal artery has been implanted into it.

The most complex problem is reoperation in the patients with fibromuscular dysplasia, since in nearly 30% of them renal arterial branches are involved and symptoms may recur not because of anastomosis stenosis, but because of uncorrected stenosis of renal branches. In these cases it is wise to do operation extracorporally with the help of optics. Under such conditions end-to-end anastomoses can be easily done by means of vein segments and then its bi- or trifurcation can be done. Present-day methods of preservation (perfusion of the cold solution) allow not to be in hurry and to do the whole operation quite meticulously.

K. Hansen and R. Dean[8] use a term "ischemic nephropathy" in case of combined extraparenchymatous occlusive renal lesions and poorly or nonfunctional kidney parenchyma or azotaemia. In such patients with present azotaemia it is wise to perform hemodyalysis before and after repeated reconstruction.

However, delayed examination of the patients with thrombosis of the reconstructed renal artery has made it impossible to make reoperation, in this case nephrectomy is feasible.

However, in the patients with azotaemia it is wise to perform revascularization only in the presence of hypertension, in normotonic patients with azotaemia revascularization of the kidney is not feasible.

While discussing nephrectomy, in the patients with atherosclerosis in particular, aggravation of stenosing process in the contralateral renal artery must be always borne in mind and therefore we must always try to attain repeated kidney revascularization. Here the decisive moments are: longitudinal size of the kidney over 8 cm and revealed free renal branches on an angiogram.

Present true autovein graft aneurysm is an indication for reoperation. Here, we must take into account, that dilatation of autovein shunt is seen in 20-44% of the children, but it doesn't aggravate (J. Stanley, 1989)[9]. Shunt aneurysms were found by the same author in only 2% of adults.

R. Dean et al.[3] described a rate of aneurysm of autovein aorto-renal shunt - 5% and in 1986[4] they presented a figure of only 4% among young patients with fibromuscular dysplasia.

In the presence of shunt aneurysm parietal thrombus formation is probable with subsequent embolization of the distal renal vascular bed. While defining indications for reoperation it should be borne in mind. However, in the presence of diffuse, but not saccular autovein shunt aneurysm in the patients with normotension it is wise to follow its size by means of duplex scanning or of repeated DSA angiography. Only in case of progressively increased aneurysm diameter reoperation is indicated.

Reoperation done for shunt aneurysm consists of repeated renal artery replacement with a graft.

False anastomosis aneurysms usually develop at the site of proximal anastomosis of a synthetic graft to the aorta. In such cases placement of the second, wider anastomosis just at the same site or interposition of a new graft segment and construction of proximal anastomosis in the new aortic area, sometimes to the iliac artery (if it is not damaged) are possible after aneurysm resection.

The last group of patients, in whom reoperation may be necessary are patients subjected to kidney transplantation. According to several data a rate of arterial anastomosis stenosis may vary from 0.6 to 16% and even to 25%[9]. However, an indication for repeated intervention is not anastomosis stenosis per se, but revealed arterial hypertension, which is related to this stenosis. Dilatation of stenosis is believed to be a method of choice. A. Raynaud et al.[14] described experience with dilatation done in 43 patients with primary success in 81% and here restenosis seen within the first 5 months after dilatation in 7 patients was redilated in 6 patients. The authors didn't remove any kidney and had good results in 67% of the patients a year after operation.

Certainly, in the patients with arterial anastomosis stenosis and hypertension dilatation must be operation of choice. In skilled hands it may be repeated in case of the restenosis development and a minimal chance of the development of complications.

In case of failed dilatation and sustained hypertension reoperation is indicated. Most often operation consists of resection of the stenosed anastomosis and its replacement with an autovein segment of a new anastomosis to iliac artery. Variants of such new reconstructions may be diverse.

A general analysis of reoperations on renal vessels confirm their efficiency with good results and a small number of complications.

REFERENCES

1. Baert, A.L., Wilms, G., Amery, A., et al., (1990) Percutaneous transluminal renal angioplasty. Initial results and long-term follow-up in 202 patients. *Cardiovasc. Intervent. Radiol.,* 13:22-26.
2. Belov, Yu.V., Kosenkov, A.N., Gavrilenko, A.V., (1990) Reoperations in the patients with recurrent vasorenal hypertension. In: Repeated reconstructive vascular operations, pp 15-16. Yaroslavl (Russian).
3. Dean, R.H., Wilson, J.P., Burko, H., Foster, J., (1974) Saphenous vein aortorenal bypass grafts. Serial arteriographic studies. *Ann. Surg.,* 180:469-478.
4. Dean, R.H., Meacham, P.W., (1986) Surgery for recurrent renal artery stenosis, edited by Bergan, J., Yao, J., pp 429-440. Grune & Stratton.
5. Dean, R.H., (1989) Management of renovascular hypertension due to atherosclerosis. In: Vascular Surgery. 3d ed., edited by Rutherford, R , pp 1245-1267. Saunders Co.
6. Dean, R.H., (1991) Management of renovascular hypertension. In: Modern vascular Surgery, edited by Chang, J., 4:371 386. PMA Publishing Corp.
7. Fiorani, P., Faraglia, V., Aissa, N., et al., (1989) Late results of reconstructive surgery for renovascular hypertension. *Intern. Angiology,* 8, 2:81-91.
8. Hansen, K.J., Dean, R.H., (1990) Renal revascularization in the Azotemic patient. Diagnostic and therapeutic implications. In: current critical problems in vascular surgery, edited by Veith, F., 2:197-203. Quality Med. Publ.

9. Lacombe, M., (1975) Arterial stenosis complicating renal allotransplantation in man. *Ann. Surg.*, 181:283-288.
10. Martin, L.G., Casarella, W.J., Alspaugh, J.P., Chuang, V.P., (1986) Renal artery angioplasty: increased technical success and decreased compilations in the second 100 patients. *Radiology*, 159:631-634.
11. Novick, A.C., Zeigelbaum, M., Vidt, D., et al., (1987) Trends in surgical revascularization for renal artery disease. *JAMA*, 257, 4:498-501.
12. Novick, A.C., (1988) Surgical correction of renovascular hypertension. *Surg. Clin. North Amer.*, 68, 5:1007-1025.
13. (1984) Percutaneous transluminal angioplasty. Council report. *JAMA*, 251, 6:764-768.
14. Raynaud, A., Bedrossian, J., Remy, P., et al., (1986) Percutaneous transluminal arterial stenoses. Angioplasty of renal transplant arterial stenoses. *AJR*, 146:853-857.
15. Stanley, J.C., (1986) Surgery of failed percutaneous transluminal renal artery angioplasty. In: Reoperative arterial surgery, edited by Bergan, J., Yao, J., pp 441-454. Grune & Stratton.
16. Stanley, J.C., Messina, L.M., (1989) Renal artery fibrodysplasia and renovascular hypertension. In: Vascular surgery. 3d ed., edited by Rutherford, R., pp 1253-1267. Saunders Co.
17. Starr, D., Lawrie, G., Morris, G., (1980) Surgical treatment of renovascular hypertension. *Arch. Surg.*, 115:494-496.
18. Stoney, R.I., Messina, L.M., Goldstone, J., Reilly, L.M., (1989) Renal endarterectomy through the transected aorta. A new technique for combined aortorenal atherosclerosis. *J. Vasc. Surg.*, 9:224-233.

Towards Fewer Biopsies: A Comparison of Pz and PI in the Non-Invasive Assessment of Renal Allograft Function Using Ultrasound

R.G. Gosling*, S.P. Ward and M.G. Taylor

Division of Radiological Sciences and Medicine, St. Thomas and Guy's Campuses,
United Medical and Dental Schools, University of London*

INTRODUCTION

Despite the advent of sophisticated Duplex Scanners, there is still considerable debate on the value of Doppler based quantitative methods of assessment of renal allograft function[4,5,8,9]. These methods are based on the observation that the arterial blood flow-velocity pattern in the graft is altered by pathological changes in renal vasculature. The blood flow-velocity changes can be measured using a number of methods, of which Pulsatility Index (PI) has proved useful.

There are two problems with the use of PI as a stand alone measure:

1) PI is time base dependant so the value of the PI measured from any artery will vary with heart rate.

2) If the transplantated kidney auto-regulates to any extent ie. alters resistance to flow in order to maintain total blood flow with varying input pressures, then PI will be dependant to some extent on systemic blood pressure.

In the original definition of PI, Gosling and King[3] described a technique which utilised the ratio of two PI values measured simultaneously in the lower limb, so that the factors 1) and 2) did not pertain.

If the pulsatile blood pressure and flow in the input artery to a low vascular impedance system are essentially in phase. A simple, ideal electrical model (Fig. 1), may be proposed[2]. Such a model is characterised by only two parameters, Pz and R the resistance of the vascular bed. When this idealised model is applied to the renal vasculature Pz can be regarded as a back pressure generated by the kidney which needs to be overcome by the arterial input pressure in order to adequately perfuse the glomeruli. In those instances when the end diastolic flow is greater than zero, Pz can be defined in terms of the mean central arterial pressure, P, the central pulse pressure, dP, and the pulsatility index, PI, of the renal artery flow-velocity sonogram waveform.

$$ Pz = \bar{P} - \frac{dP}{PI} = \bar{P} \times \left[1 - \frac{PI\,(pressure)}{PI\,(flow)} \right] $$

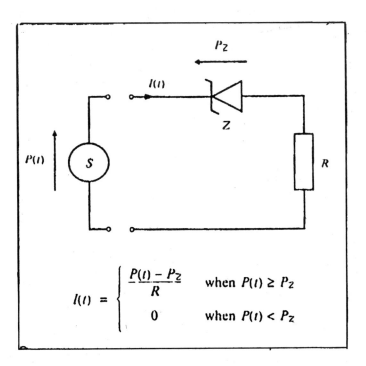

Fig. 1. Idealised electrical model of a low impedance peripheral vascular bed

This expression for Pz contains the ratio of PI's for pressure and flow and so will not be heart rate dependant, whilst PI alone does require correction. In addition equation 1 takes into account the mean central arterial pressure. Therefore it can be postulated that Pz should prove to be a more robust indicator of the haemodynamic status of the kidney than the PI of renal artery flow-velocity.

Two studies are reported here. The first a Measurement of Pz in a cohort of renal transplant recipients with well functioning grafts. Secondly, serial measurements of Pz in 16 transplant patients in the first weeks following surgery.

PATIENTS

Study 1: 40 renal allograft recipients under the care of the Renal Unit, Guy's Hospital, were recruited to the study after obtaining informed consent. A single measurement of Pz was made in each patient. All subjects had received transplantated kidneys (37 cadaveric, 3 live related donors) between 6 weeks and 66 weeks (mean 28 weeks) before the measurements of Pz. Grafts were judged to be well-functioning on the basis of the following criteria:

1) Serum creatinine was within the range 75 to 200 μmol/l on the day of Pz measurement and did not show a rise of more than 10% when compared to mean of the previous three recorded creatinine levels.

2) No evidence of a rejection episode in the 7 days prior to or after Pz measurement.

3) No indication of Acute Tubular Necrosis (ATN) or of Cyclosporin A Nephrotoxicity (CyAT).

4) No evidence of a Renal Artery stenosis.

Ten subjects were retrospectively removed from the study using these criteria.

Study 2: Serial Pz measurement were made in 16 transplant recipients, under the care of Guy's Hospital Renal Unit, over a five month period. The cohort consisted of 9 females and 7 males with an average age of 40.7 years (range 18 to 66 years). Measurements were made between day 1 and day 66 post transplant, with the majority of measurement made in the three week period following surgery. The number of scans performed on an individual patient ranged between 3 and 10 (mean 5.5). One transplant recipient received a live related organ, the remainder received cadaveric kidneys. All subjects gave informed consent prior to inclusion in the study. The study was designed to allow scans to be performed every other day in the first two weeks after surgery but individual considerations, access to equipment and individual patient wishes, did not always allow strict adherence to this protocol. Pz measurements were made in parallel to standard treatments and investigations and results were not made known to the clinical team, with the exception of occasional subjective assessments of graft perfusion based on colour Doppler images.

METHODS

All subjects were investigated with an Acuson Colour Duplex Scanner, using a 3 MHz sector probe to image the transplant kidney and to obtain Doppler signals from the renal artery. Wherever possible a Doppler signal was obtained from the portion of the renal artery between the anastomotic site and major branch. This signal was recorded and used to calculate a mean value for PI from the maximum frequency envelope of the sonogram over a period equivalent to six to ten whole heart beats, the exact number was dependent on Doppler signl quality and on the subjects heart rate.

In Study 1 the subjects blood pressure was recorded simultaneously with the Pz measurement using an Ohmeda 2300 Finapres[R] continuous monitoring system with the cuff mounted on the patients second finger[7]. The Finapres (Finger arterial blood pressure monitor) provides continuous non-invasive measurement of finger arterial pressure dispaying pressure waveform, (time interval 10 ms.), digital values of systolic, diastolic and mean pressure as well as pulse rate and a time annotated trend display. The accuracy of this system was checked against a systolic brachial pressure measurement made at the beginning and end of the procedure using a Vasoflow continuous wave 8 MHz Doppler and a sphygmomanometer. Due to reflectance of the forward-going pressure waveform from the termination of the arterial system in the finger, the Finapres gives a measure of systolic blood pressure which is usually higher than central systolic pressure. Therefore the systolic blood pressure was taken as the mean of the two manual Doppler pressure measurements and diastolic as the mean of pre, per and post (relative to Pz recordings) values measured with the Finapres. In Study 2 the subjects blood pressure was measured at the beginning and end of the Pz procedure using a long arm band cuff and standard auscultation.

In both studies it was assumed that the pulse pressure in the arterial system of the apper arm was an accurate indicator of renal artery pulse pressure. In cases where Pz measurement was not made at the bedside, subjects were asked to lie supine for 5 minutes before the first blood pressure measurement was performed.

Mean arterial pressure, $\bar{P}$, was calculated using the formula:

Mean Pressure = Diastolic Pressure + 1/3 Pulse Pressure[2]

In Study 1 the measurement of Pz was arranged to coincide with the measurement of serum creatinine levels as part of the standard clinical management of the patient group. Having calculated the PI and Pz values the well being of the allograft was established by reference to available clinical information. In Study 2 the clinical status of a graft on the day of Pz measurement was assessed independently and in retrospect, all available clinical information, including the results of biopsy, were used.

RESULTS

Study 1: A comparison of the measured PI and Pz values in each of the 30 well functioning allografts is shown in Fig. 2.

Table 1 shown the mean, standard deviation and coefficient of variance for PI and Pz data.

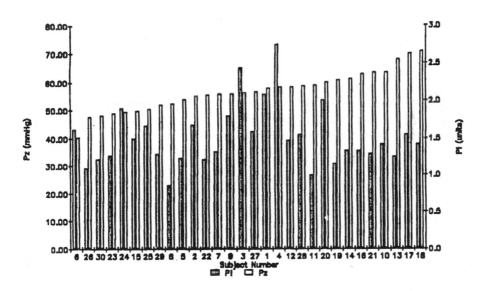

Fig. 2. PI and Pz values for 30 well functioning allografts - data sorted by ascending Pz values.

Table 1- The variability of PI and Pz

	PI (units)	Pz (mmHg)
Number of observations	30	30
Mean	1,5	56,7
Standard deviation from the mean	0,41	6,89
Coefficient of Variance	27%	12%

8 grafts were discounted from the study because of high creatinine levels or suspected renal artery stenoses. One graft dispayed rejection on biopsy ot the time of Pz measurement and demonstrated a PI of 1.6 and Pz of 87.7 mmHg. The remaining kidney was considered by the Renal Physicians to be affected by Cyclosporin nephrotoxicity and demonstrated a PI of 4.4 and a Pz of 68.3 mmHg.

Study 2: A total of 95 measurements were made. For technical reasons a Pz value could not be calculated in 7 (7.4%) of these cases - mainly due to difficulties in obtaining renal blood flow signals or reliable blood pressure in the immediate post operative period. It was established that a Pz measurement could be regularly performed in under 5 minutes, although the initial scan often took considerably longer. Although it was almost always possible to obtain an image of the transplanted kidney on day 1 post-transplant, it was not always possible to obtain noise free Doppler signals - making the day 1 Pz measurement unreliable in all but the thinnest of subjects. In most cases it was possible to obtain adequate images of the kidney without disturbing the post operative dressings - this meant that scanning did not wound infection were reported during the study.

On 14 occasions kidneys were demonstrated (on biopsy performed within 48 hours) to be affected by rejection. 26 measurements were made on ATN affected kidneys, and a further 30 measurements were made on kidneys which appeared to be functioning well. The remaining 18 measurements were made on kidneys which were non-functioning, improving or deteriorating but which were not biopsied - thus the exact status of the graft was known and this data is not presented. When a kidney dispayed primary nonfunction (ie. no immediate urine production) and was later demonstrated on biopsy to be affected by ATN, ATN was inferred for any measurements made before the biopsy was performed.

Pz and PI data for the 70 measurements recorded from grafts of known status are shown in Table 2 with kidneys grouped by clinical status. This data is also shown graphically in Fig. 3. Two examples of individual serial Pz and

Table 2 - Mean and 1 standard deviation for Pz, Pulsatility Index (PI), Calculated Mean Arterial Pressure minus Pz (P-Pz) and Calculated Mean Arterial Pressure (P) for well functioning grafts (WELL), transplanted kidneys displaying rejection (REJ) and Acute Tubular Necrosis (ATN).

Parameter		WELL	ATN	REJ
Number		30	26	14
Pz	Mean	53.60	65.79	71.29
	1 sd	11.78	18.05	5.80
PI	Mean	1.19	1.70	1.99
	1 sd	0.28	0.61	0.64
P-Pz	Mean	49.27	31.85	33.13
	1 sd	12.88	14.89	7.40
P	Mean	102.9	98.7	104.4
	1 sd	9.2	10.9	7.4

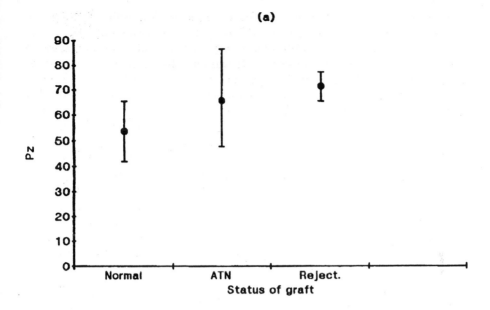

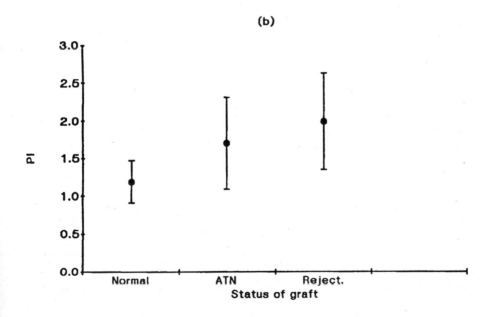

Fig. 3. Graphs showing mean and 1 standard deviation for Pz (a) and for PI (b) in well functioning, Rejection and ATN groups.

PI data have also been included in Fig. 4, which illustrate the general observation that Pz was stable when renal function remained stable, rose when renal function became impaired due to ATN or rejection and that Pz and PI values followed similar trends. This represents the first evidence that Pz does have some physiological significance.

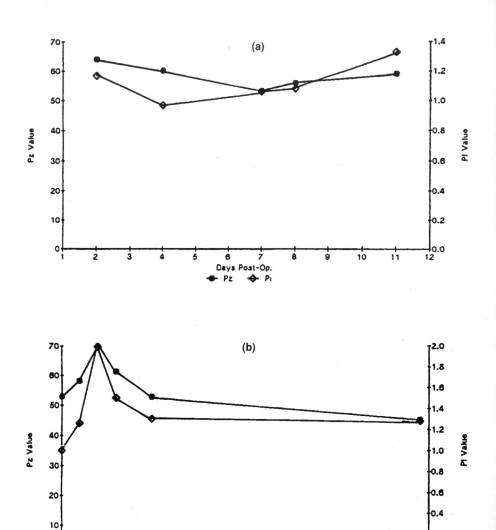

Fig. 4. Graphs showing serial Pz and PI measurement for two patients in the study.

DISCUSSION

Study 1: The mean and standard deviation for PI in this study are similar to the values obtained by Allen et al. in a study published in 1988[1]. Allen shows that PI rise in grafts affected by ATN (mean value 2.3) and is slightly higher in grafts displaying Acute Rejection (AR) (mean value 2.5). These observations are representative of the findings of other workers in this field. Evidence from the single study published in which vascular and interstitial rejection were investigated separately[9] suggests that the mean PI in vascular rejectionis higher still with the value in cellular mediated rejection similar to that obervated in the ATN affected graft. In all reported studies, the variability of PI increases as the mean value of PI rises, the coefficient of variance in a group of rejecting grafts being approximately twice the value observed in well functioning grafts. Our model predicts this observation as it may be seen from figure 5, ie. with increasing values (>2) PI becomes progressively more sensitive to chenge in Pz and diastolic pressure.

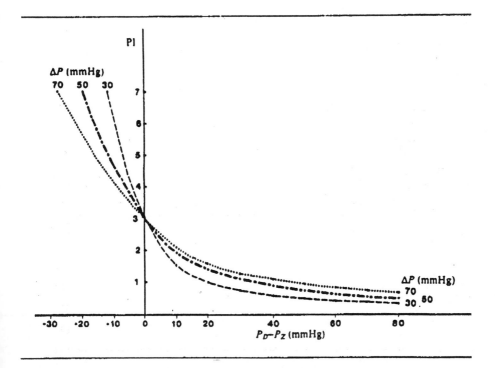

Fig. 5. Variation of PI with PD-Pz (PD = diastolic pressure), for various pulse pressures as predicted by the model of figure 1 and a standardised pressure waveform shape[2].

It is the wide variability of PI in the ATN and AR groups that makes differential diagnosis on the grounds of PI difficult. Since Pz represents the pressure which needs to be overcome to perfuse the glomeruli, it can be argued that the mean arterial pressure minus Pz will be equivalent to the glomerular capillary pressure. Further evidence in support of our model of the renal vasculature is given by the observation that the mean P-Pz observed in this study was approximately 40 mmHg, this figure is comparable with the anticipated physiological value[6].

It is clear from Table 1 that Pz is a less variable parameter than PI in the normally functioning renal allograft, with the coefficient of variance of Pz being approximately 55% lower than that of PI. Further, while PI is an indicator of downstream impedance to arterial flow, we suggest that the crucial factor in renal perfusion is the back pressure generated by the kidney and that resistance is a secondary factor.

Study 2: This study shows that Pz can be correlated to renal pathology and rises in cases of rejection. It also shows the method used to collect Pz data to be relatively simple, quick and generally reproducible. This last point is indicated by 2 patients who at no time displayed any pathology and had stable Pz's, eg. a mean value of 53.2 +/- 2.6 mmHg (n = 3) and 58.6 +/- 3.7 mmHg (n = 5) respectively. Also 3 patients with long term ATN who also gave constant Pz values, eg. 64.8 +/- 6.5 mmHg (n = 7), 82.2 +/- 8.2 mmHg (n = 6) and 68.3 +/- 1.5 mmHg (n = 5) respectively. In addition Pz has been shown to be a less variable parameter than PI, especially in the case of rejection. It is also encouraging to note the PI values shown in Figure 3 which are similar in trend to observations made by other workers, suggesting this to be representative study group.

Table 3 - Comparison the observed coefficients of variance for PI and Pz data in the various groups of kidney status including data from Study 1.

	Coefficient of variance (%)	
	PI	**Pz**
Study 1: Well	28	12
Study 2: Well	24	22
ATN	36	27
Rejection	32	8

Fig. 3 and Table 2 indicated that on the basis of the data obtained, Pz could not be used to distinguish rejection from ATN. There appears to have been a much smaller reduction in variability of Pz in ATN when compared to PI, than that observed for rejection. The reason for this anomaly is not clear, there does not appear to be any correlation to the length of individual ATN episodes, but the large spread of values may be related to the occurrence of more severe ATN episodes early in rejection. Alternatively, the observed variation of Pz in ATN may be a function of some systemic effect rather than being wholly a function of local blood flow - note the observed mean blood pressure in the ATN group, shown in table 2. Of the 26 ATN observations, 81% had a measured mean arterial pressure below the mean value of the well functioning group.

Pz and PI in the controlled, well functioning transplant group of Study 1, are higher than the values obtained from the well functioning group of Study 2. The reason for this lies in the occasional observation in Study 2 of very low Pz values, resulting from low PI's (less than 1.1) rather than a low mean arterial pressure. In one instance low Pz values were recorded throughout the observation period and this kidney remained well functioning. In addition the coefficient of variance in Study 1 was almost half that found in the well-functioning group of Study 2. This may have been - in part - due to the different methods of measuring blood pressure. The more painstaking technique of Study 1 having been abandoned in Study 2 because of the time involved.

PRE-BIOPSY SCREEN

An alternative approach to the application of Pz would be to use the measured Pz value as part of the process of deciding which grafts shoul be biopsied, ie. as a pre-biopsy screen. In the early post-transplant period (in this period cyclosporin nephrotoxicity is less frequently a problem) clinicians need to establish whether the non-function of a graft is attributable to rejection, in which case appropiate immunosoppression therapy is instigated, or to ATN. The decision to biopsy a kidney can often be a difficult one.

If were to apply a cut off criteria of 2 standard deviations below the mean Pz value for the rejection group, ie. 60 mmHg, then all 14 cases of rejection would lie above this value. Thus in predicting rejection a measured Pz level of 60 mmHg would give a sensitivity of 100%. Taking into account all situations in which graft status is known (ie. ATN and well-functioning groups) the specificity of a Pz screening test set at 60 mmHg would be 50% - this reppresents the unrealistic situation where no other clinical information is available. In realty well-functioning graft would not be considered for biopsy. The specificity for the ATN group alone is lower at 27%. While this specificity value appears poor, the application of 40 potential "decision to biopsy" episodes - would have missed no cases of rejection and lead to 7 biopsies (17.5%) not being performed. This potential reduction in biopsies, while not large, needs to be set against the risks associated with biopsy, the cost of the procedure itself and the cost of nursing care following transplant biopsy. The measurement of Pz is not only non-invasive, risk free and quick but could also be performed as part of a standard pre-biopsy ultrasound examination - potentially involving no extra cost.

The major problem with the data presented here for study 2 is the correlation to biopsy information. Not only is biopsy a poor "gold standard" but the study design employed here resulted in there being gaps of up to 48 hours between Pz measurement and biopsies. Better information on ATN and rejection will only be obtained if Pz assessments are made no more than hours before biopsy. A further study to collect data in such situations is planned.

CONCLUSION

Pz has been shown to be a function of renal perfusion status and, as predicted, a more robust parameter than PI. The evidence of the less than ideal data presented here would suggest a possible role as a cost effective pre-screening tool in the decision process leading to transplant biposy.

ACKNOWLEDGMENTS

The authors would like to thank the staff of the Guy's Hospital Renal Unit - Directors Professor JS Cameron and Dr. CS Ogg, the surgical transplant team lead by Mr CGK Koffman, the nursing staff of Astley Cooper Ward, and their patients, for their cooperation and support during these studies. Our particular thanks to Dr. I Abbs for his help.

REFERENCES

1. Allen KS, Jorkansky DK, Arger PH et al. (1988) Renal allografts: Prospective analysis of Doppler sonography. *Radiology* 169: 371-376.
2. Gosling RG, Lo PTS and Taylor MG. (1991) Interpretation of pulsatility index in feeder arteries to low impedance vascular beds. *Ultrasound. Obs. Gyn.* 3: 1-5.
3. Gosling RG and King DH. (1974) Arterial assessment by Doppler-shift ultrasound. *Proc. R. Soc. Med.* 67: 447-449.
4. Grant EG and Perrella RR. (1990) Wishing won't make it so: Duplex Doppler Sonography in the evaluation of renal transplant dysfunction. *Am. J. Rad.* 155: 538-539.
5. Kelcz F. et al. (1990) Pyramidal appearance and resistive index: insensintive and non-specific indicators of acute renal transplant rejection. *Am. J. Rad.* 155: 531-535.
6. Marchand GR. (1981) Direct measurement of glomerular capillary pressure in dogs. *Proc. Exp. Biol. Med.* 167: 428-32.
7. Molheok GP, Wesseling KH, Settels JJM, et al. (1984) Evaluation of the Penats servo-plethysmo-manometer for the continous non-invasive measurement of finger blood pressure. *Basic Res. Cardiol.* 79: 598-609.
8. Perrella RR, Duerinckx AJ, Tessler FN et al. (1990) Evaluation of Renal Transplant Dysfunction by Duplex Doppler Sonography: A prospective Study and review of the Literature. *Am. J. Kid. Dis.* 15 (6): 544-50.
9. Rigsby CN, Burns PN, Weltin GG et al. (1987) Doppler signal quantitative in renal allografts: Comparison in normal and rejecting transplants with pathologic correlation. *Radiology* 162: 39-42.
10. Taylor JW and Marks WH. (1990) Use of Doppler imaging for evaluation of dysfunction in renal allografts. *Am. J. Rad.* 155: 536-537.

Principles For Re-Operations of The Renal Artery

R.H. Dean and K.J. Hansen

Division of Surgical Sciences, Bowman Gray School of Medicine, Wake Forest University, Winstom-Salem, NC, U.S.A.

Renal arterial occlusive disease is common in the older atherosclerotic population is usually limited to isolated segments of the vessel, and development of new lesions beyond corrected disease is rare. For this reason, recurrent lesions in a previously revascularized vessel most commonly are secondary to the presence of a stenosing lesion in the anastomotic sites or the body of the graft or at the site of previous endarterectomy. In addition, since renal artery grafts have the favorable characteristics for long-term patency of short length and high flow, most instances in which a kidney becomes ischemic subsequent to an operative intervention are related to technical errors that were committed at the initial procedure. Therefore, this discussion of recurrent renal artery stenosis is divided into considerations of early and late reoperations for recurrent occlusive lesions.

EARLY REOPERATION

In general, the vast majority of causes of early recurrent renal ischemia necessitating reoperations are performed to correct errors either in operative technique or judgment committed at the initial operation and, thereby, should be entirely avoidable. Nevertheless, a brief discussion of these pitfalls is appropriate. Acute angulation, kinking and twisting of the graft can occur when graft length is inappropriate or axial orientation is not obtained. This is a particular risk with splenorenal and hepatorenal bypass. Similarly, inappropriately deep placement of sutures in the heel area of the graft will create a band-like constriction across the suture line. Further, the aortic anastomosis can be made stenotic unless a large button of aorta is excised when end-stage atherosclerosis is present. Such aortas have minimal capacity to alter their configuration and unless a large orifice for the graft is created by excision, the graft may have a stenotic origin. Suture line stenoses also can result from a "pursestring" when using a continuous suture line. To avert this problem, a spatulated anastomosis is always used in which the smaller of the two vessels being connected is opened to at least three times its cross-sectional diameter. In each of these instances, the technical error can and should be recognized at the time of operation and, when present, should prompt the surgeon to "redo" the anastomosis.

Peculiar to renal artery endarterectomy, residual intimal plaque and un-recognized intimal flap creation usually are produced by blind renal artery endarterectomy performed through the transaortic route. Stoney and as-sociates have routinely performed intraoperative angiography to exclude the presence of residual plaque or intimal flap. When found, they should be cor-rected with a counter incision in the distal renal artery to "tack down" the distal intima or complete the endarterectomy.

The use of intraoperative duplex sonography has helped identify such lesions without having to accept the risk of intraoperative arteriography. To diminish the risk of intimal flap creation and residual plaque, we prefer to perform such renal artery endarterectomies through a transverse approach, which is carried out the renal artery beyond the occluding disease. Through this incision, the entire endarterectomy is performed under direct vision and the necessity of intraoperative angiography is abolished.

Early thrombosis of renal artery reconstruction is directly attributable to faulty operative technique and thereby is preventable by employment of proper technique for small vessel anastomoses. Reported frequency of early graft thrombosis ranges from 2 per cent to over 20 per cent. We experienced a 22 per cent thrombosis of renal reconstruction in our early experience during the 1960s. Review of more recent results following implementation of modern principles of microvascular surgery has demonstrated an early failure rate of less than 2 per cent[1].

Clinical characteristics suggesting the presence of acute graft thrombosis include onset of accelerated hypertension in the early postoperative period or deterioration in renal function. Neither of these characteristics is ac-curate, however, for either can be present in spite of a functioning graft and be absent in the presence of graft thrombosis. For this reason, we routinely perform postoperative angiography to assess technical success prior to the discharge of the patient.

Although graft thrombosis can lead to clot propagation into the distal renal artery branches and lead to the necessity of nephrectomy, renal revas-cularization is frequently possible at reoperation. Since the original oc-clusion usually has prompted the development of significant collateral path-ways for renal perfusion, the kidney, though ischemic, may have retained perfusion and patent distal vessels through these collateral networks.

LATE REOPERATION

Lesions producing a need for late reoperation after an initially successful operation are relatively uncommon and have been found in less than 10 per cent of renal artery reconstructions followed angiographically from 1 to 23 years after a successful operation in our experience[2]. Causes of recurrent lesions include fibrotic stenosis of venous valves in saphenous vein grafts, tubular subendothelial fibroblastic proliferation, anastomotic lesions, and the development of new stenosing lesions beyond the initial graft.

Valves in the reversed saphenous vein do not lie against the vein wall but instead assume a nonobstructing neutral position. If such valves become fibrotic in that position and undergo contracture, a web-like stenosis of the vein graft is created. Although we have only identified four such lesions in our follow-up studies, it suggests that a valveless segment of vein should be used if possible. Percutaneous transluminal angioplasty has been used successfully in one of these patients to relieve the hemodynamic significance of the lesion. Most such lesions, however, are managed by longitudinal venotomy, excision of the fibrotic valve and patch angioplasty.

Five instances of subendothelial fibroblastic proliferation of saphenous vein aortorenal grafts have been identified in the follow-up angiographic studies in our experience. Two occurred in patients having complex branch renal artery repairs and the others occurred in patients who underwent bilateral renal artery grafts. In each of these instances, the vein was subjected to a prolonged ischemia time without the benefit of any specific measure designed to provide protection against intimal damage. Whether use of cold, heparinized blood or other preservative solutions would have prevented late tubular stenosis in these patients, however, is conjectural.

In any event, replacement of the involved portion of graft is required for management of such lesions. Frequently, the distal segment of vein is not involved and the new graft can be attached to the old graft proximal to the distal suture line, thereby not requiring definitive mobilization of the previously dissected and scar-entrapped renal artery branches.

Finally, anastomotic stenoses may represent suture line "pursestring," which went unrecognized at the initial operation or the development of neointimal proliferation at the anastomotic site when a synthetic graft had been used initially. In either circumstance, repeat bypass may be limited to insertion of an interposition graft to replace the proximal or distal anastomotic site.

Total occlusion of a previously placed aortorenal graft removes the possibility of limiting the reoperation to the offending segment of graft. Most such thromboses represent progressive sequelae of early technical errors left uncorrected or progressive stenoses that were unrecognized prior to total thrombosis.

In our experience, the development of late graft occlusion has occurred in three per cent of our patients followed by sequential postoperative angiography.

Development of new lesions in the renal artery beyond a patent graft is exceedingly rare in our experience. Each instance occurred in young patients.

Two additional problems not producing recurrent renovascular hypertension merit comments as reasons for reoperation. These are aneurysmal degeneration of vein grafts and anastomotic false aneurysms.

Aneurysmal degeneration has been a widely publicized complication of the use of autogenous saphenous vein for aortorenal bypass. Its development, however, is predictable and is primarily limited to its use in young patients. Although it has occurred in only four per cent of saphenous veins used in all age groups in our experience, all of these have occurred in relatively young patients with fibrodysplastic lesions in whom the saphenous vein was used to provide total flow to the normal kidney. The fact that all of these aneurysmal grafts occurred in such patients who were also cured of hypertension by surgery suggests an interesting hypothesis. Specifically, when the vessel and kidney beyond the stenosis are normal, cure of hypertension and relatively higher flow rates should be expected. In this situation and in children whose saphenous vein is structurally less mature, flow through the graft is disproportionately higher and aneurysmal degeneration more likely. Circumstantial support for this hypothesis is drawn from the fact that we have not seen aneurysmal degeneration of saphenous vein aortorenal grafts placed in patients with atherosclerotic lesions. Since most of these patients have some intrarenal arteriolar nephrosclerosis that results in lower graft flow rates, this group would be at reduced risk for aneurysmal degeneration of the graft. Finally, although we have replaced one aneurysmally dilated aortorenal bypass, most such dilated grafts stabilize in size and can be followed without replacement.

Although uncommonly identified, false aneurysm formation at the anastomotic suture lines can occur with aortorenal grafting. We have identified and corrected five such false aneurysms in two patients. In both instances, these were noted at late follow-up angiography and occurred in patients having synthetic graft insertion (Dacron). Since the structural integrity of synthetic to artery anastomoses is permanently dependent on suture line integrity, this complication is probably peculiar to nonautogenous grafts. Their demonstration in a patient 20 years after insertion, however, suggests that such synthetic grafts should be empirically evaluated at a point in late follow-up to exclude the presence of silent false aneurysms.

TECHNICAL CONSIDERATIONS AT REOPERATION

Finally, a few technical points are peculiar to operations on previously dissected renal arteries. Reoperation for proximal anastomotic suture line stenoses or valvular stenoses of saphenous vein grafts may be relatively simple without significantly increased technical difficulties. Mobilization of the previously dissected distal renal artery is particularly hazardous and must be performed by tedious, precise dissection. Since the renal vein is intimately associated with the renal artery, it is frequently densely adherent and easily entered in the process of its separation from the distal area, attention is first directed to the renal hilum at the edge of the kidney. By identifying each of the renal artery branches at this previously unmolested site, the surgeon can minimize inadvertent trauma to the branch points that are usually arising within the dissected scarred area of the more proximal branching sites. To carry this technical point to its logical conclusion we will usually approach the kidney and renal vasculature from an entirely new route. For instance, if the left renal artery has previously been approached through the base of the mesentery we will expose the renal hilar area by reflecting the left colon medially and approach the renal vasculature from the lateral direction.

If the previous procedure has involved the distal renal artery and a branch repair is anticipated, preparations for an ex vivo repair are always made[3] and held in "standby." Such preparations are frequently made even when branch repair is not anticipated, for removal of the kidney, ex vivo perfusion and preservation and subsequent dissection of the fused renal arterial and venous system in this controlled manner may be the only means by which precise correction, without unacceptable venous bleeding and potential irretrievable renal arterial trauma, can be obtained.

REFERENCES

1. Dean, R. (1983) Renovascular hypertension. In: Vascular surgery: a comprehen-sive review, edited by Moore, W., pp 433-463. Grune & Stratton: New York.
2. Dean, R., (1985) Renovascular hypertension. *Curr Probl Surg,*, XXII:6-67.
3. Dean, R. (1979) Operative management of renovascular hypertension. In: Surgery of the aorta and its body branches, edited by Bergan J., Yao, J., p 377. Grune & Stratton: New York.

Technical Possibilities in The Renal Arteries Reoperations

J.M. Jausseran, M. Ferdani and R. Courbier

Department of Cardio-Vascular Surgery Saint Joseph Hospital, Marseille, France

Currently, renal arterial stenosis are treated in most cases by angioplasty. Surgery being intended to this technique contraindications or to its immediate or secondary failures. Furthermore, the vascular surgeon is often faced with mixed lesions of both the aortic bifurcation and the renal arteries. However, the surgical restorations of renal arteries are not prevented from restenosis.

There are two different cases for renal arteries operations:
- further to angioplasty: the surgical anatomic conditions are slightly or not modified;
- further to surgery: the surgical anatomic conditons have been disrupted by the previous operation.

The reoperations are indicated in emergency situation for angioplasty failures, in the event of the recurrence of High Blood Pressure symptoms, further to an echographic or angiographic elective control and in the presence of restenosis further to angioplasty or surgery.

OPERATIONS INCIDENCE

In the event of renal angioplasties, the immediate failures and accidents represent 3 to 6%[4,5,6,8]. In Joffre, 210 patients multicentric study[7], serious complications represented 5%, leading to surgical procedure in 1.8% of the cases and to a mortality of 0.3%. Joffre evaluates that a stenosis recurrence superior to 50% appears in 23% of the cases (follow-up > 4 years). The recurrences appear essentially with atheromatous stenosis. They can be treated either by another dilatation with a possible endoprosthesis of by surgery.

The occurrence of peroperative thrombosis can be immediately corrected after a renal artery surgery. The restenosis or postoperative thrombosis rate is of 3% for Dean[4]. Lagnau estimates a 5 year patency at 95% over a 468 revascularization series[10].

In our departement, we estimate that the reoperation frequency is of 3% compared to direct renal surgery.

The diagnostic elements leading to a reoperation or another dilatation are the following:
- High Blood Pressure recurrence
- Renal insufficiency appearance (creatinine)
- Decreasing of the kidney size.

An increased monitoring of the patients who underwent a correction of a stenosis by angioplasty or surgery should improve the reoperation conditions.

ANATOMIC ASPECT OF RESTENOSIS AND COMPLICATIONS

Peroperative difficulties.

These can be encountered during surgery or angioplasty.

In the course of the surgery: technical difficulties can be detected with a peroperative monitoring. The blood pressure testing above and underneath the restoration has been abandoned due to its poor reliability. The peroperative angiography is much safer according to our experience. The angioscopy is interesting but only allows the distal anastomosis evaluation. Several technical faults may be avoided during bypasses:
- a distal stenosis can be avoided by using interrupted sutures rather than uninterrupted ones;
- a proximal stenosis at the anastomosis site due to a non-matching between the aortic orifice and the venous graft in aortorenal bypasses;
- graft volvulus;
- incomplete thrombo-endarterectomy (Fig. 1).
Theses various defects must be corrected during the peroperative period.

In the course of angioplasty: several cases may lead to an immediate surgical procedure, and all the authors underline the necessity of having the angioplasty room next to the operating room.

Usual complications are:
- In-situ thrombosis,
- Dissections which can be corrected by the implantation of an endoprosthesis,
- Ruptures or perforations with retroperitoneal hematoma,
- Distal branch lesions in the fibromuscular dysplasia,
- Embolisms due to cholesterol (Fig. 2).

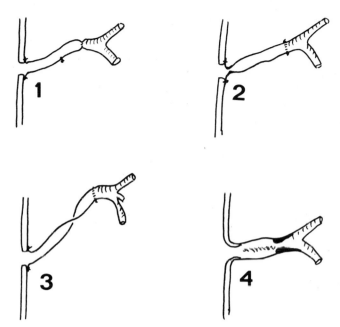

Fig. 1. Peroperative technical difficulties: 1 distal stenosis - 2 proximal stenosis - 3 bypass kinks - 4 endarterectomy sequestrum

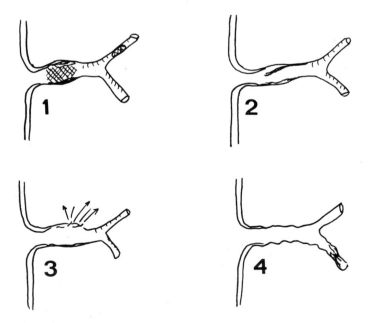

Fig. 2. Angioplasty events: 1 Thrombosis underneath embolism - 2 Dissections - 3 Arterial ruptures - 4 Dysplasia peripheral lesions.

Anatomic Aspect of the Secondary Stenosis

Further to surgical restoration with bypass, proximal or distal restenosis, alteration of the saphenous graft, stenosis or ectasia may occur. A total bypass thrombosis may appear with a reoperation probability if the distal branches are revascularized by the exorenal circle.

After a thrombo-endarterectomy or an angioplasty, the restenosis are caused by a fibromuscular hyperplasia and are generally situated at the original site. In the event of operation for fibromuscular dysplasia, an underneath extension of the lesions or some micro-aneurysms may require a peripheral restoration (Fig. 3).

For all these restenosis late from the revascularization procedure, it is necessary to evaluate the parenchyma condition. The kidney volume is to be measured by echography and the renal insufficiency by both the creatinemia and renal scintigraphy.

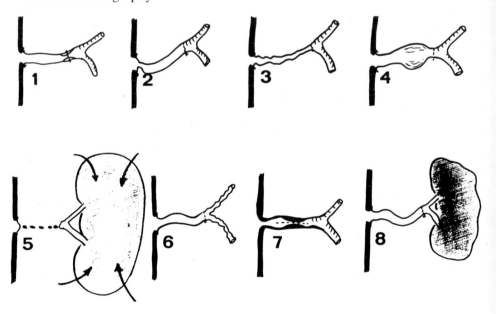

Fig. 3. Anatomic aspects of renal restenosis: 1 distal stenosis on bypass - 2 proximal stenosis - 3 venous graft diseases - 4 venous graft aneurysms - 5 total thrombosis - 6 peripheral dysplasia - 7 restenosis on endarterectomy - 8 correct bypasses, renal atrophy.

TECHNICAL POSSIBILITIES

Thrombo-endarterectomy procedures are not to be used in the course of reoperations further to renal revascularization. They should be replaced by grafting or bypassing techniques.

Access course (Fig. 4)

The parietal access course should be different from the first operation access course so to obtain a more direct access to the kidney. Likewise, if the first access to the renal pedicle was achieved in an anterior manner, it will be easier to reach the pedicle posterior side.

For a patient having undergone an operation for a more renal aortic lesion, the retroperitoneal thoraco-lumbar access over the 11th rib, will offer a sufficient access to reach the kidney and possibly implant a new bypass in an anterograde manner. If the first operation has been a renal revascularization with a retroperitoneal access, a different approach can also be selected. The subcostal access allows an efficient approach of the renal pedicle and the achievement of a right sided hepatorenal anastomosis or a left sided splenorenal anastomosis. If an aortic access is required to implant a bypass, a median or transverse laparotomy is indicated.

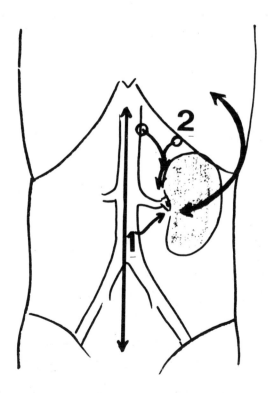

Fig. 4. Access course: 1 Usual median access and retrograde aorto-renal bypass; 2 retroperitoneal access and anterograde aorto-renal or splenorenal bypass.

Reconstruction

Simple anastomosis-resection

It is achieved in case of an anastomosis stenosis further to a renal bypass. An end-to-side anastomosis can be transformed into an end-to-end anastomosis without any added element.

For truncal restenosis further to angioplasty or thrombo-endarterectomy, the simple anastomosis resection, which is theoretically possible, must be avoided because of potential extensive lesions.

Aorto-renal bypasses

PTFE, Dacron or an autologous hypogastric artery can be used for the saphena[9]. The use of a saphenous vein may provoke ectasia. The hypogastric artery cannot be utilized for an atheromatous patient. Consequently, we choose PTFE.

For reoperations due to aortorenal bypass failures, it is possible to change only the material of the entire or segmented bypass for an anastomotic alteration or a course plication (Fig. 5). In the event of reoperations after an aortorenal bypass with laparotomy, an anterograde bypass by a retroperitoneal access will allow to avoid the already dissected areas.

The aortorenal bypass, after an angioplasty or a thrombo-endarterectomy failure, can be achieved within satisfactory anatomic conditions since the area has hardly been rearranged.

Extra-anatomic revascularizations

These techniques are of particular relevance for revascularizations. They begin at the arteries surrounding the renal artery. A complete angiographic check-up of the abdominal vessels is to be carried out prior to them.

The hepatic artery or the gastroduodenal artery can be used as a revascularization source. The first one requires an hepato-renal graft interposition. If the gastro-duodenal artery is large enough, it can be prepared and dilated to achieve a direct revascularization[11]. When the splenic artery is neither dysplasic nor atheromatous, it can be used to revascularize the left or right renal artery by carrying out a large dissection of the artery on the pancreas site (Fig. 6).

The spleen can be preserved if it is carefully mobilized with its suspending ligaments preserved[1].

The reimplantation of the renal artery over the iliac axis can also be interesting. This can be directly achieved on the primitive iliac or on the severed and turned over hypogastric artery. This technique originates from the transplantations. It requires the reimplantation of a renal vein inside the iliac one. The dissected ureter with its preserved vascularization is simply left in the iliac fossa without being shortened[9].

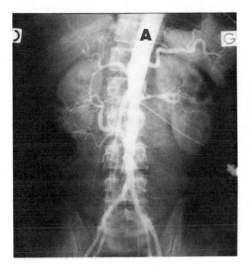

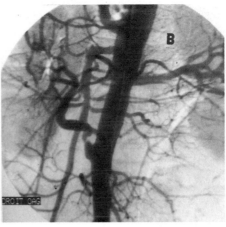

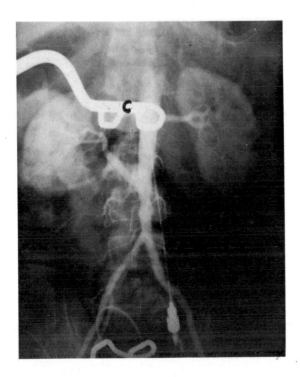

Fig. 5. A) PTFE right aorto-renal bypass; B) Stenosis on the bypass course 5 years later; C) Peroperative angiography after reoperation.

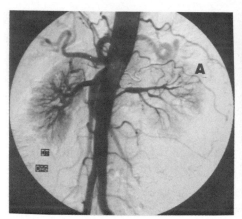
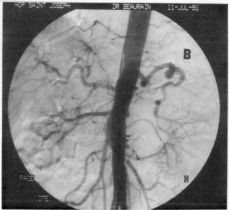

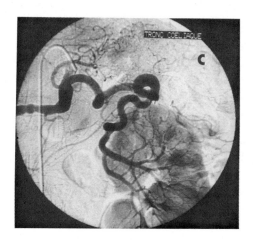

Fig. 6. A/ Tight stenosis of the left renal artery before angioplasty; B/ Acute thrombosis during angioplasty, splenorenal bypass; C/ Splenorenal bypass details.

Ex-vivo surgery

This technique varies among the various teams, according to their practice of renal transplantations. It is indicated when the reconstruction is linked to branches of the renal artery[2]. When the vessels have been severed, a perfusion of iced Collins solution is injected to the kidney. The arterial reconstruction is carried out with binocular magnifying glass. A saphenous vein with its branches, or an hypogastric artery with its dividing branches, are used. The reimplantation after restoration is achieved on the iliac vessels or on the aorta and the vena cava. This technique is usable with a retroperitoneal access.

Nephrectomy

The exeresis remains the last solution in case of a revascularization failure which caused a renal atrophy with a parenchyma no longer functional. This often happens after an iterative restoration.

DISCUSSION ABOUT INDICATIONS

Renal restenosis prevention or early detection must include a systematic control of the renal revascularization procedures. These non invasive means are efficient enough to be accepted by the patients. The renal echography provides the exact size of the renal parenchyma as well as an estimation of its function. This is also obtained with the biological tests and the renal scintigraphy. An experienced physician can monitor the arterial restorations with a renal Echo Doppler. The raising of a doubt about the vascular integrity must lead to an angiographic control which, alone, may establish the indication for a restoration procedure.

The indications for the various techniques can be simplified according to the encountered lesions. The surgical access course will be chosen so to avoid the previous operation access course.

- When facing acute cases after *angioplasty,* an extra-anatomic bypass will be chosen via a thoraco-lumbar or sub-costal access. If the hepatic or splenic arteries are of good quality, an aortorenal bypass with PTFE will be performed[3].

- *During the operation* when the angiographic control reveals a deficient restoration, it is often necessary to perform another anastomosis with separated sutures or to transform an end-to-end anastomosis into an end-to-side one. The bypass material change may be useful if the alteration is spread.

- With *restenosis further to angioplasties,* interventional radiologists advise another dilatation with or without an endoprosthesis implantation[7]. We believe that angioplasty recurrences must be surgically treated with aorto-renal bypass.

- With *bypasses alterations,* angioplasty may be useful if the lesions are limited to an anastomotic stenosis. In other cases, the best choices would be an extra-anatomic bypass or another implantation in the iliac area to avoid the already once operated area.

- The *ex-vivo surgery* is indicated for stenotic or dysplasic aneurysmal lesions occurring in the renal pedicle, in the event of angioplasty accident on a dividing branch or of anterior surgery which has reached the arterial bifurcation.

- The *indications for nephrectomy* are reserved for hypertensinogen kidneys with no or hardly any function left and for exceptional post-operative or irreparable post-angioplasty lesions.

CONCLUSION

The renal revascularization for High Blood Pressure or parenchymatous protection is achieved by angioplasty and surgery. The usual surgical techniques apply to the treatment of angioplasty acute complications. Both methods present failures as far as patency is concerned. Surgery and angioplasty are complementary to correct these failures.

REFERENCES

1. Abad C., Talbot-Wright R., Mulet J., Carretero P.: Splenorenal arterial shunt in the treatment of renovascular hypertension. *J. Cardiovasc. Surg.* 1990, 31, 706-710
2. Van Bochel J.H.,Van Den Akker P.J.,Chang P.C., J.C. Aarts, Hermans J., Terpitra J.L.: Extracorporeal renal artery reconstruction for renovascular hypertension. *J. Vasc. Surg.* 1991, 13-1,101-111
3. Mc Cann R.L., Bollinger R.R., Newman G.E.: Surgical renal artery reconstruction after percutaneous transluminal angioplasty. *J. Vasc. Surg.* 1988, 84, 389-394
4. Chiantella V., Dean R.H.: Données de base concernant les indications dans l'hypertension réno- vasculaire. *Ann. Chir. Vasc.* 1988, 2, 1, 92-97
5. Dean R.H., Callis J.T., Smith B.M., Meacham P.W.: Failed percutaneous transluminal renal angioplasty: experience with lesions requiring operative intervention. *J. Vasc. Surg.* 1987, 6, 3, 301-307
6. Hayes J.M., Risins B., Novids A.C., Gasinger M., Zelch M., Gifford R.W., Vidt D.G., Olin J.W.: Experience with percutaneous transluminal angioplasty for renal artery stenosis at the Cleveland clinic. *The J. of Urol* 1988, 139, 488-492
7. Joffre F., Nomblot C.H., Bartoli J.M., Rousseau H., Cecile J.P., Kasbarian M., Gaux J.C., Bodenard M., Lyomet D.: Résultats à long terme de l'angioplastie transluminale dans le traitement des sténoses de l'artère rénale. *J. Mal. Vasc.* 1990, 15, 239-244
8. Kazmers A., Monetta G.L., Harley J.D., Goldman M.L., Clowes A.X.: Treatment of acute renal artery occlusion after percutaneous transluminal angioplasty. *J. Vasc. Surg.* 1989, 9, 3, 487-492
9. Lacombe M., Maillard C.: Chirurgie de l'artère rénale. In: Encycl. Med Chi Paris - Techniques chirurgicales - Chirurgie Vasculaire, 9-1988, 43110, 28 p
10. Lagneau P.: Résultats des revascularisations rénales. Congrès Français de Chirurgie - Paris - 3 Octobre 1991
11. Moncure A.C., Brewster D.C., Darling R.C., Abbott W.M., Cambira R.P.: Use of the gastroduodenal artery in right renal artery revascularization. *J. Vasc. Surg.,* 1988, 8, 2, 154-159.

New Technologies in Vascular Pathology: Indications, Results and Cost-Benefit

M. Rossi, M. Bezzi, F. Orsi, P. Ricci, F. Maccioni and P. Rossi

Department of Radiology, University "La Sapienza" of Rome, Italy

INTRODUCTION

The increasing health-care costs and the growing efforts aimed at containing them within certain limits, have promoted in Italy, as in other Countries, a serious reflection on the cost-benefit ratio of the newest diagnostic and therapeutic procedures employed in the field of cardio-vascular disease.

Among all, interventional radiology offers the advantage of low invasivity, good therapeutical efficacy, limited costs, and short hospitalization, and, for these reasons, it is increasingly applied in different clinical conditions.

The recent and important contributions of the manufacturers in improving efficacy and safety of the angiographic materials have resulted in an even increased number of interventional vascular procedures.

TECHNICAL DEVELOPMENT

a. Guidewires and catheters

The new plastic guidewires available (*) are made by a Nickel-Titanium core, with an excellent torque control, covered by polyurethane and by a highly hydrophilic synthetic material or Copolymer M which continuously maintains a liquid film on the surface of the guidewire so reducing the friction during selective catheterization and the traumatic impact on the vessel's wall. Other new guidewires recently adopted in coronary and tibial artery Percutaneous Transluminal Angioplasty (PTA) (0.010, 0.014 or 0.018 inches in diameter) have a soft non-traumatic platinum tip with excellent torque control (**).

---

* Terumo Co., Tokyo, Japan.
** Target Therapeutics Co., San Jose, California.

Moreover, open-end guidewires for fibrinolytic therapy, and even guidewires extensions have become recently available.

In summary, we can say that guidewires are now available to steer through any lesion and to provide support for all catheter maneuvers during angiographic or interventional procedures. The newest catheters are usually nylon made and some of them have soft nylon-pebax tips. The main features are low traumaticity, good torque control and high flow even with small caliber; these new materials allow for easier and safer crossing of tight vascular stenoses and superselective catheterization, especially when 2-3 French (F) soft catheters are employed.

b. Angioplasty catheters

Throughout the 1980s, developments in angiographic materials have rendered PTA a safer and more effective procedure. This new technical level has been reached thanks to a strict cooperation among manufactures and interventional radiologists and cardiologists.

As regard to PTA balloon materials, one of the most important change was a shift away from polyvinylchloride (PVC) to polyethylene (PE) balloons. The relatively less compliant PE balloons provide for adequate force for PTA and permit a safer estimate of maximum balloon diameter below burst pressures. PE balloons enable the angiographer to feel confident that when selecting balloon size according to the vessel size, even if the balloon is inflated above the burst pressure, the final diameter will, always be within certain limits.

Another major development occurred in balloon catheter shafts which have now been decreased to 4-6 F. In order to reduce the size of the arterial entry and to enhance "trackability" (tendency of the catheter to advance over the guidewire up to the target location). These features are best appreciated in tortuous vessels or in tight stenoses. In addition, a variety of 4 F. balloon catheters that accept 0.014" - 0.018" guidewires are now available for tibial and segmental renal PTA. Finally, "balloon-on-a-wire" guidewires are now available for a range of vessel sizes.

Thermal angioplasty balloons have been recently used, on an experimental basis only, by inflating them with diluted contrast heated at 60-80 Celtius. The six months results obtained in an European trial on 49 pts. with peripheral vascular disease have shown a rate of 39% restenosis[6].

Therefore the theoretical benefits, based on more effective plaque remodelling and on modifications of the tunica media with reduced elastic recoil, are still to be verified.

c. Atherectomy devices

These intravascular devices are especially designed catheters able to perform ablation of atheromatous material from the arterial wall.

The most commonly used is the "Simpson Atherocath" (**); the special device on the tip of this catheter comprises an asymmetric balloon and a cutter window on the opposite side. The inflation of the balloon causes the adhesion of the cutter window onto the atheromatous plaque. At this moment the advancement of the motor-driven cutter, produces an excision, in slices, of the atheromatous material which is collected in an appropriate chamber. Short-term results seem superior to those of conventional recanalization procedures, but long-term results are comparable, since neo intimal proliferation is particularly abudant when fragments of the tunica media are excised together with the plaque.

d. Intravascular stents

Intravascular stents are generally employed in order to overcome mechanically the two most common causes of PTA failure, i.e. elastic recoil of the arterial wall and intimal dissection. Lately, vascular stenting has been proposed as primary treatment of iliac artery stenosis with good results.
Different types of vascular stents are now commercially available:
* * Palmaz: tubular mesh-work of annealed stainless steel; balloon expandable;
* ** Strecker: tantalum tubular mesh; balloon expandable;
* *** Wallstent: tubular stainless steel mesh; self-expanding;
* **** Gianturco: tempered stainless steel wire bent into a zig-zag tubular configuration; self expanding.

RESTENOSES

Surgical bypass and percutaneous angioplasty or arterial recanalization are well established therapeutic procedures with excellent results. While technical difficulties can be the cause of early failures after either surgery or vascular interventional procedures, late failures are caused by progression of the systemic disease or restenosis. Progression of the systemic disease may interest any artery above or below, while restenosis develops at the site of the anastomosis or of the PTA.
However, other factors, both in surgical and radiological procedures, do influence the long-term outcome of the different treatments: size of the graft

---

(**) DVI, distributed by PSG, California.

* Johnson & Johnson Co., Baltimore, Maryland, USA;
** Meditech, Watertown, MA, USA;
*** Medinvent, Lausanne, Switzerland;
**** Cook, Bloomington, IN, USA.

and metallic stent, flow rate, electropositive surface of the metallic stents which, in an ionic medium, attracts the elettronegative platelets, and the so called general risk factors.

The general risk factors for restenosis are the same as for the atherosclerosis[5]:

Cholesterol greater than 270 mg/dl	4.3 Fold
Smoking greater than 10 cigarettes/day	4.0 Fold
Diabetes	4.0 Fold
Obesity	3.0 Fold
Physical inactivity	3.4 Fold
Systolic/Diastolic blood press. $\geq$ 160/106 mmHg	1.8 Fold

In many necropsy studies, performed so far especially in coronary arteries, to assess the causes of restenosis after PTA, two pathophysiologic changes seem to represent the most important factors: elastic recoil of the arterial wall, 40% of early restenosis after PTA, and intimal fibrous proliferation (IFP), 60% in late restenosis, present also in arterial stenting and surgical anastomoses[16,31].

IFP, which is considered by some to be the "Achille's Heel" of PTA, is made of smooth muscle cells (SMCs) and extra-cellular matrix[4]. SMCs populate the intima by migrating from the media after any kind of arterial injury and seem to proliferate under the influence of a "platelet growth factor" (PGF). Platelet adhesion to the site of injuried site seems to initiate the PGF release.

So far, intimal fibrous proliferation is nearly impossible to predict, impossible to prevent and difficult to treat.

In order to prevent IFP through the stents, which may be mediated by thrombus deposition, many authors have proposed to apply onto the metallic stents, coats of different materials with different properties, divided into passive and active coats. Passive coats include materials of decreased thrombogenicity. Active coats involve materials that are chemically attached to anticoagulants, such as heparin[21].

Some authors have suggested also to use a string of radioactive isotope to give a small radiation dose to the tissue surrounding the stent, in order to prevent restenosis after the first stent recanalization[15].

COMPARATIVE RESULTS OF SURGICAL AND RADIOLOGICAL INTERVENTION

Aorto-iliac district

A well documented long-term study on aorto-iliac surgery, has been proposed by Szilagyi, whose series of 1647 patients had a follow-up of 30 years. The overall cumulative, primary and secondary, patency rate has been: 97.3% peri-operative; 76.6% at 5 and 10 years; 72.5% at 15 years;

67.5% at 20 years. Patients' survival, however, declined rapidly to 59% at 5 years, 33% at 10 years and 14% at 15 years[27].

PTA of iliac arteries gives excellent results as well Tegtmeyers et al.[28] reported a primary patency rate of 79% at 7.5 years and a cumulative primary and secondary patency rate, after repeated PTA, of 85.6%.

The same author, very recently, reported the results on a series of 200 patients with 340 lesions treated: initial success rate was 93% with a 5-6% of restenosis; long-term patency rate was 84% at a follow-up range of 1-90 months (92.3% with re-dilation); the complication rate was 10%[79].

In iliac artery restenosis after either PTA or surgery, repeated PTA associated with metallic stent placement seem to be the treatment of choice.

Intra-vascular stents have undoubtely improved the immediate success of PTA, mainly in case of "elastic recoil" in excentric plaque, in intimal dissection and in aorto-bifemoral anastomotic stenoses[1,20].

Long-term results of post-PTA stenting have been reported in different series. In a cumulative study reported by Palmaz[21] the total average results with two types of metallic stents were reported and are shown below (Table 1).

In this report it seems that, with the use of Wallstents, there is a higher incidence of acute occlusions of the stent due to thrombosis, but the long-term results are comparable.

In the same occasion Gaux[10], from Paris, reported the results on 105 iliac artery stenting using mainly Wallstent, which are shown below (Table 2).

Table 1

Type of stent	Patients	Acute occlusion	Patency rate	Complications
Palmaz stent	601	1%	94%	8-5%
Wallstent	175	4%	93%	11%

Table 2

F.U.	Primary patency	Secondary patency
6 months	77%	
12 months	60%	89%
30 months	56%	83%

Arterial stenting as a primary treatment for iliac artery strictures is still under evaluation, but early results seem to be very encouraging. Recently, Richter et al.[23], from Germany, reported the results of a prospective randomized trial on long-term patency, based on the measurement of the lumen size in two groups of 104 and 102 patients treated respectively with primary stenting and PTA. In this series Palmaz stents were positioned without predilation of the arterial lumen. The patency rates is reported in Table 3. These results seem to be so encouraging and if they can be reproduced by other centers, primary stenting could be considered the treatment of choice particularly in complicated irregular or ulcerated stenoses.

Infra-inguinal district

The 10 year post-surgery cumulative patency rate reported by De Weese is 45%[9]. In different series, results indicate a difference in patency rate of 10%-15% in favour of the femoro-popliteal bypass above the knee as compared to those below the knee. In a recent paper, Moore reported the experience from 1978 to 1988 with femoro-popliteal bypass with PTFE synthetic grafts[18]. Three-hundreds and twenty-two bypasses were performed in 250 patients (219 above the knee, 75 below the knee, and 23 to tibial artery); the 30-day mortality was 3.4%. The primary patency of femoropo-pliteal grafts at eight years was 63% in cases where the indication for surgery was only severe claudication but dropped to 51% in those cases with limb at risk.

Table 3

	PTA alone-104 pts.	Stent alone-102 pts.
Immediate results	86%	100%
3 years	72%	96%

It is clear that in Moore's series the surgical results are not only influenced by the technical aspect such as venous vs. PTFE graft, but also by the indications and by the clinical conditions of the patient.

In the infra-inguinal district excellent results can be obtained also by interventional procedures, mainly in those cases with limited arterial involvement and good distal out-flow. On the other hand, in long segment arterial stenoses with poor distal out-flow, particularly in patients classified as at "increased general risk", positive results are short-lived.

Capeck et al.[3] in 1991 reported the following results obtained with PTA:

periprocedural success rate of 85%; 73% at one year; 55% and 52% respectively at three and five years. Complications occurred in 10% of cases, 25% of which without clinical consequences.

Recently Graor[12] reported these results by using athecatheter, in patients with periferal vascular desease (Table 4).

These data do not really differ so much from that recently reported by Katzen in 180 patients with a patency rate, in life table analysis, of 88% at 6 months, 78 % at 12 months and approximately 50% at two years follow-up[14].

Interventional proceduers below the popliteal artery represent a true tehcnical challenge to the operator because of the size and condition of the vessels and the limited run-off.

Schwarten, in his experience with tibial and peroneal angioplasty in 96 patients, poor surgical candidates, reported an anatomical success in 87% of the occlusions and in 100% of the stenoses, with a primary patency rate of 97%[25]. Major amputations were required in four patients only with long segmental occlusion of the anterior and posterior tibial arteries and focal occlusion of the peroneal artery not amenable to recanalization.

Table 4

| | PATENCY RATE | | | |
	6 months	12 months	24 months	36 months
54 simple lesions	98%	96%	90%	82%
157 complicated lesions	90%	78.8%	77%	72.5%

Stenting of the femoral artery is also a valid alternative to PTA or atherectomy. Palmaz comparing the results of different authors[30,2,24,32,13] with different types of stents, reports the following data (Table 5).

Table 5

Stent type	Pts.	Acute occlusion	Patency rate	Complications
Palmaz stent	80	5%	87.5%	9%
Wallstent	65	21%	68%	26%

These results indicate that the femoral artery stenting, especially in long stenosis, have an high incidence of restenosis or early occlusion.

Renal district

Reno-vascular hypertension is often due to stenosis of the main renal artery or of one of its branches.

The most common causes of these strictures are fibro-muscular hyperplasia in young subjects or atherosclerosis in older patients. Symptomatic stenosis can be successfully treated by surgery or by PTA.

In recent years, PTA is considered the therapy of choice because of the excellent results obtained, the very low morbidity and the absence of procedure related mortality.

The results of surgery as reported by Dean[8] in 148 bypasses and 36 arterial reimplants are (Table 6):

Table 6

Results	Total	Non-atherosclerotic lesions	Atherosclerotic lesions
Cured	21%	43%	15%
Improved	70%	49%	75%
No change	9%	-	-
Mortality rate	3%	-	-

As already said, PTA of the renal artery gives very good results, which are better in patients with fibro-muscular hyperplasia than in atherosclerotic disease. Sos, in a review of the literature combined with his personal experience[26], reports the following results in renal PTA, which are undoubtedly better than those obtained by surgery. In addition no 30-days mortality is reported (Table 7).

Table 7

Results	Fibromuscular dysplasia	Atheromatous disease
Technical success	95%	95%
Cured	70%	25%
Improved	20%	56%
Failure	10%	19%

Metallic stents can be a valid adjunct in renal strictures not responding to PTA or in restenoses after successful PTA. The presence of ostial lesion, due to aortic plaques, is an indication for primary stenting. The combined results of different series, presented by Palmaz[21] and showed in the following table, are very good considering that the stents are used in restenosis or in difficult cases. However the number of patients treated is not sufficient for a statistically significative evaluation (Table 8).

Table 8

Stent type	Pts.	Acute occlusion	Long-term patency rate	Complications
Palmaz stent	56	0	77%	9%
Wallstent	21	4.5	81%	14%

Nephrovascular hypertension is associated also with arterial stricture in transplanted kidney. This well known complication occurs with a frequency of 25% approximately in different series, and it is more common in the "end-to-end" as compared to the "end-to-side" anastomosis[11]. These stenoses are due to different causes, including: active rejection, atheromatous plaques, trauma and post-surgical intimal fibrous proliferation or peri-vascular fibrosis.

The results of surgical correction of these lesions are satisfactory in about 50-60% of cases, but the procedure is difficult because of the extensive fibrosis surruonding the transplanted kidney[11]. Angioplasty proved to be a very effective procedure in relieving anastomotic stenoses following renal transplantation. In a review by Curry et al.[7], good control of blood pressure occurred in 76% of transplanted angioplasties.

Reported complications include segmental infarcts, renal artery thromboses and less serious complications such as hematomas, acute tubular necrosis and non-occlusive sub-intimal dissection[7].

Nephrovascular hypertension may also follow a successful renal artery PTA or a surgical procedure, with restenosis of the renal artery being the most frequent cause.

Although PTA is usually followed by an improvement of symptoms, in some cases, if the residual stenosis after dilation is more than 30% of the lumen, metallic stents may solve the problem.

CONCLUSION

The technical developments of angiographic materials, introduced in clinical practice over the last decade, have contributed to improve the safety and efficay of PTA. Most recently, the application of metallic stents, has given the interventional radiologist a valid tool to overcome most of the PTA drawbacks such as dissection, intimal flap or arterial recoil, with an increase in success rate for percutaneous revascularization procedures. These are the reasons of the worldwide diffusion of these techniques which are now available also in small centers.

Angiographic materials are very expensive, but so are the surgical ones; in addition we should consider the cost of the "intervention", and the duration of hospitalization, significantly shorter for radiological procedures. Finally, the 30-day mortality of PTA or vascular stenting, is really negligible, while this is not true for surgery.

Percutaneous revascularization can therefore offer results that are fairly comparable to those obtained by surgery.

It presents advantages of being considerably less expensive and traumatic, it gives the possibility of repeated PTA treatment or, in case of failure, surgery.

REFERENCES

1. Becker GJ, Palmaz JC, Rees CR, et al. Angioplasty-induced dissections in human iliac arteries: management with Palmaz balloon expandable intraluminal stents. *Radiology* 1990; 176:31-38.
2. Busquet J. Palmaz-Schatz stents in the treatment of iliacand femoral arterial disease. *International Congress IV,AZ,* February 13, 1991.
3. Capek P, McLean GK, Berkowitz HD. Femoropopliteal angioplasty: factors influencing long-term success. *Circulation* 1991;83(suppl I) :I-70-I-80.
4. Consigny PM. Pathophysiology of vascular disease. Proceedings of the Fourth Annual International Symposium on vascular diagnosis and intervention, Miami, Florida, February 1992:19-21.
5. Clowes AW, Reidy MA, Clowes MM. Mechanism of stenosis after arterial injury. *Lab Invest* 1983; 49:208-215.
6. Cragg AH, Smith TP, Landas SK, Nakagawa N, Barnhart W,DeJong SC. Six-month follow-up after thermal balloon angioplasty in canine iliac arteries. *CVIR* 1991; 14:230-232.
7. Curry S, et al. Interventional radiologic procedures in the renal transplant. *Radiology* 1984; 152:647-653.
8. Dean Richard H. Surgical approach to renovascular hypertension. Proceedings of the Fourth Annual International Symposium on vascular diagnosis and intervention, Miami, Florida, February 1992:197.
9. DeWeese JA. Long-term follow-up: the surgical management of femoral popliteal disease. Proceedings of the Fourth Annual International Symposium on vascular diagnosis and intervention, Miami, Florida, February 1992:103-104.
10. Gaux JClaude. Long-term follow-up of iliac artery stenting:iliac occlusion vs. dissection. Proceedings of the Fourth Annual International Symposium on vascular diagnosis and intervention, Miami, Florida, February 1992:263-265.
11. Gerlock AJ Jr, MacDonell RC Jr, Smith CW, Muhletaler CA, Parris WC et al. Renal transplant arterial stenosis: percutaneous transluminal angioplasty. *AJR* 1983; 140(2):325-331.
12. Graor RA, Whitlow P. Directional atherectomy for peripheral vascular disease: two years patency and factors influencing patency. *Abstract J Am Col Cardiol* 1991; 17(2):106A.
13. Gunther GW, Vorwerk D, Antonucci F, et al. Iliac artery stenosis or obstruction after unsuccessful balloon angioplasty: Treatment with a self-expandable stent. *AJR* 1991; 156:389-393.
14. Katzen BT. Simpson atherectomy device. Proceedings of the Fourth Annual International Symposium on vascular diagnosis and intervention, Miami, Florida, February 1992:111-113.
15. Liermann D. Proceedings of the "International Stent Symposium II". Frankfurt, October 1991.

16. Liu MW, Roubin GS, King SB III. Restenosis after coronary angioplasty. Potential biologic determinants and role of intimal hyperplasia. *Circulation* 1989; 79:1374-1387.
17. Saeed M. Ballon expandable stenting of ostial and Recurrent renal artery stenoses. Proceedings of the Fourth Annual International Symposium on vascular diagnosis and intervention, Miami, Florida, February 1992:277-278.
18. Moore WS. Femoral popliteal bypass with PTFE: a 10-years experience Proceedings of the Fourth Annual International Symposium on vascular diagnosis and intervention, Miami, Florida, February 1992:107-108.
19. Myler RK, Mooney MR, Stertzer SH, Clark DA, Hidalgo BO, Fishman J. The balloon on a wire device: a new ultra-low profile coronary angioplasty system/concept. *Cathet Cardiovasc Diagn* 1988; 14:135-140.
20. Palmaz JC, Garcia O, Schatz RA, et al. Ballon-expandable stenting of iliac arteries: the first 171 procedures. *Radiology* 1990; 174:969-975.
21. Palmaz JC. Intravascular stents: current status. Proceedings of the Fourth Annual International Symposium on vascular diagnosis and intervention, Miami, Florida, February 1992:69-79.
22. Rees CR, Palmaz JC, Becker GJ, et al. Preliminary report of a multi-center study of the Palmaz stent in Atherosclerotic stenoses involving the ostia of the renal arteries (in press).
23. Richter GM. Prospective randomized trial: iliac stenting vs. PTA. Proceedings of the Fourth Annual International Symposium on vascular diagnosis and intervention, Miami, Florida,February 992:267.
24. Rousseau HP, Raillat CR, Joffre FG, Knight CJ, Ginestet MC. Treatment of femoropopliteal stenoses by means of self-expandable endoprostheses: Mid-term results. *Radiology* 1989;172:961-964.
25. Schwarten DE. Clinical anatomical considerations for non-operative therapy in tibial disease and the esults of angioplasty. Proceedings of the Fourth Annual International Symposium on vascular diagnosis and intervention, Miami, Florida,February 1992:123-126.
26. Sos TA Techniques and long term results of percutaneous renal angioplasty for Hypertension and azotemia. Proceedings of the Fourth Annual International Symposium on vascular diagnosis and intervention, Miami, Florida, February 1992:207-216.
27. Szilagyi DE, Elliot JP Jr, Smith RF, Reddy DJ, McPharlin M. A thirty-year survey of the reconstructive surgical treatment of aorto-iliac occlusive disease. *J Vasc Surg* 1986; 3:421-436.
28. Tegtmeyer CJ, Kellum CD, Kron IL, Mentzer RM Jr. Percutaneous transluminal angioplasty in the region of the aortic bifurcation: the two ballon technique with results and long-term follow-up study. *Radiology* 1985; 157:661-665.
29. Tegtmeyer CJ, Harwell GD, Selby JB, Roberston RJr, Kron IL, Tribble CG. Results and complications of angioplasty in aortoiliac disease. *Circulation* 1991; 83 (suppl I):I-53-I-60.
30. Vorwerk D, Gunther RW. Mechanical revascularization of occluded iliac arteries with use of expandable endoprostheses. *Radiology* 1990; 175:411-415.
31. Waller BF, Pinkerton CA, Orr CM, Slack JD, VanTassel JW, Peters T. Restenosis 1 to 24 months after clinically successful coronary balloon angioplasty: a necropsy study of 20 patients. *J Am Coll Cardiol* 1991; 17:58B-70B.
32. Zollikofer CL, Antonucci F, Pfeiffer M, Redha F et al. Arterial stent Placement with use of the Wallstent: midterm results of clinical experience. *Radiology* 1991; 179:449-456.

Renal Surgery After Percutaneous Angioplasty and Surgery Failure

M. D'Addato

Department of Vascular Surgery, University of Bologna, Italy

Although still a subject for discussion, the treatment of renovascular disease is represented by the surgical therapy of revascularization and by percutaneous transluminal angioplasty of the renal arteries (PTRA).

Clinical experience has shown that surgical revascularization of the renal arteries achieves satisfactory results in 80-90% of all cases[7,11,17], as regards both arterial hypertension and improvement of renal function, often altered.

Similarly, the results reported in literature relative to transluminal angioplasty methods are satisfactory, especially if performed by expert teams. Such experiences confirm the validity of the method and make it possible to achieve, in selected cases, results that are similar to those of surgical therapy[3,24].

Both methods present immediate or later complications, or in any case therapy failures for which surgical treatment may be indicated. This "secondary" surgical therapy, which implies more difficult technical aspects with respect to a "primary" operation, presents a high risk of nephrectomy.

This report summarizes experiences in the management of complications and failures of PTRA and surgical treatment.

FAILURES OF PERCUTANEOUS TRANSLUMINAL RENAL ANGIOPLASTY

PTRA, a method introduced by Gruntzig in 1978[13] for the treatment of stenotic lesions of the renal artery, initially aroused a great deal of interest, especially among angioradiologists. This procedure, easy to perform, inexpensive, considered to have a low mortality and morbidity risk, has often been used indiscriminately in the treatment of all lesions of the renal artery, regardless of the nature of the disease, of the localization of the lesion or of its extension.

Clinical experience has, however, re-evaluated the initial enthusiasm towards PTRA, since the efficacy and harmlessness of the procedure has only been proved in selected cases, and the lesions at risk for complications or for rapid recurrence after PTRA have, on the other hand, been shown.

Among the PTRA failures, we will divide them into acute forms, which require urgent surgical treatment, and late forms, in which, on the other hand, surgical revascularization can be programmed, situations which lend themselves to different etiopathogenetic, therapeutic and prognostic considerations.

Acute failures are the major complications of PTRA, in which urgent surgery is indicated for lesions involving a risk of survival or nephrectomy.

Late failures, in which surgical treatment can be programmed, are on the other hand represented by lesions which present rapid recurrence after PTRA.

Acute failures of PTRA

Acute failures of PTRA are represented, essentially, by the complications consequent to the method.

The exact frequency of total complications after PTRA is not known, but the total percentage varies from 2.5 to 28.5%[1,5,9,22]. Renal complications, between 1 and 10%[1,9,22], are represented by dissections of the tunica intima and the tunica media, by embolization, perforation, rupture and occlusion of the renal artery.

Dissections. Lesions of the tunica intima and the tunica media represent a very frequent occurrence after PTRA. In the majority of cases, however, these are not true dissections but more or less deep fracture lines which do not represent true complications. These fractures are in fact relative to the mode of action of percutaneous dilatation which causes a limited rupturing of the artery wall[3]. These fracture zones, occasionally even quite deep, are restricted to the dilated zone and heal spontaneously, thanks to a remodelling of the artery wall[3]. Ruptures in the tunica intima are usually superficial, very focal, and often present in the sections proximal to the artery, where the vessel is more elastic.

Deeper fractures, also involving the tunica media, may be caused by the dilatation of very rigid stenotic lesions, such as calcified atherosclerotic stenoses. True dissections of the tunicae intima and media are, on the contrary, caused by the penetration of the guide or of the angiocatheters inside the arterial wall, thus creating a false lumen.

A predisposing factor for dissection is arterial spasm, present in 43% of cases during PTRA of dysplastic lesions and in 16% of atherosclerotic lesion[2]. Other conditions favouring dissection are represented by an abnormal thickening of the tunica intima, typical in patients with hypertension, and by this high arterial pressure which reinforces the effects of the intramural hemorrhage.

The majority of intimal dissections, however, are small in size and have no pathological significance, since they are apt to heal. At other times the dissected area is replaced by cicatricial fibrous tissue which may be responsible for a late stenosis.

Occasionally, the dissection of the tunica media will progress rapidly, with a consequent intramural hematoma and thus a thrombosis of the renal artery.

Embolization. A serious complication of PTRA is represented by embolization of the atheromatous or thrombotic material in the renal artery branches, with consequent renal infarct. This complication probably has an incidence of 5%[5]. There are various consequences of such embolizations; if the infarcted area is fairly small, the situation can be tolerated. At other times, being responsible for a deterioration of the hypertensive state, the renal infarct entails a nephrectomy, sometimes partial. Albeit rarely, it has been described by some as the spontaneous lysis of the thrombus [16].

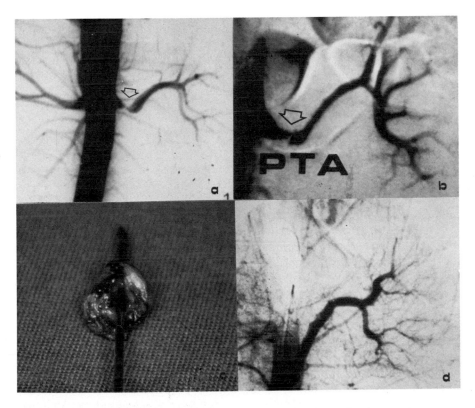

Fig. 1. Atherosclerotic ostial lesion of the left renal artery (a). The attempt at PTA causes a dissection of the artery wall (b); the intraoperative control shows the dissection with consequent thrombosis of the lumen (c); angiographic control after aorto-renal Dacron bypass (d).

Perforation of the renal artery. Perforation of the renal artery with consequent hemorrhage or thrombosis is a very rare occurrence after PTRA[24], and is generally the consequence of incorrect maneuvers during the positioning or the manipulation of the metallic guide. This results in a small perforation which does not usually require surgical treatment since the hemorrhage stops spontaneously after a few minutes.

If, however, the perforation of the artery is caused by the mechanism of dilatation itself, it is usually larger and may give rise to very extensive hematomas which require urgent surgical intervention.

Rupture. Rupturing of the main renal artery is a rare occurrence which obviously requires emergency surgery. The main cause of rupture is represented by excessive insufflation of the balloon, or by the choice of a too-large balloon. Demolition surgical is usually performed.

Occlusions. Occlusion of the main renal artery usually occurs following treatment of very extensive atherosclerotic lesions. At times the mode of action is represented by the decollement of the plaque by the guide or the catheter.

These complications occur more often when the lesions are ostial or when the atherosclerotic plaque is markedly asymmetrical and the arterial lumen is extremely restricted and situated in an eccentric position.

Some authors report, with favorable results, attempts to re-enter the true lumen, with subsequent dilatation of the artery[22]. In most cases, surgical treatment is necessary.

LATE FAILURES OF PTRA

Late failures of PTRA include rapid recurrences of renal artery lesions after initial dilatation of the lumen.

Recurrence after PTRA is reported in various case studies with a percentage between 5 and 8%[24], although some authors report percentages of 22%[19] and even of 42%[14].

In a recent review of 202 cases treated with PTRA, Baert reports a recurrence in 16 cases, equal to 8%, in an average follow-up of 11.3 months[1]. Twelve (75%) of these patients had a recurrence of the stenosis, while in 4 cases (25%) the stenosis developed into a complete occlusion of the artery.

The majority of the recurrences occur in the first year after PTRA[5], but according to Flechner the incidence increases proportionally with the increase of the follow-up, especially for atherosclerotic lesions[9].

Common experiences of various authors confirm that there are some lesions with a greater and even early risk of recurrence.

The lesions which present less favorable results right from the start are ostial or paraostial atherosclerotic type lesions, dysplastic type unifocal stenoses, dysplastic stenoses which have spread to the renal artery branches, and, finally, Takayasu type inflammatory lesions.

In particular, ostial or paraostial atherosclerotic plaques of the renal artery are in reality aortic lesions which have spread to the renal ostium. This plaque is often incompressible, so that the stenosis appears to be unaltered when the balloon is deflated, or it presents a rapid recurrence. Studies on this problem show that only 25% of the ostial lesions subjected to PTRA present favorable results over a period of time[20].

As regards dysplastic lesions, those of a focal type, frequently congenital, localized in the intima and subadventitia, have a high incidence of recurrence. The abundant elastic tissue in the lesion is responsible for the easy distension of the wall after PTRA, but also causes a rapid recurrence.

As far as the treatment of the recurrences is concerned, according to some authors a secondary PTRA is favorable in 80% of the cases[24], while other authors prefer to resort directly to surgical revascularization[15] since after secondary PTRA recurrence re-occurs in 22% of the cases[24].

SURGICAL TREATMENT OF PTRA FAILURES

Surgical treatment of PTRA complications and failures may be demolitive or reconstructive. Nephrectomy is performed in situations in which the artery presents lesions that are not susceptible to reconstruction, or in cases of irreparable parenchymal damage.

Sometimes a partial nephrectomy is sufficient, as in cases of renal infarct consequent to embolization. In these cases, delimitation of the damaged tissue with respect to the healthy tissue can be made with the help of vital dyes, but usually a preoperative selective angiograph makes it possible to correctly identify the frankly ischemic area.

Operations to reconstruct the renal vessels are technically more difficult than primary revascularization. Regardless of the acute complications, the actual trauma suffered by the arterial wall, following forced distension, is responsible for the obliteration of the periadventitial surfaces, which therefore makes the exposure and mobilization of the renal artery and its branches difficult. This results in a greater risk of nephrectomy and a greater incidence of operative morbidity and mortality.

As regards surgical technique, the aorto-renal bypass is usually the reconstruction technique of choice for damaged renal arteries. The prosthetic material used varies, in the various authors' experiences, from an autologous vein to synthetic prostheses in Dacron or PTFE.

In our experience, renal revascularization after PTRA failure was performed in 12 patients, 4 of which were treated for immediate complications of the procedure and 8 for late PTRA failures.

In the early failures surgery was performed for medial dissection, with consequent thrombosis of the renal artery in 2 cases (50%). Both these cases presented lesions consequent to attempts to dilate the ostial atherosclerotic plaque. Revascularization of the kidney was possible in both cases by means of bypass with synthetic prostheses, obtaining positive results (Figs. 1,2).

In the third case, an attempt to perform PTRA of an ostial atherosclerotic lesion caused not only an immediate recurrence of the stenosis but also an embolization, with consequent infarct of the lower pole of the kidney. In this case too, a Dacron reconstruction of the renal artery was performed, while the infarcted area, being small, was not removed.

In the fourth patient, the early PTRA failure was the result of treatment of an extensive atherosclerotic lesion, with consequent thrombosis of the main renal artery. In this patient, the presence of a valid distal collateral circulation made it possible to carry out renal revascularization with a Dacron bypass, associated with an aortobisiliac bypass for the concomitant presence of an abdominal aortic aneurysm.

Positive results (cured + improved) were obtained in all the surgically treated cases.

Considering the late PTRA failures, surgery was indicated for a recurrence of the lesion in 8 cases. These were atherosclerotic lesions which presented a recurrence of the symptoms, with restenosis after PTRA at a varying distance of time of 3 to 10 months. In six cases dilatation was performed to correct the ostial stenosis, and in two cases due to the presence of a distal atherosclerotic stenosis of the renal artery. Surgical treatment, reconstructive in all cases, was performed with Dacron bypasses. Positive results were obtained in the 6 cases of revascularization after recurrence of the ostial stenosis, while one of the patients with distal renal stenosis presented an early occlusion of the bypass.

Positive results were obtained in 91% of the cases treated surgically for early and late PTRA failures.

FAILURES OF PREVIOUS RENAL SURGERY

The percentage of surgical failures, both early and late, is reported in literature with a wide range, between 4 and 39%[4,10], although the true incidence is however difficult to establish.

Only a few of the studies reported in literature, on the follow-up of operated patients, were performed with angiographic methods. From these experiences, it emerges that the percentage of surgical failures, for which redo surgery is indicated, is between 12 and 15.5%[21,26].

As with PTRA failures, it is also possible to distinguish between early and late surgical failures.

Early surgical failures

Early stenoses and occlusions are reported in literature with a frequency varying between 2 and 20% of the cases.

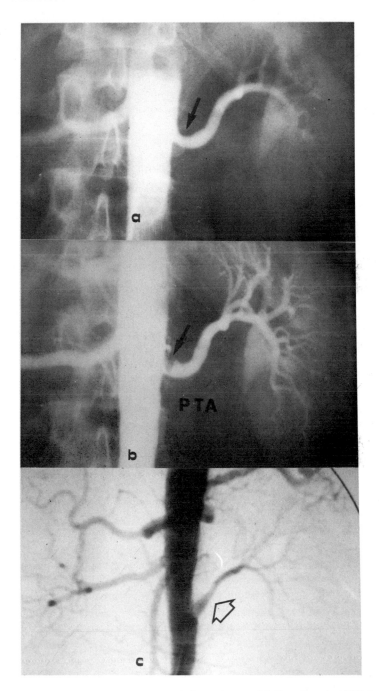

Fig. 2. Atherosclerotic ostial stenosis of the left renal artery (a); the attempt at PTA is responsible for the parietal dissection (b); intravenous digital subtraction angiography after left PTFE aorto-renal bypass (c).

These complications can be attributed, in most cases, to surgical technique errors. Many of these can therefore be identified intraoperatively and, thus, corrected.

In renal revascularizations carried out with an autologous saphenous vein or prosthetic implant, an excessively long prosthesis or its incorrect orientation can lead to angulations, kinking or twisting, conditions which predispose early thrombosis.

Similarly, anastomotic, proximal and distal defects represent conditions at risk for thrombosis, although in some cases the disappearance of the anastomotic stenoses over time has been demonstrated[6,21]. Such a favorable evolution is present above all in anastomoses between the aorta and the prosthesis, which may appear stenotic at an early angiographic follow-up. Nevertheless, these lesions must not be underestimated, and, if not treated, they require careful control to evaluate their evolution.

Acute thrombotic complications after endoarterectomy of the renal artery present an average incidence of 9%[18], but this seems to be lower in the case reports of authors who perform this procedure as the method of choice in renal revascularization[25].

Technical defects, such as flaps, intimal ledges, residual plaque and dissections represent the most frequent causes of thrombosis after endoarterectomy, especially if performed as blind endoarterectomy. For this reason, Stoney suggests that an intraoperative angiography should always be performed[23].

Clinical aspects which arouse suspicion of an acute occlusion are represented by an abrupt increase in arterial pressure and by a deterioration of renal functionality in the early post-operative period. Both clinical aspects are not however characteristic, since they may also occur in patients with bypass perviousness and there are also cases of completely asymptomatic acute occlusion. It is therefore necessary for the patient to undergo an early angiographic study.

Late surgical failures

Late failures after renal revascularization are mainly represented by bypass stenoses and occlusions, or by aneurysmatic dilatations of the prosthesis. Prosthetic infections with enteric fistulation, pseudoaneurysms and thromboses of the renal veins are less frequent.

Late bypass stenoses are caused mainly by anastomotic stenoses due to technical defect, especially at the distal level. Other important factors which, however, concern only autologous vein prostheses are represented by an accumulation of dysplastic fibrous tissue at the site of the anastomosis, by mural fibrosis phenomena, secondary to trauma from the clamp on the venous prosthesis, and by subintimal fibroblastic proliferations which may widely involve the vein.

Graft stenosis of autogenous saphenous veins was reported in 41% of the cases[8], and stenosis of the suture line in 17%[6]. However, only 8% of these stenoses had hemodynamic characteristics[6].

As regards synthetic prostheses, Dacron or PTFE, the studies published in the literature report a higher percentage of late complications with respect to the use of autologous vein prostheses[10,17]. On the contrary, in our experience, using mainly synthetic prostheses (Dacron), a study performed with duplex, scintigraphic and angiographic controls showed the presence of late anastomotic stenosis in 14.2%[12].

With regard to late occlusions, the majority of authors agree that these are occlusions which in fact occurred in the early post-operative period, as the result of incorrect technical defects, since they were disregarded or underestimated[17,21].

Aneurysmatic dilatation is another negative characteristic of the autologous vein prostheses. A limited expansion of the vein is reported with a frequency between 20 and 40% of the cases[6,21]. True aneurysmatic dilatations have an incidence of 6%, rising to 20% if they are venous prostheses implanted in pediatric age[21]. The cause of this degeneration is unknown, but it is presumed that in infancy the structurally immature saphenous vein is inadequate for the high flow present in the aorto-renal bypass.

REDO OPERATIONS FOR FAILED SURGERY

In the event of persistence or recurrence of symptoms correlated with renal ischemia, the cause of failure must be identified. Before resorting to a redo operation, the coexistence of other causes of renal ischemia, such as parenchymal nephropathy or the presence of untreated stenotic lesions, must in fact be excluded.

Considering the technical difficulties of redo surgery and the high risk of nephrectomy, a second operation is generally only performed in cases in which the persistence or recurrence of the symptoms is undoubtedly correlated with a failure of the first operation.

Technically, in redo surgery of the renal artery, the presence of cicatricial fibrous tissue makes it difficult to isolate the vessels, especially in late redo operations. For this reason, the intraoperative use of ultrasound or angiographic methods, which can help to avoid irreparable lesions in the renal vessels, has been suggested[21].

Reconstruction of the distal anastomosis on the remaining segment of renal artery, often very short, may be equally difficult. This aspect is present above all in redo operations performed in dysplastic lesions, in which the percentage of redo operations is more frequent[10]. Another aspect which limits the efficacy of redo surgery procedures is represented by the delayed recognition of the lesion.

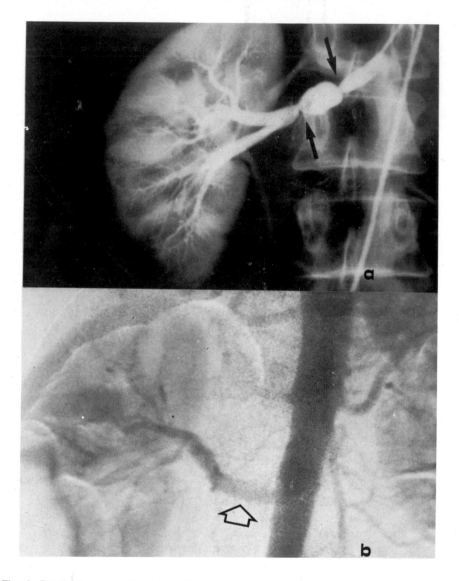

Fig. 3. Proximal and distal anastomotic stenosis of an autologous saphenous vein graft 12 months after the implant for a dysplastic stenosis of the right renal artery (a); angiographic follow-up of the new PTFE graft (b).

Renal revascularization for acute occlusion or stenosis is generally performed with in situ methods. Replacement of the prosthesis or angioplasty with a patch is the procedure most commonly used.

Finally, in selected cases of stenosis, percutaneous transluminal angioplasty may be indicated, especially in patients with a high surgical risk.

In our experience, surgical treatment of surgical failures was performed in

15 cases out of a total of 211 patients who had undergone renal revascularization, with an incidence of 7.1%. In particular, redo surgery was indicated in 8 patients (53%) due to early failures, and in 7 cases (47%) due to the presence of late complications.

Acute complications, present in 8 patients, were represented by early occlusion of the bypass in all cases. These patients presented dysplastic lesions in 66.6% of the cases. Nephrectomy was performed in 6 patients (75%).

The thrombectomy of the bypass with a subsequent angioplasty was performed in two patients (25%), with favorable results.

Reoperations for late surgical failures were carried out in 7 patients, with 2 cases (28.5%) undergoing nephrectomy and the other 5 (71.5%) reconstruction surgery.

Of the two patients who underwent demolition surgery, both atherosclerotic, one presented a thrombosis of the bypass two years after the first operation, while in the second patient the redo-surgery was performed for stenosis of a right aorto-renal bypass, 5 years after the first operation, associated with a stenosis of the contralateral artery. In this latter case, the presence of dense cicatricial fibrous tissue made it impossible to correct the stenosis; a right nephrectomy was therefore performed, associated with revascularization of the contralateral kidney.

As regards the reconstructive operations, performed in 5 patients, redo surgery was indicated in 3 patients for the presence of a stenosis of the bypass. These patients, all atherosclerotic, presented a recurrence of the disease after a period of time varying from 5 months to 5 years since the first operation.

In the last 2 cases of redo surgery, both females with dysplasia, the reconstruction operation was performed due to the deterioration of the vein used as the prosthesis. In particular, one case presented a stenosis of the vein in correspondence with the proximal and distal anastomoses, 12 months after the first operation (Fig. 3), while the second case presented a recurrence of the symptoms caused by a valvular stenosis of the saphenous vein, after a period of 5 years. In both cases revascularization was performed, replacing the vein with a PTFE prosthesis.

Considering all the redo operations for surgical failures together, the operative mortality was 6.6% (1/15). In particular, one patient who underwent nephrectomy and contralateral revascularization died from myocardial infarct.

The most favorable results were obtained in the treatment of the late forms of failure, especially considering the lower percentage of nephrectomies (28.5% versus 75% in the early failures).

The patients who underwent revascularization obtained positive results as regards arterial pressure and renal functionality in 71.4% of the cases (5/7).

REFERENCES

1. Baert, A.L., Wilms, G., Amery, A., Vermylen, J., Suy, R., (1990) Percutaneous transluminal renal angioplasty: initial results and long-term follow-up in 202 patients. *Cardiovasc. Intervent. Radiol.,* 13:22-8.
2. Beinhart, C., Sos, T.A., Saddenky, S., et Al., (1983) Arterial spasm during renal angioplasty. *Radiology,* 149:97-100.
3. Castaneda-Zuniga, (1983) Transluminal angioplasty, edited by Castaneda-Zuniga. Thieme-Stratton Inc., New York.
4. Chung, W.B., Salvian, A., (1979) Surgical treatment of renovascular hypertension. *Am. J. Surg.,* 138:143-48.
5. Colapinto, R.F., Stronel,l R.D., Harries-Jones, E.P., et Al., (1982) Percutaneous transluminal dilatation of the renal artery: follow-up studies on renovascular hypertension. *A.J.R.,* 139:727-32.
6. Dean, R.H., Wilson, J.P., Burko, H., Foster, J.H., (1974) Saphenous vein aortorenal bypass grafts: serial arterographic study. *Ann. Surg.,* 180:469-78.
7. Eigler, F.W., Dostal, G., Montag, H., Jakubowski, H.D., (1983) Results of ten-year period of reconstructive surgery for renovascular disease. *Thorac. Cardiovasc. Surg.,* 31:45-8.
8. Ekelund, L., Gerlock, J., Goncharenko, V., Foster, J.H., (1978) Angiographic findings following surgical treatment for renovascular hypertension. *Radiology,* 126:345-9.
9. Flechner, S., Novick, A.C., Vidt, D., Buoncore, E., Meaney, T., (1982) The use of percutaneous transluminal angioplasty for renal artery stenosis in patients with generalized atherosclerosis. *J. Urol.,* 127:1072-75.
10. Foster, J.H., Maxwell, M.H., Franklin, S.S., et Al., (1975) Renovascular occlusive disease: results of operative treatment. *J.A.M.A.,* 231:1043-48.
11. Fry, R.E., Fry, W.J., (1982) Renovascular hypertension in pateints with severe atherosclerosis. *Arch. Surg.,* 117:938-41.
12. Gargiulo, M., Cifiello, B.I., Rossi, C., Dondi, M., Tarantini, S., Stella, A., (1991) La sintesi anastomotica nelle rivascolarizzazioni aorto-renali. Studio ecotomografico ed angiografico. *Arch. Chir. Torac. e Cardiovasc.,* 3:215-19.
13. Gruntzig, A., Kuhlman, U., Vetter, W., et Al., (1978) Treatment of renovascular hypertension with percutaneous transluminal dilatation of a renal artery stenosis. *Lancet,* 1:801-2.
14. Harrington, J.T., Sommers, S.C., Kassierer, J.P., (1968) Atheromatous emboli with progressive renal failure. Renal arteriography as the probable inciting factor. *Ann. Intern. Med.,* 68:152-60.
15. Hovinga, T.K.K., de Jong, P.E., de Zeeuw, D., et Al., (1986) Restenosis prevalence and long-term effects on renal function after percutaneous transluminal renal angioplasty. *Nephron.,* 44(suppl 1):64-7.
16. Katzen, B.T., Chang Lukowsky, G.H., et Al., (1979) Percutaneous transluminal angioplasty for treatment of renovascular hypertension. *Radiology,* 131:53-8.
17. Lawrie, G.M., Morris, Jr. G.C., Soussou, I.D., et Al., (1980) Late results of reconstructive surgery for renovascular disease. *Ann. Surg.,* 191:528-33.
18. Pechan, B.W., Npovick, A.C., Stewart, B.H., Straffon, R.A., (1979) Endarterectomy and patchgraft angioplasty in treatment of atherosclerotic renovascular hypertension. *Urology,* 14:487-90.
19. Schwarten, D.E., (1984) Percutaneous transluminal angioplasty of the renal arteries: intravenous digital subtraction angiography for follow-up. *Radiology,* 150:369-73.
20. Sos, T.A., Pickering, T.G., Sniderman, K., et Al., (1983) Percutaneous transluminal angioplasty in renovascular hypertension due to atheroma or fibromuscolar dysplasia. *N. Engl. J. Med.,* 309:247-9.
21. Stanley, J.C., Whitehouse, W.M., Zelenock, G.B., et Al., (1985) Reoperation for complications of renal artery reconstructive surgery undertaken for treatment of renovscular hypertension. *J. Vasc. Surg.,* 2:133-44.
22. Stanson, A.W., (1985) Complications of transluminal angioplasty of renal arteries. In: Complications in vascular surgery. Ed 2 Orlando, Grune & Stratton.
23. Stoney, R.J., (1977) Transaortic renal endaterectomy. In: Vascular Surgery, edited by Rutherford, R.B. W.B. Saunders, Philadelphia.
24. Tegtmeyer, G.J., Kellum, D., Ayers, C.A., (1984) Percutaneous transluminal angioplasty of the renal artery. Results and long-term follow-up. *Radiology,* 153:77-84.
25. Thevenet, A., Mary, H., Boennec, M., (1980) Results following surgical correction of renovascular hypertension. *J. Cardiovasc. Surg.,* 21:517-28.

26. Van Bockl, J.H., van Schilfgaarde, Overbosch, E.H., et Al., (1988) The influence of the surgical technique upon the short-term and long-term anatomic results in reconstructive operation for renovascular hypertension. *Surg. Gyn. Obstet.,* 166:402-8.

Secondary Renal Revascularization For Recurrent Renal Artery Stenosis

A.C. Novick

Department of Urology, Cleveland Clinic Foundation
Cleveland, Ohio, U.S.A.

INTRODUCTION

Surgical renal revascularization is well established as an effective form of treatment for patients with severe hypertension, renal insufficiency, or both, resulting from renal artery disease.

The incidence of stenosis of a surgically repaired renal artery is less than 10%. with current techniques[8]. This is typically a late complication occurring weeks, months, or even years following revascularization.

The causes are myriad and include faulty suture technique, intimal trauma, incomplete excision of primary vascular disease, tension on the vascular suture line, wide disparity in vessel size, torsion or kinking of the vessels, devascularization injury of a saphenous vein graft, and recurrent or de novo primary vascular disease. There have been relatively few reports on the approach to management in such cases[2,3,4,13].

We believe that secondary revascularization is the treatment of choice in patients with functionally significant recurrent renal artery stenosis and a viable kidney.

PATIENT SELECTION

All patients who have undergone surgical renal revascularization should be followed at six to twelve month intervals with blood pressure measurements, determination of renal function, and isotope renography. Postoperative renal artery stenosis that is more than 75% occlusive is invariably accompanied by an elevation in the blood pressure, and not uncommonly, deteriorating renal function.

When either of these conditions is present, or if there is serial isotope renal renographic evidence of diminished renal perfusion, repeat arteriography is indicated to evaluate the status of the repaired renal artery. Other possible causes of persistent or recurrent post-reconstructive hypertension include renal parenchymal disease, essential hypertension, and untreated renal artery disease.

In patients with recurrent renal artery stenosis, the therapeutic options are medical management, percutaneous transluminal angioplasty (PTA), and surgical reoperation.

If hypertension is severe and the involved kidney has suffered irreversible ischemic damage, then a simple nephrectomy should be done. If the involved kidney is functionally salvable, then an attempt to restore normal renal arterial flow is indicated. There has been scant experience with PTA in this setting, however, this may be an appropriate initial approach for focal stenotic lesions.

SURGICAL TECHNIQUES AND RESULTS

Recurrent renal artery stenosis is usually located at a vascular suture line but may present anywhere along the course of the repaired renal artery. Secondary surgical revascularization in such cases may be technically complicated. Reoperation often entails dissection in a surgical field obliterated by fibrous scar tissue, which may be particularly problematic when attempting to mobilize the renal artery distal to the primary revascularization site. The most efficacious approach is to employ a reconstructive technique which avoids the site of previous surgery. In patients with recurrent renal artery stenosis following an abdominal aortorenal bypass, alternate approaches which may be used for secondary revascularization include hepatorenal bypass[1], splenorenal bypass[6], iliorenal bypass[9] and thoracic aortorenal bypass[10]. With extensive renal hilar fibrosis or branch arterial involvement, extracorporeal revascularization may provide the optimum technique for mobilizing and repairing the distal renal arterial circulation[11]. Following extracorporeal revascularization, autotransplantation is performed into the iliac fossa.

We have performed secondary renal revascularization for recurrent renal artery stenosis in ten patients. The initial pathologic diagnosis was fibrous dysplasia in five patients and atherosclerosis in five patients. All patients had initially undergone a successful aortorenal bypass operation. Recurrent renal artery stenosis and hypertension developed 11-120 months later (mean 58 months). Secondary revascularization operations included renal autotransplantation, hepatorenal bypass, iliorenal bypass, and aortorenal bypass. Hypertension was relieved and renal function was stabilized or improved in all cases.

SURGICAL REVASCULARIZATION FOR TRANSPLANT RENAL ARTERY STENOSIS

Hypertension following renal allotransplantation is common and may be. secondary to rejection, ischemic allograft damage, retained native kidneys, steroid therapy, cyclosporine therapy, recurrence of primary renal disease in the allograft, or renal artery stenosis. Renal artery stenosis has been reported in 1-12% of transplant recipients, and can occur at the site of anastomosis, in the donor renal artery, or in the recipient hypogastric artery[12]. The causes include faulty suture technique, damage to the donor arterial intima during perfusion, intimal damage from rejection, improper apposition of the donor and recipient vessels with torsion, excessive length of the renal artery leading to angulation, or atherosclerosis in the recipient artery.

Renal arteriography is indicated whenever an allograft recipient has severe hypertension or unexplained deterioration in renal function. A change in the intensity of an allograft bruit or development of a diastolic component further suggests the possibility of renal arterial stenosis. Revascularization is indicated when arterial stenosis is considered the cause of intractable hypertension or renal dysfunction. Percutaneous transluminal angioplasty has yielded good results in this setting and is an appropriate initial option[5]. Secondary surgical revascularization is indicated if PTA cannot be done or is unsuccessful. These are technically complex operations which are best performed through a midline transabdominal incision. Although a variety of reconstruction procedures have been described, saphenous vein bypass from the common or external iliac arteries and segmental resection with reanastomosis are the preferred methods of repair.

SURGICAL RENAL REVASCULARIZATION AFTER FAILED PERCUTANEOUS TRANSLUMINAL ANGIOPLASTY

Percutaneous transluminal angioplasty (PTA) currently provides effective therapy for patients with certain types of renal artery disease. Patients treated with PTA may have persistent or recurrent renal arterial obstruction that necessitates subsequent surgical revascularization. There is controversy concerning whether the prior performance of PTA increases the technical difficulty or compromises the outcome of surgical renal revascularization.

To address this issue, we recently reviewed our experience with surgical treatment of renal artery disease in 53 patients who previously underwent PTA from 1980 to 1989[7]. Renal artery stenosis was due to fibrous dysplasia in 17 patients and atherosclerosis in 36 patients. The reasons for failure of PTA were inability to completely dilate the stenotic lesion (32 patients), acute renal arterial occlusion[2] or dissection[8] from attempted PTA, and the development of recurrent renal artery stenosis after initially successful PTA[11]. Three patients underwent nephrectomy due to the finding of a non-viable kidney at operation. Successful surgical revascularization was achieved in 50 patients.

Our experience suggests that surgical renal revascularization is not more technically difficult to perform after PTA. At operation, we did not observe significant fibrosis or inflammation around the previously dilated renal artery. Specifically, surgical dissection and mobilization of the diseased renal artery were not rendered more difficult by the prior performance of PTA. PTA necessitated a more complicated vascular reconstruction in only 1 of 50 patients. This patient required extracorporeal revascularization and autotransplantation due to involvement of renal artery branches from a dissection induced by PTA. Notwithstanding these results, our data also emphasize that PTA is an invasive technique that can result in loss of the kidney. Three patients in our series underwent nephrectomy due to irreversible ischemic damage caused by a complication of PTA. However, if the kidney is viable at operation, renovascular reconstruction does not appear to be more technically difficult than when done primarily and the same satisfactory clinical results can be achieved

REFERENCES

1. Chibaro EA, Libertino JA, Novick AC: Use of hepatic circulation for renal revascularization. *Ann Surg,* 199:406, 1984.
2. Ekestrom S, Liljegrist L, Nordhus O, Tidgren B: Persisting hypertension after renal artery recon-struction. *Scan J Urol Nephrol,* 13:83-88, 1976.
3. Erturk E, Novick AC, Vidt DG, Cunningham R: Secondary renal revascularization for recurrent renal artery stenosis. *Cleve Clin J Med,* 56:427, 1989.
4. Fowl RJ, Hollier LH, Bernatz PE, Pairolero PC, Vogt PA, Cherry KJ: Repeat revascularization versus nephrectomy in the treatment of recurrent renovascular hypertension. *Surg Gyn Obstet,* 162:37-42, 1986
5. Hayes JM, Risius B, Novick AC, et al: Experience with percutaneous transluminal angioplasty for renal artery stenosis at the Cleveland Clinic. *J Urol,* 139:488, 1988.
6. Khauli RB, Novick AC, Ziegelbaum M: Splenorenal bypass in the treatment of renal artery stenosis: experience with 69 cases. *J Vasc Surg,* 2:547, 1985.
7. Martinez AG, Novick AC, Hayes JM: Surgical treatment of renal artery disease after failed percutaneous transluminal angioplasty. *J Urol,* 144:1094, 1990.
8. Novick AC, Ziegelbaum M, Vidt DG, Gifford RW, Pohl MA, Goormastic M: Trends in surgical revascularization for renal artery disease. Ten years experience. *JAMA,* 257:498-501, 1987.
9. Novick AC, Banowsky LH: Iliorenal saphenous vein bypass: an alternative for renal revascularization in patients with a surgically difficult aorta. *J Urol,* 122:243, 1979.
10. Novick AC, Stewart R: Use of the thoracic aorta for renal revascularization. *J Urol,* 143:77, 1990.
11. Novick AC, Jackson CL, Straffon RA: The role of renal autotransplantation in complex urologic reconstruction. *J Urol,* 143:452, 1990.
12. Palleschi J, Novick AC, Braun WE, Magnusson M' Vascular complications of renal transplantation. *Urology,* 16:61, 1980.
13. Stanley JC, Whitehouse WM, Zelenock GB, Graham LM, Cronenwett JL, Lindenauer SM: Reoperation from complications of renal artery reconstructive surgery undertaken for treatment of renovascular hypertension. *J Vasc Surg,* 2:133-42, 1985.

REDO SURGERY IN AORTO-ILIAC AREA

"Redo" After Vascular Surgery in The Aorto-Iliac Area

R. Courbier

Department of Cardio-Vascular Surgery
Saint Joseph Hospital, Marseille, France

Redo after vascular surgery is unavoidable whenever a complication occurs. As the figures that will be presented during this Symposium will show, redo is a high-risk procedure with high morbidity and mortality.

Late stenosis and thrombosis are the consequences of the atherosclerotic process. Only long-term medical treatment can prevent or postpone their appearance. In contrast, early thrombosis, infection, and anastomotic aneurysm result from surgical flaws and thus can be considered as avoidable.

Prevention of redo is the subject of this introductory session. Rather than overlap on the topics that will be dealt with by the speakers in this session, we would simply like to present our personal experience in this domain. This experience has led us to gradually modify our strategy in an attempt to lower our redo rate.

PREVENTION OF EARLY THROMBOSIS

Obviously the best insurance against early thrombosis consists in careful patient selection, accurate assessment of the extent of the lesion and reconstruction in a healthy segment of the artery. In our experience we were able to avoid a certain number of technical faults using routine per-operative x-ray control and controlled anti-coagulation followed by normalization.

Per-operative arteriography

Allows detection of surgical flaws. However, for routine use, an ordinary x-ray device to visualize the progression of contrast material is not sufficient.

A specialized system is needed to allow visualization of the vasculature from the aorta to the leg arteries.

The x-ray tube, film exchanger and operating table must be aligned in the vertical plane. A trackway in the floor of the operating room allows alignment of the film exchange. The x-ray tube can be mounted over the exchanger by means of a boom or secured to the ceiling above the center of the operating table.

In our experience, x-ray control allowed detection of 4.5% of surgical flaws[1]. It was particularly useful during procedures involving the femoral artery and leg arteries, but also allowed detection and correction of flaws at the aortic level. Use of per-operative x-ray lowered our redo rate from 8.5% to 2%[1] in the first two years.

Anticoagulant therapy

Allows management of clotting during surgery. We use a standard dose of 5000 IU since a lower dose of 1 mg per kg doubles coagulation time for about 90 minutes. In obese patients we inject 7500 IU.

We long ago established[2] that normo-coagulation could be safely used to prevent thrombosis in the post-operative period provided that the daily dose was maintained below 10000 IU of heparin. Vascular surgery results in the activation of the fibrinolytic system[2].

When the procedure is performed for aneurysm of the abdominal aorta in a patient with a patent peripheral arterial network, clotting in the ilio-femoral artery is frequently observed. Routine use of heparinotherapy has lowered the need for passage of a Fogarty catheter. In patients with Leriche syndrome, collateral circulation maintains a higher flow rate during clamping thus reducing clot formation. Heparin is neutralized by an equal dose of protamine sulfate at the end of the procedure.

Postoperatively 10000 IU of heparin per day are administered intravenously for 48 hours. Thereafter anticoagulant therapy using subcutaneous injections of heparin at an appropriate dose is continued until the patient is released from the hospital. If the condition of the peripheral artery bed is poor, anticoagulant therapy using coumadin is pursued for several years. Several American groups concur in advocating coumadin after vascular surgery. This is a change from previous years in which only platelet therapy was recommended.

INFECTION

Infection usually results from per-operative contamination. The high rate of positive bacteriology of lymph node specimens in the inguinal region confirms this observation especially in cases involving peripheral trophic disorders. Bacterial specimens have also been collected from clinically uninfected bypasses during redo. Electron microscopy reveals bacteria colonies oin the wall of the prosthesis[4]. It is impossible to pinpoint the exact moment of contamination. An infection occurring several years after the procedure may be due to per-operative contamination that remained latent or to secondary infection of the prosthesis by transient bacteriemia. In view of this fact, several precautions can be proposed.

The surgeon and his assistants must operate "cleanly". It is sometimes well to recall the importance of asepsis, careful hand scrubbing, disinfection, etc... These simple measures are easy to overlook. We always impregnate the prosthesis with an antibiotic agent (e.g. Rifacydine) and administer short-term antibiotic therapy (cephalosporin = 3 injections). As we will discuss below, to prevent anastomotic aneurysm, we wrap femoral anastomoses with a free omentum graft. Omentopexy may also play a role in preventing infection.

In 1981, we began working in an operating theater equipped with a laminar airflow system and since that time our infection rate has decreased. The sterility of the operating room is regularly checked by placing culture dishes in the operating room. Limiting staff movement in the operating room and filtering out dust particles has practically eliminated minor subcutaneous infection in the inguinal region.

We advise all patients with prostheses to undergo antibiotic treatment at the least sign of infectious disease, even years after surgery. This is standard practice after placement of a heart valve.

In our group, operating room sterility and routine short-term local and systemic antibiotic therapy have helped reduce per-operative contamination. Our infection rate is now less than 1%.

PREVENTION OF ANASTOMOTIC ANEURYSM

Numerous factors can cause anastomotic aneurysm (without infection). The quality of the suture, the type of prosthesis, and association of endarterectomy have been implicated with certainty. Anticoagulants and arterial hypertension are only general causes. A combination of factors is necessary for anastomotic aneurysm to occur.

Several findings in our series should be emphasized :

- the incidence of anastomotic aneurysms at various levels varies from 0.3 to 0.7% (with a follow-up of 9 years). The rate of femoral artery anastomotic aneurysm ot a aorto-bifemoral bypass was 5 times higher (2.4%) than in other locations;

- when the prosthesis is placed in front of the inguinal ligament (axillofemoral bypasses), the number of anastomotic aneurysms decreases and the incidence returns to 0.5% as in other locations;

- anastomotic aneurysm (except immediate hemorrhage) never occurs after end-to-end suture of two prosthesis made of the same material.

- in almost all cases of anastomotic aneurysm, it is the wall of the artery that tears. The suture is usually intact.

These observations have led us to speculate that the inguinal ligament plays a central role in the formation of femoral anastomotic aneurysms. The passage of the prosthesis is narrowed by the inguinal ligament. Fibrous adhesions develop between the ligament and the prosthesis. Flexion and extension movements of the hip place stress on the junction between the prosthesis and artery, especially if the anastomosis is end-to-side but also if it is end-to-end. The wall of the artery eventually tears especially when the prosthesis dilates with age. The suture thread usually remains intact.

After verification of this concept by histologic studies[7], we have added the following two procedures to our surgical technique :

1) enlargement of the diameter of the opening through which the prosthesis is passed. This is achieved by sectioning the fibrous part of the inguinal ligament as previously proposed by Lord.

2) placement of a free omental graft between the inguinal ligament and the prosthesis. The whole prosthesis and the anastomosis down to the healthy segment of the artery are covered by omentopexy. We have never noted necrosis or rejection of this graft and tolerance has always been excellent[6]. This was verified by biopsy specimens taken in 12 cases in which redo was performed to extend the bypass. Vacuoles form in adipose omental tissue which undergoes a progressive fibrous transformation.

This fibrous sheath protects the prosthesis during movements of flexion and extension of the hip. The shear stress is no longer applied to the junction between the prosthesis and the artery but rather to the "healthy" artery wall which being elastic is more physiologically apt to support the strain.

Out of 115 aortofemoral bypasses performed between October 1981 and December 1986 with omentopexy, no femoral anastomotic aneurysm was recorded (mean follow-up: 7.30 years). Out of 2173 patients operated on between 1965 and 1981 before use of the omentopexy, there were 77 femoral anastomotic aneurysms. The peak incidence of anastomotic aneurysm noted in the first 4 years in the first series was not observed in the second series. Use of omentopexy eliminated femoral anastomotic aneurysm in the first 8 years. It is likely that late anastomotic aneurysms will occur with the same incidence as in other locations but at least the rate of immediate anastomotic aneurysm has been "normalized".

In our experience, the frequency of complications requiring redo after peripheral vascular surgery was reduced. However, in case of complication and even though the prognosis is poor, re-operation remains a necessary and effective procedure in case of complication.

REFERENCES

1. Courbier R, Jausseran, JM, Reggi M: Detecting complications of direct arterial surgery. The role of intra-operative arteriography. *Arch Surg,* 1977: 112; 1115-1118.
2. Courbier R: Intra-operative use of heparin. *J Card Vasc Surg,* 1975: 16; 346 - 349.
3. Courbier R, Vairel E, Brunel-Atlan F:Etude comparative de la plasminemie dans deux séries de malades opérés d'arteriopathie périphérique. Congrés du Coll. Franc. de Path. Vasc.Sandoz Edit. Paris, 1970, pp 300 - 306.
4. Formichi M., Jausseran JM, Guidoin R, Marois M, Bergeron P, Gosselin C, Courbier R: Analyse des prothèses arterielles en teflon microporeux aprés exérèse chirurgicale. *J. Maladies Vasc.,* 1986: 11; 248- 255.
5. Courbier R, Ferdani M, Jausseran JM, Bergeron P, Reggi M: Role of omentopexy in the prevention of femoral anastomotic aneurysm. *J Card Vasc Surg,* (in Press).
6. Courbier R, Larranaga J: Natural history and management of anastomotic aneurysms. In: Bergan J, Yao JST (eds). Aneurysms: Diagnosis and Treatment, Orlando, Grune & Stratton 1981, pp. 567 - 580.
7. Courbier R, AbouKhater R: Progress in the treatment of anastomotic aneurysms. *World J. Surg,* 1988:12; 742 - 749.

Detection of Failing Graft After Aorto-Femoral Revascularization

G.P. Deriu, G.P. Signorini *, D. Cognolato, F. Verlato *,
D. Milite and G.P. Avruscio *

Department of Vascular Surgery, University of Padua, Italy
* Service of Angiology, Padua Hospital, Padua, Italy

INTRODUCTION

Aorto-femoral bypass is a well established procedure for aorto-iliac revascularization and its results are satisfactory[1].

The most frequent long term complication is mono or, more rarely, bilateral branch thrombosis[2].

This complication is usually secondary to the development of a stenosis (due to myointimal fibroplasia or neoatherosclerosis) on the so called outflow segment which is the common femoral artery or more frequently the profunda femoral artery since the majority of aorto-femoral revascularization concern patients with a sequential femoro-popliteal block.

Branch thrombosis may be a compensate situation that allows a deferred evaluation but can present it self as an acute severe ischemia with a sensible risk of major amputation.

The aim of this paper is to study the ability of Eco Doppler Color Flow to detect graft-threatening outflow stenoses before thrombosis happens in patients with aorto-femoral bypass; the correction of these stenoses is a relatively minor procedure and, besides improving the long term patency of the graft can prevent in a subpopulation of patients an emergency situation.

MATERIALS

Two hundred twelve patients operated on from January 1980 to December

1990 for aorto-bifemoral bypass at the Departement of Vascular Surgery of Padua University were checked between October 1991 and January 1992.

They were 169 males (79,71%) and 43 females (20,29%); the mean age was 62,03 years. The risk factors were smoking, diabetes and hypertension.

The indications for surgery was atherosclerotic occlusive arterial disease with absolute indication for surgery (severe claudication, rest pain, gangrene, ascending aortic thrombosis) or relative indications (mild or medium claudication, but intolerable for the social or working requirement of the p., with a technically favourable situation).

The p. were checked with clinical and strumental follow-up (mean 58,5 mo.; range 11-120 mo.) (Table 1). Evaluation consists of clinical history, physical examination, measurement of the Winsor index and Echo Doppler Color Flow scans ferformed with a PHILIPS Quantum. The examination consisted of imaging the inguinal segment of the graft including the distal anastomosis and the femoral tripod by use of a 7,5 or 5 MHz linear array probe. The criteria assumed to detect the stenosis degree were the Strandness ones[3] modified on the basis of previously retrospective comparison study with angiography.

Table 1 - Echo Doppler Color Flow of distal anastomosis of p. with aorto-bifemoral bypass - Materials

---

* Angiography in all p. with stenosis > 80% at Echo Doppler Color Flow

* Redo surgery for all p. with stenosis > 80% at Angiography

Stenosis greater than 80%, defined by a velocity systolic peak > 300 cm/sec and with a 300% velocity increase, was the indication for angiography considered in this study the "gold standard" for definitive diagnosis.

Angiography confirmed the presence of an hemodinamically significant > 80% stenosis with prevision of impending thrombosis the patient underwent reoperation to restore a good runoff (usually with an endarterectomy of the profunda femoral artery and great saphenus vein angioplasty of this vessel)[4].

RESULTS

At the follow-up 70 p. were dead (33%) and 30 (14%) were not available. Our checked series is therefore of 112 p. (Table 2).

Seventheen have previously showed a branch thrombosis, well compensated in 4 cases and 13 cases needed a reoperation (3 of these patients, all presented

Table 2 - Results of 112 p.-221 distal anastomoses (3 major amputations)

Graft thrombosis	4 (3,5%)	well compensated
Stenosis > 80%	7 (6,2%)	
Stenosi < 50%	1 (0,9%)	
Profunda femoral a. occlusion	1 (0,9%)	

with a clinical picture of severe acute ischemia, required major amputation). Of the remaining 95 p., 86 did not have significant alterations while 9 p. (8%) showed asymptomatic outflow stenosis: all these p. did not show any particular clinical symptomatology capable to draw attention on the disease evolution.

The angiograms confirm the hemodinamically significant stenosis in 8 cases (in one case the stenosis was < 50%).

Seven stesosis underwent a revision (in one case with a profunda femoral artery occlusion a large circumflex femoral artery, completely patent, was considered a sufficient runoff).

In 5 limbs lesions of the common femoral or profunda femoral artery were relieved by endarterectomy and profundoplasty; in one limb by a profunda femoral artery bypass; in one limb it resulted technically impossible to revascularize the profunda femoral artery and a PTFE femoro-popliteal bypass was performed to revascularize the limb (Figs. 1-2).

All p. had a perfect restore of the runoff without morbidity and mortality.

DISCUSSION

The role of Echo Doppler Color Flow in detecting critical stenosis of infrainguinal bypass graft is well established[5] but also the postoperative monitoring with Echo Doppler Color Flow of distal anastomosis and femoral biforcation in p. with aorto-femoral bypass is very useful. In fact in these p. symptomatology and clinical examination cannot detect disease progression and impending graft failure. Winsor index in useless because it is a test only for patients with very advanced progression of the disease and this usually appears only after complete runoff occlusion and retrograde thrombosis of the graft.

In conclusion in p. with aorto-bifemoral bypass a brach thrombosis may be well compensated allowing the problem to be resolved adeguately in time.

If there is no compensation the situation may be critical not only for technically reasons but with high risk of major amputation. The identification of high risk stenosis of the distal anastomosis od aorto-bifemoral bypass can prevent graft thrombosis in both groups of p. avoiding the risk of major amputation in the second group.

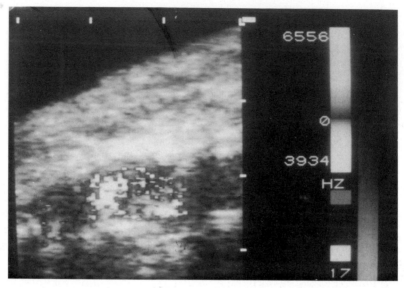

Fig. 1. Patient with aorto-bifemoral bypass. Outflow stenosis due to a diaphragm at the distal anastomosis site. A) Echo Doppler Color Flow shows a stenosis > 80%;

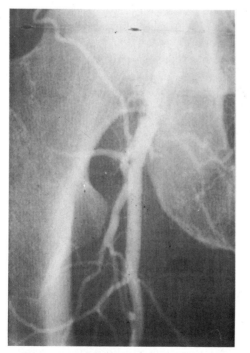
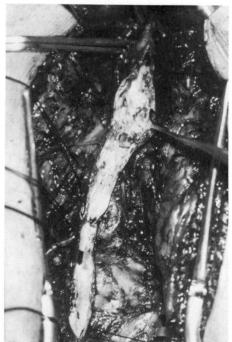

Fig. 1. (suite) B) Angiogram confirms at the end of the anastomosis; C) Redo surgery. The longitudinal arteriotomy of the profunda femoral artery show the diaphragm. This p. underwent profunda endarterectomy and saphenous vein patch graft angioplasty.

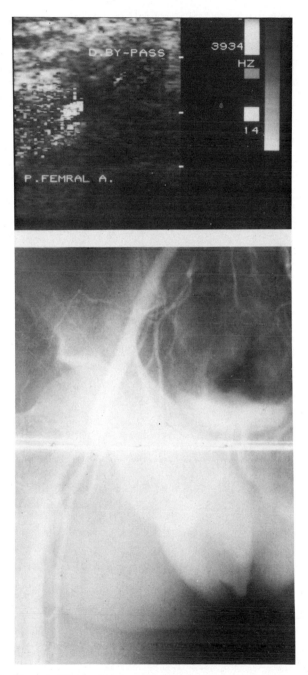

Fig. 2. Patient with aorto-bifemoral bypass. Outflow stenosis due to lesion of the profunda femoral artery. A) Echo Doppler Color Flow show the colour change representing increased flow velocity within the stenosis; B) Angiogram confirms the stenosis of the profunda femoral artery.

REFERENCES

1. Nevelsteen A., Wouters L., Suy R.: Long-term patency of the aorto-femoral dacron graft. *J Cardiovasc Surg.*, 1990; 32:174-180.
2. Malone J.M., Moore W.S., Goldstone J.: The natural history of bilateral aortofemoral bypass grafts for ischemia of the lower extremities. *Arch. Surg.*, 1975; 110:1300-1306.
3. Jager K.A., Richetts H.S., Strandness D.E. jr.: Duplex scanning for the evaluation of lower limb arterial disease. In: Non-invasive diagnostic techniques in vascular disease. 3rd Ed., Edited by E.F. Bernstein, pp. 619-631 C.b. Mosby . St. Louis.
4. Deriu G.P., Ballotta E., Grego F.: Emergency surgery in late occlusion of aortobifemoral bypass reconstructions. *Vasc. Surg.*, 1985; 19: 329-342.
5. Londrey G.L., Odgson K.J., Spadone D.P., et al.: Initial experience with Color-Flow Duplex Scanning of infrainguinal bypass grafts. *J. Vasc. Surg.*, 1990; 12: 284-90.
6. Neumyer M.M., Thiele D.S.: Evaluation of lower limb extremities occlusive disease with Doppler-ultrasound. In: Kenneth J.W. Taylor et al.: Clinical application of Doppler ultrasound; 1988. Ed. Raven Press, pag. 317-337.

Detection of Failing Procedures in Aorto-Iliac Area: Role of Magnetic Resonance

R. Passariello, E. Di Cesare * and C. Spartera **

Department of Radiology, University "La Sapienza" of Rome, Italy
* Department of Radiology, University of L'Aquila, Italy
** Department of Vascular Surgery, University of L'Aquila, Italy

INTRODUCTION

Many complications, such as hemorrhage, graft thrombosis, aortoenteric fistula, anastomotic pseudoaneurysm and infection, may arise in the post-surgical period in patients operated for aorto-femoral by-pass graft[8]. The post-surgical status of the prosthesis is currently evaluated by means of Ultrasound and CT, and eventually, in suspected infections, with fine needle aspiration, though limitations of US in providing an accurate evaluation in all patients and the need of contrast media injection and high exposure to ionizing radiation in CT. Actually, CT scans cannot distinguish periprostetic hematoma from infected fluid collections without gas or septation, and the borders between the fluid collection and the surrounding tissues are not clearly detectable[5,7,9]. Recently, MRI has been proposed as alternative method for an accurate evaluation of the prosthesis in the early as well as in the late stage. Multiplanar imaging and non-invasiveness of this technique provide more detailed information and allow a repeated follow-up[1,2,3,6]. Purpose of our study was to evaluate the possibility of MRI to detect the presence of complications and the normal evolution of the perigraft hematoma in comparison with the appearance of the perigraft infected collection.

MATERIAL AND METHODS

By means of MRI, we studied 30 patients who underwent a graft implantation for infra-renal aortic aneurysm (16 patients) and aorto-iliac obstructive arteriopathy (14 patients); the patients, 26 males and 4 females, ranged in age between 52 and 74 years, with a mean of 62.6. In the 16 patients who underwent surgical repair for aortic aneurysm, the graft was placed end-to-end at the level of the proximal and distal anasthomosis and the native aorta was wrapped around the implanted graft.

In the remaining 14 patients, surgically treated for aorto-iliac obstructive arteriopathy, the proximal and distal anasthomosis was end-to-side and the graft was positioned ventral to the native aorta.

MRI studies were performed with a superconductive magnet operating at 0.5 T. We used T1 weighted spin-echo sequences (TR 480-520 msec, TE 20 msec) and T2 weighted sequences (TR 1800 msec, TE 70 msec) on axial planes; we employed coronal and sagittal planes in 8 cases only.

The slice thickness was 10 mm, the acquisition matrix was 256x256 on T1 weighted sequences and 128x256 on T2 weighted sequences. The field of view 41 cm.

We performed 96 examinations, 30 at 1 week after graft implantation, 16 at 1 month, 26 at 3 months, 24 at 6 months and 10 after 6 months.

We evaluated the presence and the size of the periprosthetic fluid collection and the intensity of MRI signal at 1 week, 1, 3 and 6 months after the operation. In 1 patient with clinical signs of infection we performed examination with T1 w.s. 20 minutes after injection of 0.2 mmole/Kg of gadolinium-DTPA.

The size was classified in "minimal" (diameter 0-1.5 cm), "moderate" (diameter 1.6-3.5 cm) and "large" (diameter > 3.5 cm) according to the parameters proposed by Qvarford[9].

In 16 patients operated for aneurysmatic condition, quantitative evaluation was carried out by measuring the signal intensity of the perigraft fluid collection versus the ileopsoas muscle. The signal intensity was calculated using a ROI (Region Of Interest) of 8x8 pixels.

RESULTS

In 28 of 30 patients examined at 1 week after surgical treatment, we found presence of periprosthetic fluid collection. The size was minimal in 8 of 14 patients operated for aortoiliac obstructive arteriopathy; in the remaining 6 patients, the size was classified as moderate. In patients who underwent operation for aneurysmatic aortic condition, the size was classified minimal in 1 case, moderate in 12 and large in 3.

The signal intensity of perigraft collection, related to the ileopsoas muscle, was medium-low on T1 w.s. (S.I. 1.14±0.19) and high on T2 w.s. (S.I. 2.92±0.41) in 16 patients studied for aneurysmatic condition. In 8 of these, we found little areas of high signal intensity on T1 w.s. and low on T2 w.s.

Table 1 - Signal intensity of perigraft collection, related to ileopsoas muscle, in patients operated for anerysmatic aortic condition

	PFC/Muscle	
	T1	T2
1 Week	1.14±0.19	2.92±0.41
1 Month	1.11±0.05	2.42±0.18
3 Months	1.06±0.11	2.51±0.40
6 Months	0.89±0.11	1.52±0.37

At 1 month control, we found a slight size reduction and persistent medium-low signal intensity on T1 w.s. (S.I. 1.11±0.05) and high on T2 w.s. (S.I. 2.42±0.18).

At 3 months control, in patients operated for obstructive disease, we found disappearance in 9 patients and minimal entity of residual areas in the remaining 5 patients, who presented low signal intensity on both T1 and T2 w.s. (Fig. 1). On the other hand, in those patients who received end-to-end anasthomosis to repair an abdominal aortic aneurysm, we found size reduction, but persistence of low signal intensity on T1 w.s. (S.I. 1.06±0.11) and high signal intensity on T2 w.s. (S.I. 2.51±0.40).

We classified the hematoma in 1 case as "large", in 5 cases as "moderate" and in 11 as "minimal".

In 14 patients, at 6 months control, we found little areas of low signal intensity on T1 w.s. (S.I. 0.89±0.11), medium-low on T2 w.s. (S.I. 1.52±0.37) and size reduction of perifluid collection. In 1 case, the patient, who was operated for primary aorto-duodenal fistula, presented clinical signs of infection. MRI in serial study revealed presence of signal intensity of perifluid collection comparable with the values of normal graft healing, but areas of high signal intensity were evident also in the ileopsoas muscles. Moreover, at 3 months control, we noticed no perigraft collection on the proximal anasthomosis; a little area of hematoma,however, was evident at the level of the graft links and the signal analysis on T1 w.s. after gadolinium-DTPA injection revealed a signal intensity increase of the perigraft collection and the psoas muscle. Clinical signs (back pain, increase white blood cells count and high fever) lasted two days only and the patient was not operated but treated with a specific antibiotic therapy.

At 6 months, the patient did not present clinical signs and MRI control showed unreduced size and high signal intensity of perigraft collection. This patient developed diffuse infection of the retroperitoneal space at 9 months (Fig. 2). Very similar findings were found in another patient. We evidentiated the infective evolution, at an early stage, as absence of size reduction at successive controls and for the presence of a small area of signal void inside the perigraft collection, presumably related to gas content. The signal intensity analysis carried out in the first six months did not prove useful in

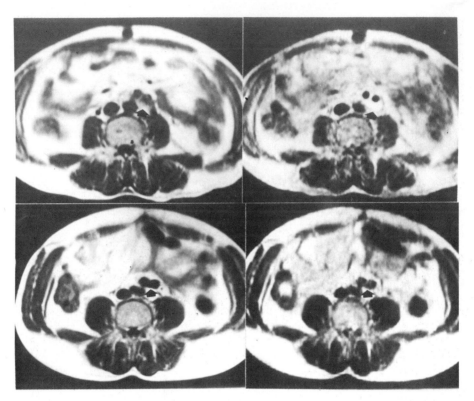

Fig. 1. Surgical repair in the patients operated for peripheral vascular disease. A-B: moderate hematoma was evident on both T1 and T2 w.s. at one week control (arrows). B-C: only a small amount of residual fibrotic material was evident at 3 week control (arrows).

the differentiation between infected and non infected perigraft fluid collection, since it showed very similar signal intensity values (Fig. 3).

Distal pseudoaneurysmatic anastomosis was evident in two patients (after 6 and 12 months from surgery) of our series. MRI was useful in the detection, side and size characterization. In both patients, sagittal and coronal scans were useful to define the cranio-caudal extension and the presence of thrombotic deposition (Fig. 4).

At last, one patient presented at two year control presence of thrombotic deposition at the level of the right branch of the prosthesis, that was suspected on T2 w.s. and well evidentiated by means of gradient rephased echo sequences with short TR/TE (Fig. 5).

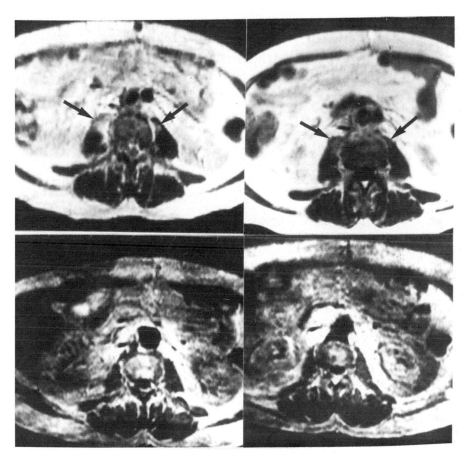

Fig. 2. Infective evolution of the periprosthetic collection. A: T2 w.s., three months control in patients operated for aortic aneurysm. There were no significative differences in the signal of the perigraft collection as compared to non-infected patients, but inside the psoas muscle areas of high signal intensity were evident (arrows), as confirmed after Gd-DTPA injection (B). B-C: at three months control, a diffuse area of high signal intensity was evident in the retroperitoneal space, close to the proximal anastomosis.

DISCUSSION

Our study was useful to define the role of MRI in the evaluation of the suspected complications after aortic graft surgery[10]. The major advantages were related to the possibility of detecting perigraft collections as infection or hematoma, of evaluating pseudoaneurysms of the anastomotic site, and of providing much more information than angiography[11].

MRI showed very clearly the retroperitoneal spaces, the graft prosthesis, the native aorta and the presence of the perigraft collection. The multi-parametricity of this technique was particularly helpful for the morphologic analysis on T1 w.s. and for the detection of even small areas of fluid collections on T2 w.s.[12].

MRI examination provided valuable information in the detection of the suspected endoprosthetic thrombotic deposition on T2 w.s., where the signal loss of the flowing blood allowed a good evaluation of the wall. However, the presence of artifacts at long TR/TE sequences could lead to misinterpretation in some cases. To improve the signal to noise ratio, in these cases, we used gradient rephased echo sequences with short TR/TE by means of which the high signal intensity of the flowing blood allowed easy differentiation with the wall and the thrombotic deposition that appeared of medium-low signal intensity[4].

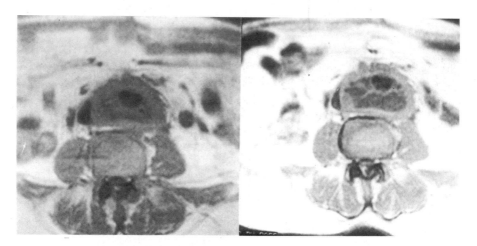

Fig. 3. A: at one month control in patients operated for aortic aneurysm, large hematoma is evident. B: no size reduction was evident at three months control; this was related to infective evolution and confirmed by needle aspiration.

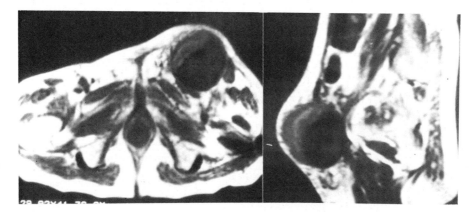

Fig. 4. Large pseudoaneurysmatic evolution at the level of the left distal anastomosis. The thrombotic material was well differentiated from the flowing blood.

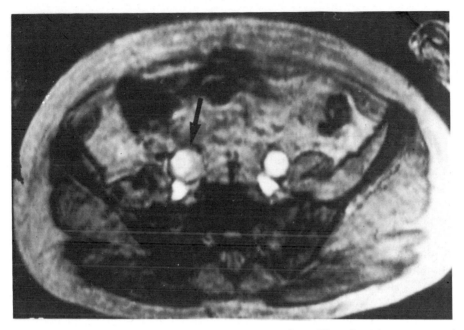

Fig. 5. Gradient rephased echo sequences were used to differentiate the presence of stenosis of the prosthesis (arrows).

Our study was particularly focused on the evaluation of the possibility of differentiation between periprosthetic hematoma and infection. In fact, it can be difficult to assess aortic graft infection, whose occurrence is sometimes revealed by presence of aspecific signs, such as fever and/or lumbar pain[8].

Perigraft hematoma is quite common at an early stage and can cause fever even if there is no infection[10].

MRI can evidentiate periprosthetic collections[1,6].

We performed serial axial scans to assess the normal appearance and course of the perigraft incorporation. In accordance to other studies, we also found that peri-prosthetic hematoma is usual at an early stage[9].

We distinguished patients operated for peripheral vascular disease from those treated for aneurysmatic condition[8].

In the first group, we observed dissappearance or minimal entity of the hematoma after only 3 months. At this period, the hematoma showed low signal intensity on both T1 and T2 w.s., probably related to a more easy reabsorption of the perigraft fluid in the retroperitoneal space.

On the other hand, in patients treated for abdominal aortic aneurysm, we found that, at an early stage, the hematoma between the graft and the native aorta was larger than the hematoma evident in patients treated for peripheral vascular disease. The evolution of the perigraft collection was slower than in peripheral vascular disease. This finding could be ascribed to the localization of the perigraft collection, that was contained between the graft and the native aorta. In fact, in our series, only 18% of patients had minimal size or disappearance and low signal intensity on both T1 and T2 w.s. after 3 months. At this time, in the remaining cases, we found a partial size reduction and persistence of high signal intensity on T2 w.s. due to an incomplete reabsorption.

Only after 6 months, we found a complete fibrotic evolution of the perigraft collection.

In our series, only 2 patients had clinical signs of a post surgical infection, 3 and 4 months after operation respectively. The signal intensity analysis on T1 and T2 w.s. did not show significant differences from non infected patients at an early stage. In our study, the only evident sign of infection was the involvement of the psoas muscle presenting a region of high signal intensity on T2 w.s. After gadolinium-DTPA injection, we found signal intensity increase of the perigraft collection and of the anterior region of the psoas muscle on T1 w.s. The contrast enhancement between infected and non involved muscle after Gd-DTPA injection was less on T1 w.s. than on T2 w.s., but the contrast-to-noise ratio was much better on T1 w.s. The antibiotic therapy was enough to "fridge" the infection for six months, until the final evolution. At this stage, MRI was able to define the presence of diffuse phlogistic involvement of the retroperitoneal space. In the second patient, MRI showed the persistent large size of the collection at three month control and the presence of a small area of signal void related to gas, as confirmed by CT. The fine needle aspiration confirmed the diagnosis suspected with MRI. In conclusion, MRI was able to evidentiate the presence of the prosthesis and the normal evolution of the perigraft collection versus the infection. In our study of patients surgically treated for aorto iliac stenosis we found disappearance or minimal entity of perigraft collection and low signal intensity on both T1 and T2 w.s., after 3 months.

On the other hand, in patients treated for abdominal aortic aneurysm, we found a progressive reduction of size and low signal intensity only after 6 months. As a result of this serial study and also according to literature, therefore, we can say that hematoma is not easily distinguishable from infection at an early stage[14]. In our experience, only indirect signs like unreduced size, psoas involvement or presence of gas were considerable.

The high signal intensity of the perigraft collection on T2 w.s. is a signal of infection only after 3 or 6 months depending upon the surgical treatment.

ACKNOWLEDGEMENT

The Authors wish to thank Anna Avitabile for photographs, Carmelita Marinelli for secretarial assistance and Angela Martella for translation of the manuscript.

REFERENCES

1. Auffermann W, Olofsson PA, Rabahie GN, Tavares NJ, Stoney RJ, Higgins CB. Incorporation versus infection of retroperitoneal aortic: MR imaging features. *Radiology*, 1989; 172: 359-362.
2. Auffermann W, Olofsson PA, Stoney RJ, Higgins CB. MR imaging of complications of aortic surgery. *JCAT*, 1987; 11: 982-989.
3. Di Cesare E, Di Renzi P, Pavone P, Marsili L, Ventura M, Spartera C, Passariello R. Evaluation of hematoma by MRI in follow-up of aorto femoral by pass. *MRI*, 1991 9: 247-253.
4. Di Cesare E, Occhiato R, Pavone P, Di Renzi P, Michelini O, Ventura M, Morettini G, Passariello R. :Risonanza Magnetica: utilità delle sequenze gradient echo refocusing nella diagnostica degli aneurismi dell'aorta addominale. *La Radiologia Medica*, in press.
5. Hilton S, Megibow AJ, Naidich DP, Bosniak MA. Computed tomography of postoperative abdominal aorta. *Radiology*, 1982; 145:403-407.
6. Justich E, Amparo EG, Hricak H, Higgins CB. Infected aortoiliofemoral grafts: magnetic resonance imaging. *Radiology*, 1985; 154: 133-136.
7. Mark A.; Moss A.A.; Lusby R.; Kaiser J.A. (1982). CT evaluation of complications of abdominal aortic surgery. *Radiology*, 145:409-414.
8. O'Hara PJ, Hertzer NR, Beven EG, Krajewsus LP. Surgical management of infected abdominal aortic grafts: rewiew of a 25-year experience. *J Vasc. Surg.*, 1986; 3:725-731.
9. Qvarfordt PG, Relly LM, Mark AS, et al. Computerized tomographic assessment of graft incorporation after aortic reconstruction. *Am. J Surg*, 1985; 150:227-231.
10. Reilly LM, Ehrenfeld WK, Goldstone J, Stoney RJ. : Gastrointestinal tract involvement by prosthetic graft infection. *Ann Surg*, 1985; 202:342-348.
11. Wesbey G.E, Higgins CB, Amparo EG, Hale JD, Kaufman L, Pogany AC. Peripheral vascular disease: correlation of MR imaging and angiography. *Radiology*, 1985; 156:733-739.
12. Yeager RA, McConnell DB, Sesani TM,Vetto RM. Aortic and peripheral prosthetic graft infection: differential management and causes of mortality. *Am J Surg*, 1985; 150:36-43.

Strategies in The Management of Aorto-Femoral Graft Limb Occlusion

M.D. Colburn * and W.S. Moore

* Department of General Surgery, Division of Vascular Surgery, UCLA School of Medicine, Los Angeles, California, U.S.A.

INTRODUCTION

Most patients with significant aorto-iliac disease are middle-aged to elderly, and usually possess one or more of the general risk factors for atherosclerosis including: cigarette smoking, hypertension, hypercholesterolemia, and diabetes. The initial manifestations of occlusive disease in the distal aorta and iliac arteries is most often intermittent claudication involving the muscles of the hip, buttock, thigh and occasionally the calf.

Calf muscle involvement is usually an indication that concomitant superficial artery disease is present. In addition, male patients with aorto-iliac occlusive disease, with significant involvement of the internal iliac arteries, will often complain of the inability to achieve or maintain an erection. This symptom complex, which combines the typical manifestations of aorto-iliac occlusion (hip, buttock and thigh claudication, decreased femoral pulses and leg muscle atrophy) with impotence, is called the Leriche syndrome[10].

Of all the vascular procedures performed for atherosclerotic occlusive disease, the aorto-bifemoral bypass is perhaps the most satisfying to both the patient and the surgeon. This is because of the uniformly prompt relief experienced by the patient and the high degree of early technical success and long-term patency enjoyed by both.

The perioperative morbidity and mortality for this procedure have been excellent and are reported by several authors to be less then 2%[14]. Furthermore, the long term durability of these procedures for the last 40 years has been exceptional. Reported patency rates for bypass grafts in the aorto-bifemoral position range from 81-92% at three years and from 78-92% at five years[8,11,17,20]. Despite the above successes, complications from these procedures have not been totally eliminated and their management continues to be among the more challenging cases that a vascular surgeon is asked to treat. Such complications include: graft infection, anastomotic aneurysms, aorto-enteric fistulas, as well as graft limb thrombosis. The first three of these important complications will be covered elsewhere in the proceedings of this symposium. The purpose of this chapter is to review the current strategies in the management of aorto-femoral graft limb occlusion.

INCIDENCE

Bypass grafts placed in the aorto-femoral position are perhaps the most durable of all the reconstructions performed for atherosclerotic vascular disease. Thrombosis of an aortic graft limb is not common, but can occur at any interval following implantation. If one takes into account all graft limb occlusions occurring anytime following aortic reconstruction, the over all graft limb thrombosis rate has been estimated to be between 10-20%[3,5]. However, it is well recognized that early (within thirty days of operation) and late graft limb occlusion, represent the manifestations of very different pathophysiologic mechanisms. For this reason, it is useful to separate the overall graft limb occlusion rate into those which occur perioperatively and those which represent late thrombotic complications of a previously functioning bypass. When one dissects the overall 10-20% graft limb thrombosis rate following all bifurcated aortic reconstructions, only 18-28% of these occlusions occur early where as the great majority (72-82%) occur as late complication[3,5,9].

ETIOLOGY OF AORTIC GRAFT LIMB THROMBOSIS

The pathophysiology of aorto-femoral graft limb occlusion can have many causes and is often multifactorial. A knowledge of these mechanisms is critical because many can be avoided if appreciated at the time of graft implantation, and the remainder can only be properly managed with a thorough understanding of their likely etiologies. It is convenient to divide the discussion of the mechanisms of aortic graft limb thrombosis into those which occur perioperatively, and those which present as late occlusions.

Early Graft Limb Thrombosis

Although no prospective randomized data related to the complication of early aortic graft limb thrombosis has been reported, traditional teachings have generally separated these occlusions into two groups: grafts placed in extremities with inadequate outflow, and technical errors made at the time of graft implantation.

The two key hemodynamic requirements for any vascular bypass graft are satisfactory inflow and outflow. Almost by definition, the adequacy of the inflow is assured by the placement of the bypass graft in the aorto-femoral position. Certainly, any proximal defect which threatens perfusion of the proximal graft would ordinarily be repaired at the time of the original grafting procedure. On the other hand, failure to recognize a preexisting compromised and inadequate outflow tract continues to be a frequent cause of early aorto-femoral graft limb occlusion.

In an attempt to identify any factors that might predict those patients with a high risk of subsequent graft limb thrombosis, Malone and associates reviewed their experience in all patients who had received an aorto-femoral bypass graft during a 15 year period[13]. During this interval, 180 patients underwent bilateral aorto-femoral bypass grafting for a total of 360 femoral anastomoses. Post-operative graft limb thrombosis occurred in 44 limbs (12%), approximately half of which occurred in the first year following the operation. A correlative analysis of all factors that might identify those patients with a predisposition to graft limb thrombosis revealed that the presence of arterial occlusive disease distal to the site of the femoral anastomosis was associated with a significantly increased rate of graft thrombosis. Specifically, in those limbs with distal arterial occlusive disease, the thrombosis rate was 32/119 (27%). In contrast, when there was no distal disease noted, the thrombosis rate was 12/241 (5%). This difference was statistically significant (p=0.001). Further analysis of the 32 graft which had thrombosed in association with distal arterial occlusive disease demonstrated that 15 had solitary profunda femoral disease, 9 were associated with isolated tibial trifurcation disease and 8 had combined or tandem lesions. Statistical analysis, based on these groups, revealed a highly significant correlation between the presence of tandem lesions in the profunda femoral and tibial trifurcation vessels and the subsequent risk of aorto-femoral graft limb thrombosis.

Thus, it is essential to assess both the common and deep femoral arterial vessels, prior to the placement of an aorto-femoral graft. Specifically, the origin and patency of the profunda femoral vessel should be analyzed as well as the condition of the superficial femoral and distal outflow arteries at least to the level of the tibial branches. When the outflow vascular tree is considered inadequate to support a proximal aorto-femoral bypass, the addition of a distal procedure such as a local common femoral endarterectomy, profundaplasty or simultaneous distal reconstruction should be considered.

Many technical problems, which occur during the implantation of an aorto-femoral graft, have been described and are well known causes of early perioperative graft thrombosis.

First, precise measurement of each aorto-femoral graft limb is very important and can prevent inadvertent redundancy in the length of the graft limb. This redundancy usually occurs in the mid-section of the graft limb just proximal to the passage of the graft beneath the inguinal ligament. Depending on the type of graft used, and the degree of graft kinking, this configuration can lead to decreased flow and ultimately thrombosis of the graft limb.

A second cause of perioperative graft limb thrombosis is twisting of the graft limb. This usually occurs when the graft is tunneled from the abdominal to the groin incision without due care taken to ensure proper alignment of the graft limb segment. Severe twisting can lead to a significant compromise in the lumenal diameter and subsequently to thrombosis.

A third cause of early aorto-femoral graft limb occlusion is the failure to perform a technically perfect distal anastomosis. This portion of the procedure is of critical importance and many early failures can be attributed to an imprecise distal anastomosis. Most patients with symptoms related to aorto-iliac disease have some degree of atherosclerotic involvement in the groin as well as more distal levels. If possible, a soft portion of the artery should be selected for the distal anastomosis and any inadvertent intimal cracks or flaps must be repaired immediately. Care should be taken not to compromise or reduce the lumenal diameter during the anastomosis, and the angle of the end to side anastomosis should optimally be as tapered and gradual as possible to avoid excessive turbulence at the anastomotic site.

Unusual types of errors which can also lead to early perioperative graft limb occlusion include: trapping of the graft limb beneath the inguinal ligament (usually caused by a improperly placed subcutaneous tunnel), incomplete removal of autologous clot used to preclot certain types of aorto-bifemoral grafts, and a previously present but undiagnosed systemic hyper-coagulopathy.

With awareness of these pitfalls and careful attention to precise surgical technique most, if not all, of these errors can be consistently avoided.

Late Graft Limb Thrombosis

Like early aorto-femoral graft limb thrombosis, the etiology of graft limb thrombosis which occurs months to years following graft implantation, is multifactorial. By far the most common causes of late graft thrombosis are distal anastomotic intimal hyperplasia and worsening of outflow disease due to the progression of atherosclerosis.

Intimal hyperplasia can be defined as the abnormal proliferation of cells and extracellular connective tissue substances which occurs as the result of an arterial wall injury. Histologically, the important cell in this proliferative process is the medial smooth muscle cell[18]. In response to an arterial injury these cells undergo a series of changes beginning with active replication. Following this replication the activated myofibroblasts migrate across the internal elastic lamina into the intima where they continue to proliferate and begin to deposit connective tissue elements[10]. The resulting intimal proliferation forms the basis of the hyperplastic cellular changes seen in the lumen of a traumatized vessel. In the case of an aorto-bifemoral bypass graft, these changes most often occur at the site of the distal graft to native vessel anastomosis and leads to the progressive stenosis of the outflow tract. It has been well established in animal models that the most active period of hyperplastic change occurs between 4 weeks to 2 years. Thus the vast majority of graft limb thromboses which occur within 2 years of operation are likely to be due to this intimal proliferative process.

Those grafts which continue to function beyond 2 years but ultimately occlude within 5 to 10 years following operation, are likely to have failed because of progressive atherosclerotic occlusive disease that develops in the distal extremity.

Several rare causes of late aorto-femoral graft occlusion, although uncommon, should be mentioned. Low flow states (such as the development of congestive heart failure, certain cardiac arrhythmias, thyroid dysfunction or dehydration) can alter a grafts hemodynamic balance and lead to thrombosis. Unexpected late graft thrombosis can also occur due to the onset of an acquired hypercoagulable state, as in the patient who develops a primary neoplasm years following graft insertion.

Distal anastomotic aneurysms are a well described complication of aorto-femoral bypass grafts and secondary thrombosis of these aneurysms can lead to to subsequent graft limb occlusion. Lastly it should not be overlooked that, just as the distal arterial tree is prone to progression of the atherosclerotic occlusive process, so is the distal aorta and bifurcation.

For this reason, it is the preference of most surgeons to position the aortic anastomosis proximally, close to the origin of the renal vessels. Widespread practice of this technique has led to the diminished role of progressive distal aortic and bifurcation atherosclerotic disease as a significant cause of late aorto-femoral graft failure.

CLINICAL MANIFESTATIONS / INDICATIONS FOR INTERVENTION

The clinical presentation of patients who develop aorto-femoral graft limb occlusion varies greatly and is dependent on several factors. The most important factors are related to the duration from, and the indication for, the original operation. Most patients, following an aortic graft limb thrombosis, complain of the acute onset of ipsilateral extremity ischemic symptoms. When the occlusion occurs early, and the indication for the graft insertion was aorto-iliac occlusive disease, many patients will describe a return to their preoperative level of ischemic symptoms. On the other hand, if the original graft was implanted for aneurysmal disease, the patient often reports an abrupt onset of ischemic symptoms which were not present preoperatively. Late occlusions can also present with different clinical manifestations. Patients whose graft occlusion results from the gradual stenosis of the distal anastomosis, and have acquired a well developed collateral circulation, will often exhibit a progressive degree of ischemic symptoms. When these patients present with these complaints, it can be difficult to pinpoint the precise time of thrombosis. It is not unusual for patients with late graft occlusions to report symptoms of extremity ischemia that are more severe then those experienced preoperatively. This certainly will be the case when the graft was implanted for aneurysmal disease but can also be due the progressive atherosclerotic occlusive disease in the distal extremity outflow tract.

As in all vascular surgical procedures, the indications for intervention in the case of aortic graft limb thrombosis should be individualized. Most patients who present with acute graft failure will have limb-threatening ischemic symptoms that require urgent therapy. In a series reported from the Massachusetts General Hospital, 81% of acute graft limb failure patients presented with severe limb-threatening symptoms and approximately half received an operation within 48 hours following admission. However, it should also be recognized that reoperation is always technically more difficult and is associated with a greater risk of complications and unsatisfactory outcomes. Keeping this in mind, it may be appropriate to elect to use a more conservative, nonoperative approach, in selected patients. The poor risk patient with gradual aortic graft limb thrombosis, who has developed sufficient collateral circulation to prevent limb threatening ischemia, is an example of a situation in which intervention may not be mandatory.

PRE-OPERATIVE EVALUATION

The pre-operative evaluation in patients being considered for all types of vascular surgery is very important and should be directed to address two general questions: a) what is the general condition of the patient?, and b) what is the anatomy of the lesion under investigation?

As always, each patient should undergo a thorough history including the identification of important risk factors. Likewise, the physical exam should be complete, with particular emphasis on the vascular system.

Atherosclerosis is a systemic disease and involvement in other vascular beds is likely and must be identified. Carotid and coronary involvement with peripheral atherosclerotic changes is well described and should always be specifically addressed. Evidence of carotid disease should be worked up with appropriate non-invasive studies and operative therapy pursued if indicated. Any patient with a history of coronary artery disease, suggestive symptoms, or silent abnormalities on a routine electrocardiogram (EKG), should undergo a comprehensive cardiac work-up prior to any vascular reconstruction.

MANAGEMENT

Early Graft Limb Thrombosis

Aortic graft limb occlusion which occurs in the early perioperative period most often leads to severe ischemic symptoms and immediate intervention is usually required. Angiography in this situation is generally not necessary and only rarely adds important clinical information. The commonly excepted method of treatment in this situation is reoperation. Inspection of the distal graft anastomosis is accomplished by reopening the involved groin incision. Any technical abnormalities are then identified and corrected. A transverse incision can be made in the hood of the distal graft to facilitate complete inspection of the lumen of the distal anastomosis. A retrograde graft limb thrombectomy can be performed with a Fogarty balloon catheter through this same graft incision. In the setting of early graft limb thrombosis, this is almost always successful in restoring inflow. If following thrombectomy, the inflow remains inadequate, retrograde intraoperative angioscopy may be helpful in identifying proximal technical defects or any residual thrombus. If the inflow is sufficient and no technical errors are identified at the distal graft anastomosis, poor outflow should be considered as a possible primary cause of the graft limb failure. In this instance, intraoperative angiography can be very helpful. If correctable disease exists at the orifice of the profunda femoral artery, addition of a femoral profundaplasty may be the easiest and most expeditious method of improving outflow. On the other hand, if the profunda femoral artery has significant distal disease, a distal bypass graft to the popliteal or tibial level may be required to achieve adequate outflow. Thrombolysis is generally not considered safe following a recent surgical procedure and should not be considered in the setting of early aortic graft limb thrombosis.

Late Graft Limb Thrombosis

The selection of the appropriate management of late graft limb occlusions is guided by the consideration of three factors: a) the current status of the arterial inflow, b) an evaluation of the present status of the outflow vessels, and c) a determination of the probable cause of the graft limb thrombosis.

For these reasons, preoperative angiography is required in almost all instances of late graft limb occlusion. Depending on the preference of the surgeon, an angiogram can be accomplished by the percutaneous puncture of either the contralateral graft limb, or through a transaxillary approach. The angiogram should be performed with the intention of addressing several specific questions which are important in the management of these patients.

First, the proximal anastomosis should be visualized, preferable in two planes. This will document the unilateral graft limb thrombosis and allow evaluation of the arterial inflow. Next, the collateral pathways, point of reconstitution, and status of the distal runoff vessels should be carefully examined.

Specific attention should be given to the condition of the profunda femoral artery and the presence of any adequate outflow target vessels in case a concomitant distal bypass is required.

Lastly if possible, the distal anastomosis should be thoroughly evaluated. The presence of a distal anastomotic aneurysm or any evidence of a hyperplastic intimal reaction should be noted. If necessary, a CT scan can be useful if uncertainty remains regarding the presence of a distal anastomotic aneurysm.

It should be emphasized that the failure to visualize any vessels at the femoral or distal level, in the setting of an acute unilateral graft limb thrombosis, should not preclude an attempt at revascularization.

It is not uncommon that, following exploration of the groin and intraoperative angiography, such patients are found the have a usable profunda or more distal outflow vessel.

The approach to the operative management of a patient with late graft limb occlusion can not be standardized. Each case must be individually analyzed by the careful assessment of several variables.

These include the probable age of the thrombotic occlusion, the anatomic detail demonstrated by preoperative angiography, the presumed cause of the occlusion as well as the degree of limb threatening ischemia and the overall condition of the patient. If the degree of ischemia and condition of the patient suggest that intervention is indicated, the surgeon must conceive a therapeutic plan. Specifically, attention must be directed to establishing both adequate inflow and outflow.

Several techniques are currently available to aide the surgeon in achieving these goals. It is convenient to divide these therapeutic approaches into those which provide restoration of arterial inflow, and those which enhance the quality of the distal outflow.

THERAPEUTIC TECHNIQUES

A) Inflow

Graft Limb Thrombectomy

Most unilateral aorto-femoral graft limb occlusions can be managed by a combination of retrograde graft limb thrombectomy and outflow reconstruction. General anesthesia is preferred for this procedure and the patient should be prepped and draped from the neck to the toes bilaterally. This is important should it be necessary to perform an extraanatomical inflow procedure or a distal bypass to improve the outflow.

A vertical incision is made over the involved groin and the distal portion of the occluded bypass graft is exposed with a combination of sharp dissection and lateral retraction. Continued sharp dissection is used to identify and mobilize the native common femoral, superficial femoral and profunda femoral arteries. Care should be taken not to divide any major collateral branches particularly when dissecting around the profunda femoral artery where the lateral or medial circumflex arteries can easily be damaged. When the scar tissue due to the previous groin incision is particularly dense it is often helpful to begin this dissection distally, over a previously undissected area of the superficial artery, and then carry the sharp dissection of the scarred fibrous capsule back to the common femoral artery. Once these vessels are identified and mobilized, proximal control of the native common femoral artery should be obtained in case it remains patent proximal to the graft anastomosis. The thrombosed graft can then be divided just proximal to the femoral anastomosis. The distal portion of the detached graft can be further opened longitudinally to expose the orifices of the outflow vessels, determine the mechanism of obstruction, and predict the likely reconstructive procedure necessary for repair.

If the occlusion is recent, removal of the clot from the proximal portion of the graft can almost always be easily performed with an embolectomy balloon catheter. When the catheter is inserted retrograde into the graft, the contralateral groin pulse should be obliterated by manual compression. This minimizes the risk of distal embolization of dislodged thrombus into the patent uninvolved graft limb. After the successful removal of the occluding thrombus and the establishment of forceful arterial inflow, the absence of residual clot should be documented by one of two available methods. An angiogram of the graft limb can be performed, in a retrograde fashion, by injecting contrast through a small catheter secured within the thrombectomized graft. Alternatively, the completeness of the graft limb thrombectomy can be evaluated by direct vision using angioscopy. The proximal graft limb is reoccluded with a balloon-tipped catheter, and an appropriate size angioscope with an irrigating channel is introduced into the graft lumen. Any identified residual thrombus can be removed with biopsy forceps or additional passes of the embolectomy catheter.

If satisfactory inflow is not achieved by the passage of an embolectomy catheter, then it is likely that an older organized thrombus is present and additional maneuvers will be required. One such technique is the use of a loop endarterectomy stripper. A Balloon-tipped catheter is passed through the loop of the endarterectomy stripper and advanced up the occluded graft limb into the body of the aortic graft. After inflating the balloon, the catheter is pulled back gently until the balloon occludes the orifice of the occluded graft limb. Next, using the balloon catheter for countertraction, the loop endarterectomy devise is carefully passed up the occluded graft limb over the balloon catheter. When resistance is encountered, the loop is carefully advanced a few more centimeters with a twisting motion using the balloon catheter as a guide. By holding traction on the balloon, and advancing the loop, the organized proximal thrombus can be loosened. Once the thrombotic plug is mobilized, the inflated balloon and the loop endarterectomy catheter are removed together along with the disengaged clot. If brisk arterial inflow is achieved, the completeness of the thrombo-endarterectomy should again be documented with either angiography or angioscopy. When the loop endarterectomy devise fails to provide adequate inflow, then a new bypass graft will generally be required.

Bypass Graft Reconstruction

There are several options for providing alternative inflow to the femoral level and each may be appropriate in a particular situation. The degree of the involved limb ischemia, the condition of the contralateral patent graft limb and runoff vessels, as well as the age and condition of the patient must all be considered before choosing which method of reconstruction is indicated. In the poor risk patient with limb threatening ischemia and a patent but unsuitable contralateral graft limb, an axillo-bifemoral bypass graft may be the safest and most expeditious method of achieving inflow. On the other hand, in the same patient, if the contralateral system is both patent and uncompromised, a crossover femoral to femoral bypass graft can be constructed with similar ease and better expected long term patency. Lastly in the good risk patient, particularly if the adequacy of the contralateral system is uncertain, direct replacement of the occluded graft limb can be accomplished often through a retroperitoneal approach. This technique has the advantage of better expected long-term patency then an extraanatomical bypass, but is more technically difficult due to the previously operated area.

Role of Thrombolytic Therapy

A recent addition to the therapeutic options for reestablishing inflow through an occluded aorto-femoral graft limb is the direct intraarterial infusion of thrombolytic agents. Although this technique has been shown to be a safe and reliable alternative to surgical thrombectomy[6,19], the procedure can take up to 48 hours and should be reserved for the patient with a relatively recent occlusion in whom the degree of extremity ischemia is not felt to require urgent revascularization. The procedure is usually performed immediately following the preoperative angiogram. A guide wire is passed into the graft limb thrombus and advanced through the occlusion under fluoroscopy. The ease with which the wire can be advanced through the thrombotic occlusion provides clinical information regarding the age and character of the thrombus and has become a reliable predictor of therapeutic success. When the wire passes through the occlusion easily, it is likely that the graft is occluded by fresh thrombus and the chances of successful thrombolysis are quite high. On the other hand, if the wire cannot be advanced through the graft limb occlusion the thrombus is probably older with a large degree of fibrotic organization and, in this instance, the likelihood of complete lysis is more uncertain. Once the guide wire is in place, an infusion catheter is advanced over the wire and the lytic therapy is begun. Several different agents and dosing protocols have been developed and proposed as techniques for enhancing the chances of thrombolysis. Unfortunately, no prospective randomized trails have been completed to compare these methods.

At UCLA we use a high-dose urokinase protocol which usually begins with 4000 IU/min of urokinase[15,16]. The drug is delivered by a coaxial catheter system in which the lytic agent is delivered simultaneously into both the proximal and distal portions of the clot. The drug is delivered into the distal clot through an open-ended infusion guide wire. At the same time, a second catheter with multiple side holes, delivers the agent around the wire into the proximal portion of the clot. The urokinase dose is split equally between the two ports. The graft occlusion is then reassessed with digital subtraction angiography after 4 hours of drug infusion. If little or no improvement is seen at that time, the chance of successful lysis with continued infusion is unlikely and most patients will proceed with operative intervention. In many instances the initial reexamination at 4 hours shows considerable improvement often with reestablishment of significant flow. When residual thrombus remains present, the infusion is continued with a dose of 4000 IU/min for 4 hours or 1000 IU/min delivered overnight. The specific protocol in each patient is individualized based on the degree of ischemia, the condition of the patient and the amount of improvement following the proceeding interval. Baring any complications, the infusion is continued until complete clot lysis is achieved. Following the completion of the thrombolysis, the vessels are carefully examined looking specifically for any flow limiting lesions which may be the presumed etiology of the graft limb occlusion. On occasion, a focal lesion is identified which can be successfully treated with endovascular techniques, such as balloon angioplasty, and no further therapy is required. More commonly, following complete clot lysis and restoration of flow through the graft, some form of distal outflow obstruction which requires operative repair is revealed. Regardless, in this instance, the patient has still benefited as the operative therapy is limited to an outflow procedure and can be directed by the specific anatomical findings demonstrated by the completion angiogram.

It should be emphasized that patients who undergo thrombolysis as a method of establishing inflow through an occluded aorto-femoral graft limb should be carefully selected. Thrombolytic agents should not be used within two weeks of a operative procedure. In addition, because of the duration of therapy required, some patients with severe limb threatening ischemia that requires urgent revascularization are better served with operative intervention. Lastly, certain diagnoses such as a history of gastrointestinal bleeding, recent stroke, or the clinical suspicion of the presence of a anastomotic pseu-doaneurysm, are contraindications for thrombolytic therapy and these patients should be primarily treated surgically.

B) Outflow

Femoral Artery Reconstruction

As mentioned, the key to success following intervention for aorto-femoral graft limb occlusion is the establishment of both adequate inflow and outflow. By far the most common cause of graft failure, in this setting, is outflow obstruction at the distal femoral anastomosis. Whether this obstruction is due to a hyperplastic intimal reaction, thrombosis of an anastomotic aneurysm or progression of distal atherosclerotic disease, reconstruction at the femoral level is mandatory for a successful long-term outcome.

Following the groin dissection, transection of the graft just proximal to the femoral anastomosis, and establishment of satisfactory inflow by one of the methods described above; the distal graft is opened longitudinally and the orifices of the runoff vessels carefully inspected.

If there is significant stenosis in one or both runoff vessels, either from intimal hyperplasia or progressive atherosclerotic disease, the arteriotomy should be continued onto either the superficial femoral or profunda femoral artery, or both, and an angioplastic repair constructed. Several techniques have been described for performing this repair. A short segment of graft can be bevelled and anastomosed to the newly opened femoral artery bifurcation.

For a short stenotic lesion limited to the orifice of the runoff vessel, this is the method of choice. Alternatively, when the lesion in the runoff vessel extends beyond the orifice, the arteries should be patched opened with the use of an autologous reconstruction.

The preferred autogenous patch material is a short segment of the superficial femoral artery provided this vessel is found to be chronically occluded. Otherwise a patch can be made from the adjacent saphenous vein. The importance of outflow reconstruction of the femoral bifurcation, particularly of the profunda femoral artery, cannot be overemphasized[11,12].

Role of Concomitant Distal Bypass

Rarely, when the profunda femoral artery is severally diseased, and judged to provide an insufficient degree of outflow, it may be necessary to perform a synchronous distal bypass to the popliteal or tibial level. This determination is most often made at the time of the groin exploration and can be aided by the use of intraoperative angiography. As mentioned previously, a preoperative angiogram should not be used to rule out the possibility of a distal reconstruction. The choice of conduit and the most suitable target outflow vessel must be individualized to each particular patient. Regardless, as always, the general principle remains that adequate outflow must be established if any long-term patency is to be derived from the newly reconstructed aorto-femoral bypass graft.

RESULTS

The operative mortality rates following intervention for an aorto-femoral graft limb occlusion are reported to be between 0-3%[1,3,5,7,11]. This is quite low considering the age of these patients and the fact that a large proportion also have advanced cardiovascular disease.

Thrombectomy combined with femoral artery bifurcation reconstruction is successful in restoring graft limb patency in between 65-100% of cases[1,3,5,7,9,11]. In those few instances where this method is not successful, the vast majority can be reconstructed with the use of extraanatomic inflow procedures and concomitant distal outflow bypasses when necessary.

With attention to the time honored principles outlined in the text above, long-term patency following reoperation for aorto-femoral graft limb occlusion can be expected to approach 75-85% at three years[1-3,5,7,9,11]. Although it should be acknowledged that some patients will require repeated procedures to achieve these results.

REFERENCES

1. Bernhard VM, Ray LI, Towne JB, (1977) The reoperation of choice for aortofemoral graft occlusion. *Surgery,* 82: 867-874.
2. Brewster DC. (1989) Reoperation for aortofemoral graft limb occlusion. In: Current Critical Problems in Vascular Surgery, edited by Veith FJ, pp 341-351. Quality Medical Publishing, Inc., St. Louis.
3. Brewster DC, Meier GH, Darling RC, et al, (1987) Reoperation for aortofemoral graft limb occlusion: optimal methods and long-term results. *J Vasc Surg,* 5: 363-374.
4. Clowes AW, Clowes MM, Fingerle J, Reidy MA, (1989) Regulation of smooth muscle cell growth in injured artery. *J Cardiovasc Pharmacol,* 14(Suppl. 6): S12-S15.
5. Ernst CB. (1991) Aortic graft limb occlusion. In: Current Therapy in Vascular Surgery, edited by Ernst CB, Stanley JC, pp 449-454. B. C. Decker, Inc., Philadelphia.
6. Gardiner GA, Harrington DP, Koltun W, et al., (1989) Salvage of occluded arterial bypass grafts by means of thrombolysis. *J Vasc Surg,* 9: 426-431.
7. Hyde GL, McCready RA, Schwartz RW, et al, (1983) Durability of thrombectomy of occluded aortofemoral graft limbs. *Surgery,* 94: 748-751.
8. Johnson WC, LoGerfo FW, Vollman RW, et al, (1977) Is axillo-bilateral femoral graft an effective substitute for aorto bilateral iliac/femoral graft? *Ann Surg,* 186: 123.
9. LeGrand DR, Vermillion BD, Hayes JP, et al, (1983) Management of the occluded aortofemoral graft limb. *Surgery,* 93: 818 821.
10. Leriche R, Morel A, (1948) The syndrome of thrombotic obliteration of the aortic bifurcation. *Ann Surg,* 127: 193.
11. Malone JM, Goldstone J, Moore WS, (1978) Autogenous profundaplasty: The key to long-term patency in secondary repair of aortofemoral graft occlusion. *Ann Surg,* 188: 817-823.

12. Malone JM, Moore WS. (1982) Aortoiliac and aortofemoral grafts: management of early and late occlusive complications. In: Vascular Emergencies, edited by Haimovici H, pp 441-458. Appleton-Century-Crofts, Norwalk.
13. Malone JM, Moore WS, Goldstone J, (1975) The natural history of bilateral aortofemoral bypass grafts for ischemia of the lower extremities. *Arch Surg,* 110: 1300-1306.
14. Mannick J, Whittemore AD, Donaldson MC. (1991) Aortofemoral bypass for atherosclerotic aortoiliac disease. In: Current Therapy in Vascular Surgery, edited by Ernst CB, Stanley JC, pp 391-394. 2nd ed. B. C. Decker Inc., Philadelphia.
15. McNamara TO, (1990) The use of lytic therapy with endovascular "repair" for the failed infrainguinal graft. *Seminars in Vascular Surgery,* 3(1): 59-65.
16. McNamara TO, Fischer JR, (1985) Thrombolysis of peripheral arterial and graft occlusions: improved results using high-dose urokinase. *American Journal of Roentgenology,* 144(4): 769-775.
17. Papadopoulos CC, (1976) Surgical treatment of aorto-iliac occlusive disease. Journal of Cardiovascular. *Surgery,* 17: 54.
18. Spaet TH, Stemerman MB, Veith FJ, Lejnieks I, (1975) Intimal injury and regrowth in the rabbit aorta: Medial smooth muscle cells as a source of neointima. *Circ Res,* 36: 58-70.
19. VanBreda A, Robison JC, Feldman L, et al, (1984) Local thrombolysis in the treatment of arterial graft occlusions. *J Vasc Surg,* 1: 103-112.
20. Vantinnen E, Inberg MV, (1975) Aorto-iliac femoral arterial reconstructive surgery. *Acta Chir Scand,* 141: 600.

Indication to Monolateral Versus Bilateral Aorto-Femoral Reconstruction and Long-Term Post-Operative Results

G.M. Biasi and P.M. Mingazzini

Department of Vascular surgery, University of Milan, Italy

Aorto-femoral reconstruction using a bypass bifurcation graft is perhaps the most successful procedure in the treatment of lower limb ischemia ever performed by vascular surgeons and the long-term results are most satisfactory.

The notable improvements in vascular prostheses, operative techniques and instrumentation has progressively increased the results of this procedure, whereas the related surgical morbidity and mortality has greatly decreased.

We are therefore able to consider bilateral aortofemoral grafting as the treatment of choice of aorto-iliac occlusive and aneurysmal disease.

Furthermore, the knowledge of the natural history of the atherosclerotic disease, as well as of the connected risk factors have ameliorated the correct indication to the bypass procedure, producing in such way better results.

Nevertheless, the vascular surgeon, when dealing with the single clinical case, should always think in an eclectic way, without rejecting prior alternative surgical procedures. In addition to this, other technical procedures such as iliofemoral, femoro-femoral (cross-over) bypass or axillo-femoral grafting, and more recently the radiologic interventional procedures such as percutaneous transluminal angioplasty (PTA), laser, atherectomies, etc., represent other options as surgical solutions for aorto-femoral steno-obliterative lesions.

If we have to state the correct indication to monolateral rather than bilateral aorto-femoral reconstruction, we should take into consideration the advantages and the disadvantages of the two techniques.

First of all there are some conditions that undoubtedly require a single sided reconstruction, such as a previous amputation of one limb, or an aneurysmal disease involving a single iliac artery.

Doubt can arise in case of a symtomatic lesion of one iliac artery with unaffected contralateral vessel (Table 1). As a matter of fact truly unilateral iliac disease is uncommon, whereas atherosclerosis is well known as a systematic process, generally diffused and more often bilateral. Moreover, the disease is progressive and the deterioration of flow in the aorta or in the contralateral iliac artery will necessitate later a bilateral revascularization.

The adequacy of the flow on the opposite side should therefore be checked not only by angiographic visualization and by non invasive study, but also with a papaverine test. The arterial pressure in the femoral and brachial arteries is measured at the same time; in basal condition the pressure gradient between brachial and femoral arteries should not exceed 15 mm of mercury. A drop of more than 10 mm Hg or 20% of the initial value after 20 mg papaverine injection means a significative disease in the iliac artery[15, 17]. Furthermore the arterial lesion should not be amenable to percuta-neous transluminal angioplasty. The PTA technique has to be addressed only to focal stenotic lesions; a surgical procedure may be required in case of complications and long-term results of PTA seems not to be so good, even with the use of stents[17].

Table 1 - Indications for single sided aorto-femoral bypass

– Previous amputation of one limb
– Monolateral iliac artery aneurysm
– Symptomatic steno/occlusive lesion of one iliac artery with unaffected controlateral vessel.

In retrospective reviews higher patency rates follow bilateral bypass procedures, with a percentage of long-term patency of about 80% up to 99% [6, 12]. When a unilateral aortofemoral or aorto-iliac bypass is carried out, the figures suggest that thrombosis is at least twice as common as it is for the limbs of aortobifemoral bypass, and may occur in over 40% of unilateral bypasses[2, 13]. Moreover, if the operation is carried out for arteriosclerosis on one side only, between 20 and 50% of patients require a second operation on the contralateral side[2]. On the contrary some Authors report similar late patency rates for single sided reconstructions (87%) with lower incidence of evolution of atherosclerotic lesions in the contralateral iliac artery (12%)[12].

Other factors in favour of bilateral reconstruction are the little added morbidity and mortality associated with a bilateral rather than a unilateral repair and the technical ease of performing the second side at the same time[7]. If we consider also the technical problems associated with the possible need for a later operation on the contralateral side, caused by difficulties in approaching the aorta due to extensive scarring, which usually follows a previous prosthetic implantation, we should give our preference to a bilateral procedure.

Besides this we should also take into account other alternative procedures such as iliac endoarterectomy and femoro-femoral cross-over bypass.

The endartectomy procedure can be easily performed with an extra-peritoneal approach; it may also be accomplished with a ring-stripper, semi-closed technique, which avoids extensive exposure of the artery and does not necessitate the use of alloplastic material, thus excluding extensive scarring and unfavourable complications related to infection, and especially stimulation of diffuse and extensive intimal hyperplasia.

On the other hand there are contraindications to this procedure, such as extensive calcification of the vessels and possible post-operative sexual malfunction in males. The use of the technique of femoro-femoral grafting has progressively increased because of the ease of the procedure, which avoids abdominal incision and is consequently indicated also in poor-risk patients[8].

Long-term results of cross-over grafting are also good and approach those of aorto-bifemoral grafting[9, 11]. Relative contraindications are exposure of the unaffected femoral artery and the possibility of infection involving the prosthesis, although infection in a superficial graft is less threatening than that involving an abdominal implant.

Here we have to remember also the possibility of axillo-femoral bypass, but this procedure has not as good long-term results and has a different indication, in fact it is reserved to high risk patients in which the controlateral side cannot offer a good flow, or if the abdomen cannot be approached owing to infection.

On the other hand the single sided grafting procedure gives some advantages: it is amenable using a safer unilateral extraperitoneal approach with minimal dissection, and consequent minimal post-operative sexual malfunction problems. The inflow vessel may be the lower aorta, with a side anastomosis or the same common iliac artery if still patent. The superior portion of the infrarenal aorta, most often free of disease, may remain untouched and easily accessible for a secondary bifurcation grafting procedure should it become necessary[16, 19] (Table 2).

Table 2 - Criteria of choise for monolateral aorto-femoral bypass

---

PROS

- Unilateral extraperitoneal approach
- Rare post-operative sexual malfunction problems
- Patent common iliac artery used as inflow vessel
- Large diameter inflow vessel, with low angled anastomoses and short and straight anatomic pathway (as compared to femoro-femoral bypass)

CONS

- Focal stenotis lesions amenable to PTA
- Lower patency rates (as compared to bilateral bypass procedures)
- Little added morbidity and mortality associated with bilateral repair
- Progression of atherosclerotic disease with deterioration of flow in the controlateral iliac artery, requiring a second operation
- Difficult approach to the aorta for scarring due to previous prosthetic implant

---

Having discussed the advantages and the disadvantages of monolateral and bilateral aorto-femoral reconstructions, we should compare the results of the different procedures, in order to state the indications.

Several unappropriate experiences using the different surgical techniques have been reported with varying results, but the frequent lack of documentation regarding general conditions of patient, risk factors, inflow and outflow vessels and individual indications for surgery make a reliable comparison quite impossible.

Besides, the aorto-femoral monolateral by-pass procedure is now rarely performed (and consequently reported) by most Vascular Surgical Centers.

We reviewed the literature in search of comparative techniques and found few articles[24] comparing aorto-bifemoral, femoro-femoral and iliofemoral by-pass procedures. Examining their experiences these Authors conclude that aorto-bifemoral by-pass is preferable to femoro-femoral by-pass whenever aortoiliac atherosclerosis is accompanied by unilateral occlusion in good-risk patients with a reasonable life expectancy. They reserve femoro-femoral by-pass to patients at prohibitive risk, or with abdominal disease presenting serious technical difficulties, while iliofemoral by-pass, because of poor long-term results, is no longer considered an appropriate option.

Based on our own experience we came practically to the same conclusion: during the course of the years we have slightly modified our indication delaying the insertion of an aortobifemoral graft. Considering the natural history of the atherosclerotic disease and the clinical observation that, mostly in case of unilateral iliac disease, with appropriate control of risk factors and physical exercise, the onsetting claudication may be reduced or even disappear owing to the increased collateral blood flow.

We therefore reserve aortobifemoral grafting to the disabling claudication and have nearly completely abandoned unilateral procedures such us ileofemoral endoarterectomies or by-pass procedures.

Femoro-femoral grafting is performed by us only in poor risk patients with short life expectancy.

REFERENCES

1. Ameli F.M.,Stein M.,Pravan J.L.,Aro L.,Praser R. Predictors of surgical outcome in patients under-going aortobifemoral by-pass reconstruction. *J.Cardiovasc.Surg.,* 31(3) 333-339,1990
2. Charlesworth D. The occluded aortic and aortofemoral graft in reoperative arterial surgery. Bergan J.S., Yao J.S.T., Grune & Stratton 271-278; 1986
3. Christenson J., Eklof B. Synthetic arterial grafts: General complications Scand. J. Thor. Cardiovasc. *Surgery,* 11: 37-42; 1977
4. Crawford S.E., Bomberger R., Glaeser D.H Aortoiliac occlusive disease: Factors influencing survival and function following reconstructive operation over a twentyfive year period. *Surgery,* 90: 10055-1067; 1981
5. Crawford E.S., DeBakey M.E., Morris G.C. Jr. Evaluation of late failures after reconstructive operations for acclusive lesions of the aorta, iliac, femoral and popliteal arteries. *Surgery,* 47: 79-104; 1960

6. Crawford E.S., Manning L.G.,Kelly T.F.. Redo surgery after operations for aneurysm and occlusion of the abdominal aorta. *Surgery,* 81: 41-52; 1977
7. Dale A.W. Management of vascular surgical probelms. McGraw-Hill, N.Y., 138-164; 19
8. DeVolfe C., Adelaine P. Ilio-femoral and femoro-femoral cross-over grafting analysis of eleven years' experience. *J. Cardiovasc. Surg.,* 24: 634-640; 1983
9. Dick L.S., Brief D.K., Alpert J. A twelve-year experience with femoro-femoral cross-over grafts. *Arch. Surg.,* 115:1359; 1980
10. Duncan W.C., Linton R.R., Darling R.C. Aortoiliofemoral atherosclerotic occlusive disease: Compara-tive results of endarterectomy and dacron bypass grafts. *Surgery,* 70: 974; 1971
11. Eugene J., Goldstone J., Moore W.S. Fifteen-year experience with subcutaneous bypass grafts for lower extremity ischemia. *Am. Sug.,* 186: 177; 1977
12. Fiorani P. Single sided iliac reconstruction in the maintenance of arterial reconstructions. Ed. R. Greenhalgh - London : 373-380; 1991
13. Fulenwider J.T., Smith R.B., Johnson R.W. Reoperative abdominal arterial surgery. A ten year experience. *Surgery,* 93: 20-27; 1983
14. Hepp W., de Jonge K., Pallua N. Late results following extra-anatomic bypass procedures for chronic aorto iliac occlusive disease *J. Cardiovasc. Surg.,* 29(2); 181-185,1988
15. Kadir S., White R.I., Kaufmen S.H. Long-term results of aorto-iliac angioplasty. *Surgery,* 94: 10; 1983
16. Kalman P.G., Hosang M., Johnston K.W., Wallacr P.M. Unilateral iliac disease: The role of iliofemo-ral bypass. *J. Vasc: Surg. &*: 139-43; 1987
17. Katzen B.T. Percutaneous transluminal angioplasty for arterial disease of the lower extremities. *Am. J. Roentg.,* 142: 23; 1984
18. Knudson J.A., Downs A.R. Reoperation following failure of aortoiliofemoral arterial reconstruction. *Canad. J. Surg.,* 21: 316-319; 1978
19. Levison S.A., Levison H.J.,Hollorar G. Limited indication for unilateral aortofemoral or iliofemoral vascular grafts. *Arch. Surg.,* 107: 791-796; 1973
20. Mozersky D.J., Summer D.S., Stradness D.E. Long-term results of reconstructive aortoiliac surgery. *Am. J. Surgery,* 123: 503-509; 1972
21. Najafi H., Dye W.S., Javid H. Late thrombosis affecting one limb of aortic bifurcation graft. *Arch. Surg.,* 110: 409-412; 1975
22. Neverlsteen A.S., Suy R., Daenen W., Boel A., Staelpaert G. Aortofemoral grafting: Factors influen-cing late results. *Surgery,* 88: 642-653; 1980
23. Perdue G.D., Long W.D., Smith R.F. Perspective concerning aorto-femoral arterial reconstruction. *Ann. Surg.,* 173: 942-944; 1971
24. Piotrowski J., Pearce W., Jones D.N. Aortobifemoral bypass: The operation of choice for unilateral iliac occlusion. *J.Vasc. Surg.,* 8: 211-218; 1988
25. Szilagyi D.E., Elliot J.P., Smith R.B. Secondary arterial repair. The management of late failures in reconstructive arterial surgery. *Arch. Surg.,* 110: 485-493; 1975
26. Szilagyi E., Joseph P.E., Smith R.F. A thirty year survey of the reconstructive surgical treat-ment of aortoiliac occlusive disease. *J. Vasc. Surg.,* 3: 421-436; 1986
27. Waibel P.P., Dunant J.H.Late results of aorto-iliac reconstructive surgery. *J. Cardiovasc. Surg.,* 42: 492-494; 1972

Thrombolytic Treatment of Late Graft Occlusion

D. Bertini, C. Pratesi and S. Michelagnoli

Department of Vascular Surgery, University of Florence, Italy

The incidence of acute and sub-acute graft thrombosis is increasing due to the larger number of graft implantation, and to the improvements of vascular surgery techniques that made possible more vascular procedures.

Since recurrent ischemia is the main problem of vascular surgery, is obvious that a close and effective follow-up study that may find out a progression of distal atherosclerotic disease or a miointimal hyperplasia at anastomosis before the onset of thrombosis is required. The treatment in this phase is more easy and has more probability of success.

When the occlusion is present the choice between surgical and medical management is difficult and usually guided by personal ability, etiologic elements, associated pathology, and clinical status. Vascular graft may be savaged with thrombolytic therapy after an acute occlusion as an alternative to thrombectomy. The possibility of success depends on detection of the reasons for the thrombosis. In these challenging situations lytic therapy may be able to achieve the patency of the graft, and so it may be considered as a therapeutical and diagnostic step, usually followed by adjunctive procedure like surgery or PTA.

METHODS AND RESULTS

Our experience is based on 151 treatments of which 60 were related to late graft occlusions (54 men and 6 women, mean age 57 years), in whom we used urokinase.

In all cases the lytic drug was administered locally by Seldinger method, directly into the clot. The authors are nowadays using this protocol: 100.000 U. bolus of urokinase and then 35.000 U/hour. During the application of this

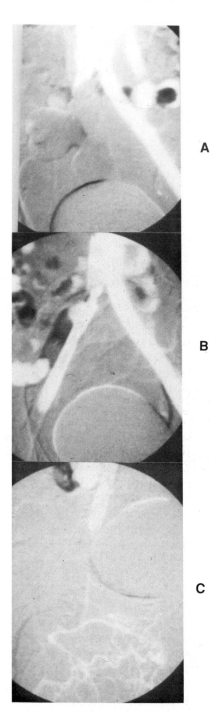

A

B

C

Clinical Case N.1

A 55-years old male returned 3 years postoperatively (Aorto-bifemoral bypass) with an ischemic right limb.

Arteriography immediately performed showed the complete occlusion of the right branch (A). Occlusion was present on anamnestic data from 96 hours.

The infusion catheter was positioned, the thrombolytic drug somministred, and a complete patency achieved after 48 hours (B, C, D).

Final angiographic control (E) showed the presence of a residual stenosis. A "limitated surgical" intervention was performed, the presence of a stenotic and calcific lesion was detected as the cause of thrombosis (F).

protocol some laboratory parameters are monitored (fibrinogen, activated partial thromboplastin time, thrombin time, fibrinogen degradation products) in order to evaluate the coagulation system during therapy. Our protocol also includes serial controls by means of clinical evaluation, Doppler examination at least every 6 hours, and angiography every 12 hours or every time required. Angiography can be considered at the end of the therapy as a means of final evaluation and can detect those cases that need adjunctive therapy (i.e. see clinical case N. 1).

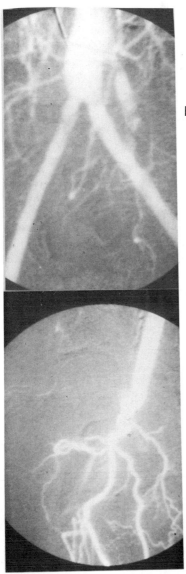

D

E

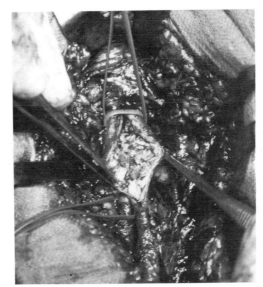

F

The clinical results were good in 71.6% of cases. The overall lysis as determined by angiography was complete in 44 patients (73.3%), partial in 5 cases (8.3%), and no lysis was achieved in 11 patients (18.3%) (Table 1).

The mean occlusion time in this group was of 387 hours.

We divided the patients with late graft occlusions into two subgroups according to the occlusion level.

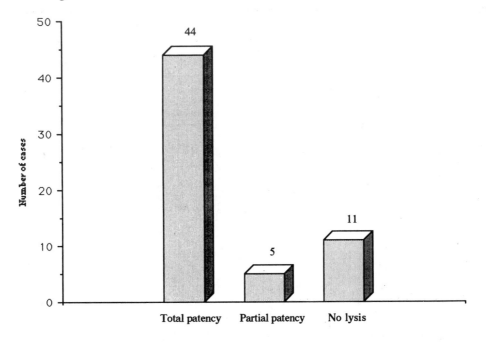

Table 1 - Thrombolytic treatment of late graft occlusion : personal experience (60 cases)

Concerning particularly patients with proximal graft occlusion we considered 42 cases in which a good clinical results was obtained in 85.7%; a total recanalization was obtained in 36 cases (85.7%) (mean I.W. from 0.21 to 0.62), 2 cases of partial recanalization (4.7%) and 18 cases of distal obstruction in which the clinical results was good in 38.8%. There was complete recanalization in 8 cases (44.4%) and 4 cases of partial recanalization (22.2%) (mean I.W. from 0.20 to 0.55) (Table 2).

We have also evaluated our results concerning occlusion time.

If we consider only the 41 patients treated within 240 hours from occlusion we achieved a good clinical results in 78%, a complete angiographic lysis in 80.4% (33 pts), a partial 9.7% (4 pts) and no recanalization 9.7% (4 pts). In this subgroup the increase of the mean Winsor Index rose from 0.17 to 0.65.

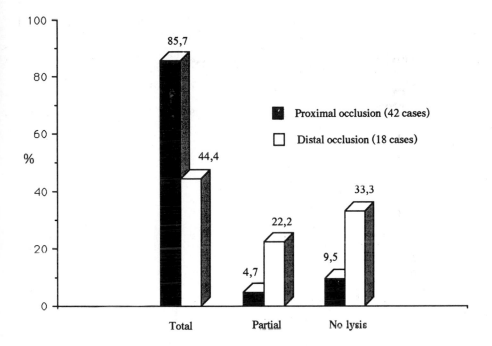

Table 2 - Angiographic patency

In the 19 patients with more than 240 hours a good clinical results was achieved in 61.1%; a complete recanalization was obtained in 57.8% (11 pts), a partial patency was achieved in 5.2% (1 pts); (mean I.W. from 0.27 to 0.51). In 7 cases we didn't achieve the patency (36.8%) (Tables 3 and 4).

In 50% of 6 patients treated after 900 hour of occlusion we obtained a good graft recanalization (i.e. see clinical case N. 2).

Concerning complications, we haven't notices common reactions or major haemorrhages. It has been recorded 2 distal embolisms that were completely resolved continuing thrombolytic therapy.

For that regards the trans-graft extravasation we have to notice that in one case the complications has been caused by the too short period elapsed (45 days) after graft installation and the start of thrombolytic therapy.

At last we have to signalize 7 cases of bleeding during arterial catheterization managed with local compression.

In no cases it has been necessary blood transfusion.

As concern haemorrhagy far from the catheter insertion point or from the infusion site of drug we have signalized 2 cases macroscopic haematury.

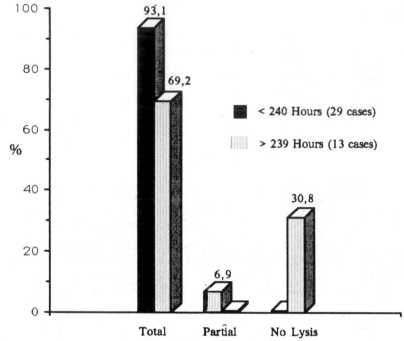

Table 3 - Angiographic patency - Proximal Occlusion (42 cases)

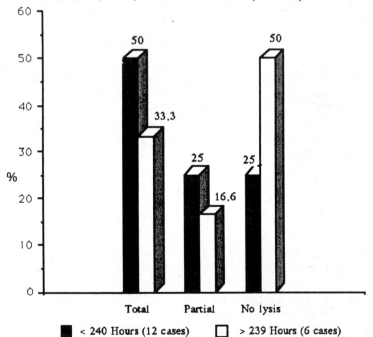

Table 4 - Angiographic patency - Distal Occlusion (18 cases)

Clinical Case N.2

A 55-years old male was hospedalized for an ischemic symptomatology lasting from 140 hours. This patient was surgically treated 30 months before in an other hospital for an iliaco-femoro-popliteal bypass.

A transbrachial arteriography was performed and showed a complete graft occlusion (A). The infusion catheter was positioned into the clot (B), the thrombolytic drug somministred, and a complete patency of the iliaco-femoral graft achieved after 48 hours (C, D, E). The infusion catheter was then positioned into the obliterated femoro-popliteal graft, and a complete patency was achieved after 48 hours of adiunctive therapy. The final angiographic control showcd thc patency of proximal (G) and distal anastomosis (H) and also of tibial vessels (I). On anamnestic data the occlusion of the femoro-popliteal bypass was present from more than 30 days.

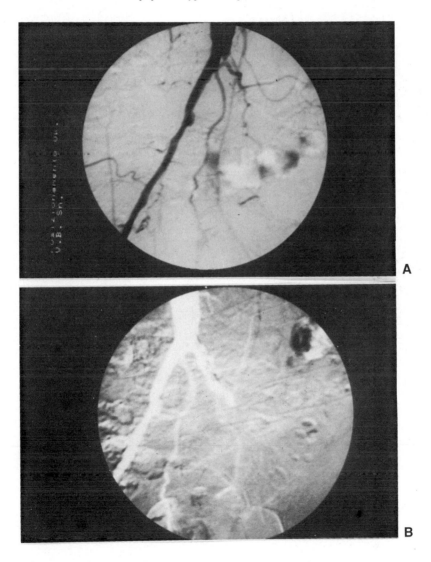

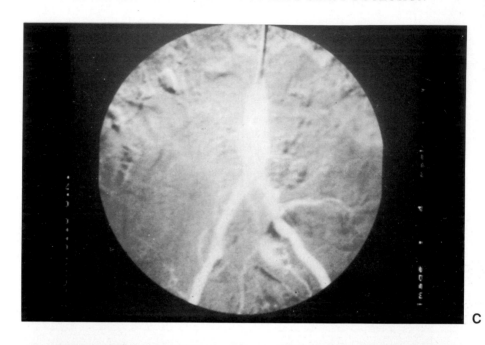

C

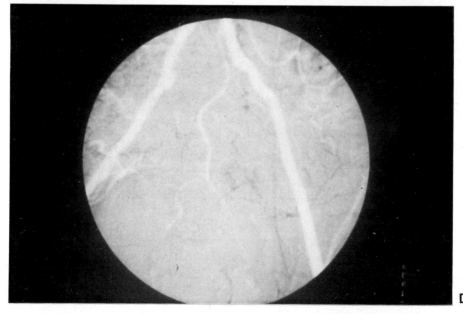

D

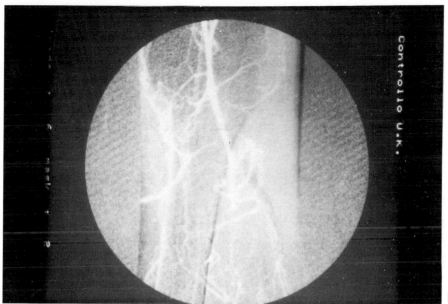

E

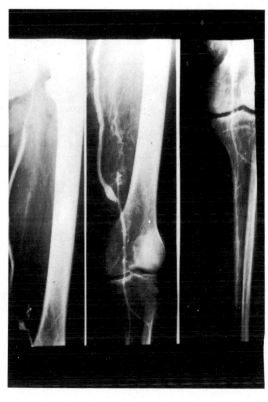

F

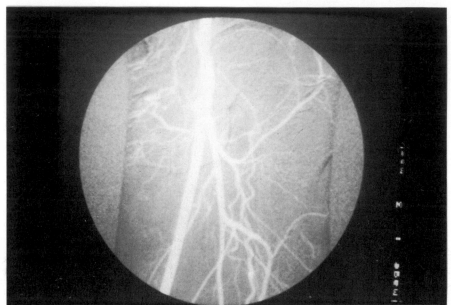

G

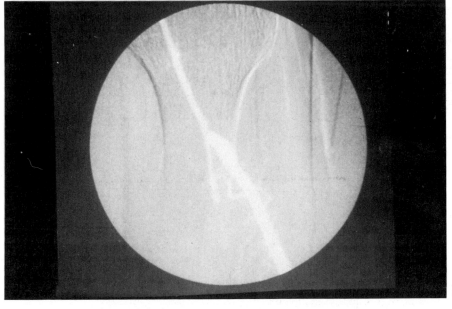

H

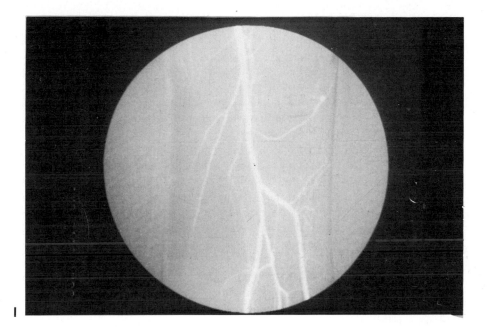

DISCUSSION

Analyzing the different problems concerning thrombolytic therapy, we must evaluate the indications of this kind of therapeutical approaches.

In the group of lower limbs ischemic pathology, extreme distal embolism, evolutive episodes of occlusive disease, acute aneurysm and late graft thrombosis may be successfully treated with thrombolytic drugs. They have been also employed in the immediate post procedural period in patients with critical distal "run off".

All these applications have been made possible by the local administration technique, reduction of doses, improvement of the "know how" to prevent complications, but a careful evaluation of contraindications is fundamental[15].

Analyzing the role of thrombolytic infusions in late graft thrombosis we must also consider the possible development of complications.

Are universally accepted as absolute contraindications:

1) Current active bleeding
2) Recent cerebral accidents (less than 30 days)
3) Intracranial disease
4) Pregnancy, or menstrual period
5) No drugs controllable hypertension (diastolic 120 mmHg)
6) Endocarditis
7) Substance idiosyncrasy
8) Deep hepatic failure

9) Occlusion of an infected vascular graft

10) and finally hyperacute lower limbs ischemia. In these cases we prefer an emergency thrombectomy with associated intra and post-operative lytic infusion. This is due to the incapability for the ischemic limb to tolerate hours needed for the initial clot lysis.

By contrary it is still contraindicated to delivery thrombolytic drugs in course of early grafts occlusions for the well know problem of trans-graft blood extravasation on true haemorrhage.

The rare cases of peripheral ischemia arising in the immediate post-surgical period of a proximal revascularization performed in an aneurysmal pathology or in an obliterating pathology represent a completely different group. In these situations there are many problems to be solved before deciding the therapy, particularly in cases of worsening ischemia in the extreme distal vascular bed. Till recently, the treatment of such cases was limited to an embolectomy with a balloon catheter. Considering the extreme peripheral site, the success rates were less than optimal and, therefore, recently endothrombotic thrombolysis has been applied in appropriate doses with good results. Such an approach clearly contrasts with one of the contraindications of thrombolytic therapy, the application of a graft in the aorto-iliac area within the 15 preceding days and therefore concerns only select cases to be followed with particularly close attention, positioning the catheter in the most possible distal seat, if possible via the popliteal artery and with lower initial doses paying attention to reduce the doses afterward according to angiographic results and close checks of the coagulative parameters.

Another possible application of thrombolysis in limb saving is its use during the intraoperative phase.

Some of the authors maintain that the use during this phase is dangerous while others report good results without particular complication[38,43]. It must be born in mind that these are situations in which it is impossible to obtain a good distal back flow during the surgical procedure. In this condition an angiographic check can indicate the presence of endoluminal thrombosis in distal vessels, which cannot be removed through surgical thrombectomy. In such circumstances thrombolytic therapy can be applied with the possibility of lysing small distal thrombi[36,37]. The modality of the intraoperative application can consist, in the course of a surgical thrombectomy, of a pharmacological distal completion of the proximal surgical removal, limited to the moment of the operation, mediating repeated or continuous infusions with a distal angiographic catheter or an irrigating balloon catheter, or even a continuous infusion in the immediate post-surgical period through small catheters left in situ[9,13]. Intra-operative thrombolysis can be useful not only together with surgical thrombectomy, but also in interventions of distal revascularization. In such circumstances the distal bed is of poor quality. The aim of this therapy is to clean the distal bed during the intraoperative phase in order to improve run-off. The therapy with thrombolytics may be continued in the perioperative phase via a catheter positioned during the intervention through a collateral or introduced through the common femoral in order to avoid early reocclusion. Such a procedure has been applied recently in personal experience with encouraging results; it was possible to maintain the graft patency (in some cases with very poor distal vascular conditions) and because it was possible to evaluate daily the process of prosthetic healing and particularly the evolution of the thrombotic apposition at the distal anastomosis site.

In choosing thrombolytic drugs, we must remember the better results and the poor risks of urokinase versus streptokinase and the advantages of the local way of administration[4].

Urokinase (UK) has now become the preferred agent for intra-arterial fibrinolytic infusion therapy for peripheral vascular disease. UK is superior and safer fibrinolytic agent than Streptokinase (SK) because it is an human protein and a direct plasminogen activator complex. UK is cleared rapidly by the liver. It has a half life that is relatively short, averaging 20 minutes or less[9]. This fact may by important in planning a complemental therapy.

Recently rt-PA seems to have the same effectiveness as urokinase and shorter therapy duration[6]. Because of its better affinity for thrombotic fibrin, rt-PA might also be administered by systemic infusion.

Berridge et al.[7] have compared three randomized groups of 20 (both arterial and graft occlusion) patients each treated respectively with intra-arterial recombinant tissue plasminogen activator, intravenous recombinant tissue plasminogen and intra-arterial streptokinase. Limb salvage at 30 days was achieved in 80, 45 and 60 per cent respectively. Haemorrhagic complications occurred in 6 patients following SK, and in 13 following I.V. rt-PA; only one minor hemorrhage occurred following a catheter arterial perforation in a patient who received I.A. rt-PA. The authors conclude that I.V. route of infusion is not as successful as I.A. even with rt-PA, and carries more risks of haemorrhagic complications.

Meyerovitz et al.[28] reported a randomized trial concerning the use of rt-PA (10 mg in bolus and 5mg/hours up to 24 hours) versus UK (60.000 U.I. in bolus followed by 240.000 U.I./h for 2 hours, 120.000 U.I./h for 2 hours, and 60.000 U.I./h up to 20 hours) in a group of 32 patients. They conclude that hemorrhagic complications were more prevalent in the rt-PA group, although the difference did not reach statistical significance. rt-Pa tended to cause a more rapid thrombolysis than UK, but 24 hours the lysis rates were similar.

In our experience recombinant tissue plasminogen activator seems to be of high efficacy in recent occlusion, but in older thrombosis it may carry an higher rate of complications. This fact may be due to the extreme selective action of this drug that may be active in high concentration also after one step run throughout the ischemic limb. In other words with actual protocol of infusion this kind of therapy in old thrombosis may be assimilate to a loco-systemic infusion.

As concern occlusion time also in our series best results are obtained when thrombolysis is started within 240 hours from occlusion, but it is possible to obtain good results also after more time.

Concerning this problems there are a lot of different view also among these physician that usually employ this kind of therapy.

Usually an ischemic symptomatology lasting more than 10 days was not considered an indication for thrombolytic therapy, in more recent time this period of time was widened even if with less results, and a lot of physician utilize this approach till two months[7, 24, 32, 34, 42, 45, 46, 47].

Barr et al.[2] achieved a complete recanalization in 90% of patients with symptoms lasting less than 1 week (31 Pts.), in 60% of 12 patients with symptoms greater than 1 week and less than 4 weeks, and in 40% of patients with symptoms greater than 4 weeks (12 Pts.)

However are reported a lot of contribution in which several authors achieved good results with extimated occlusion time lasting more than 1 year, both in arterial and graft occlusion[29, 40, 50]. The problem in these cases is that the occlusion time is usually calculated on clinical ground, and so when the occlusion is lasting for more than 1 month it is difficult to achieve reliable data from the patients; only anecdotical data are reported in literature. Risius et al.[40] reported a successful recanalization in a case of arterial occlusion, angiographically documented lasting more than 7 years. To overcome this problem Cragg et al.[10], propose for chronic ischemia to reserve the decision to perform thrombolysis to be based on the ability to traverse the occluded artery or graft with a guide wire, regardless to the extimated occlusion time.

For a rational evaluation of therapeutical indications of thrombolysis we must evaluate the relations between this kind of therapy and surgery. If we consider the indications of surgery for graft occlusions we must underline the important role of the secondary patency rate, that is 16% in three years for reoperations on a femoropopliteal bypasses, decreasing to 8% in a year for femoropopliteal bypasses set on isolated segments of the popliteal artery, according to Ascer et al.[1].

The "post-primary" patency rate changes according to different authors from 39%[18] to 37%[3,49], and to 31%[8].

Late thrombectomy of an autologous saphenous vein graft is particularly complicated and a new bypass is usually necessary to assure an adequate revascularization. Analyzing many reports, it is possible to assume that the long-term patency rate of thrombectomized autologous vein bypasses is very low, even after a well accomplished operation. Percutaneous angioplasty or complementary surgical interventions can, however, improve the patency of these bypasses.

Results are obviously better when we deal with occlusion of vascular segments in more proximal districts (aorto-femoral).

Local thrombolysis has a specific role in late thrombosis therapy using both prosthetic and autologous vein grafts, and usually permits a complete rccanalization. Analyzing the local and general conditions of each patient, we have to consider the eventual complementary treatments of the thrombolysis. Naturally, when a thrombosis appears, its cause is a proximal and/or distal anastomosis with intimal hyperplasia or a peripheral atherosclerotic progression. During thrombolysis is also possible to detect occlusive lesions by means of angiographic studies and proceeding to an eventual appropriate therapy[46]. In a recent contribution of Durham et al.[12] in the 51% of cases of a group of 53 patients the probable cause of graft failure could be attributed to a single lesion. If surgery is utilized sometimes the cause of thrombosis may be not find out in course of emergency thrombectomy, especially if it isn't possible to perform an intraoperative angiographic study.

Graor et al.[22] referred an experience about a comparative study between thrombectomy and thrombolysis during prosthetic thrombosis. They studied 22 patients who had thrombolysis (rt-PA) and 32 who had thrombectomy with the same risk factors and type of bypass in the two groups. The most significant data are: after thirty days the patency rate was 86% in the thrombolysis group compared to 42%; the indication of complementary surgical treatment was 91% and 86% respectively; finally, they found a lower amputation rate in the thrombolysis group.

Thrombolytic agents have been shown to have the potentials to reduce skeletal muscle damage after acute ischemia. This phenomenon is probably due to improved patency of the distal vessels, and in particular the microvasculature, allowing watershed areas to survive[7]. In a recent contribution Van Der Wall et al.[48] demonstrated using gadolinium DTPA in association of NMR, the presence of reperfused areas in myocardium in patient treated with thrombolytics drugs in course of myocardial infarction, even if with current techniques it is difficult to discriminate acutely infarcted from reperfused areas.

Moreover, Graor's study demonstrates that complications are less frequent with rt-PA (2.5% vs.15-17% of the streptokinase). It has a higher and faster lytic power (4 or 5 hours), and finally there is a relationship between thrombus age and lysis time, i.e. the older the thrombus, and the longer the infusion time.

Delaying with thrombolytic complications we must discriminate the arterial catheterization complications such as spasm, dissection, embolisms and sepsis from drugs complications such as anaphilactoid reactions and hemorrhages.

Distal embolism as an asymptomatic syndrome which, according to the experience of Graor et al.[21] has a rate of 48%, demonstrate with angiography; it can be easily treated with good evolution continuing the thrombolytic therapy.

The risk of an ascendent thrombosis by means of the catheter that achieves with a variable from 5% to 30% rate[14,16] is also referred to. This is a dangerous situation that could develop a massive embolism often needing surgical treatment (in 4 cases out of 15 as referred by Eskridge[16]. Many techniques were proposed to prevent this complication: the use of smaller catheters with lateral windows, higher doses of thrombolytic drugs and heparin association. Embolic complications rate decreases drastically by heparin association. Otherwise authors reported that even using correct doses of heparin i.v., the pericatheter thrombosis rate is not reduced. Pernes et al.[35] trying to reduce the rate of this incident, propose the use of a coaxial system constituted by a short external catheter (5 F) placed proximally to the occlusion and by a longer internal catheter (3 F), placed in the thrombotic site. Urokinase perfuses through both the catheters so that external proximal catheter infusion allows the progressive lysis of a potential distal thrombus. Also, Van Breda et al.[47] suggested the use of a coaxial system; thrombolytic drug passed through the longer internal catheter and heparin at 250 U/h through the shorter external one. Moreover, the anterograde approach must be preferred, as referred to by Katzen and Van Breda[26]. We often use this method as well.

Hemorrhage is the most dangerous complication, both as haematoma in the place of catheter introduction, which is developed in 10-30% of cases (it often has poor clinical importance except in particular sites as above the crural arch with a possible retroperitoneal hemorrhage, or next to the axillary site with plexus paralysis), and a much more dangerous complication such as cerebral and digestive hemorrhages (their prevention is included in the same absolute contraindications of this therapy). The hemorrhage is probably linked to circulating plasmine increase which exceeds the neutralizing capacity of its inhibitors, in particular alfa 2-antiplasmin.

McNamara and Fischer[27] assessed that hemorrhage is correlated to the degree of systemic biological fibrinolysis; these authors recommended the suspension of treatment when the fibrinogen level is under specific values. On the contrary, Mori et al.[30] attributed the hemorrhage with thrombolytic therapy duration. In this view, looking the relation between different type of drugs we have considered two groups, the first composed of 317 cases treated with streptokinase[30,21,25,45], and the second 297 cases treated with urokinase[11,19,27]. We found an hemorrhage rate of 9% for the second group versus 30% of the first, and 15% of major hemorrhage in the streptokinase group was demonstrated.

Seabrook et al.[44] recently reported in a group of 30 cases of graft occlusion in which they used UK 5 episodes of bleeding (16.6%), 3 of which needed a blood administration and surgical treatment.

Therefore, we must affirm that hemorrhage is a very important problem, because many studies report serious cerebral hemorrhages although there is always a careful evaluation of the neurological contraindication. Many mechanisms contribute to cause serious complications such as embolisms, preexistent asymptomatic ischemic lesions, and the difficult prevention of systemic effects of local thrombolysis.

Quinones-Baldric et al.[36,37] suggests that these hemorrhagic complications may be due to associated antiplatelet and anticoagulant postoperative therapy. They also recommend limitation of lytic infusion to very distal vascular districts. Parent et al.[31] recommend close monitoring of patients during intraoperative lytic infusion with particular regard to the fibrinogen level, which should not fall below 100 mg/dl. Above this limit they have never recorded bleeding.

Fennerty et al.[17] have mentioned the dilemma that exists between the risk of hemorrhage during thrombolytic therapy and plasmatic proteolysis induced by the plasmin as reported by several groups studying the use of rt-PA or streptokinase in ischemic heart attack and in deep venous thrombosis. They speak of a higher incidence of bleeding complication with fibrinogen lower than 150 mg/dl and values of fibrin degradation product higher than 400 microg/ml. They conclude that lysis of the fibrin in the haemostatic coagulum in the wound is the most important factor in bleeding induced by thrombolytic agents.

We have never found any important variation in these parameters, especially in the fibrinogen value as related by several authors who have used urokinase in local treatment.

Cerebral or digestive hemorrhages may also be possible. These complications may be originated by an increase in circulating blood plasmine, enough to saturate the inhibitory capacity. According to McNamara and Fischer[27] this complication is linked to an surplus of thrombolytic substances, and they propose that therapy be reduced or stopped if fibrinogen falls below certain critical values. Mori et al.[30] do not agree with this interpretation and propose infusion time as the critical factor. There are also fewer complications with urokinase than with streptokinase as found by several authors.

Recently Haber et al.[23] talking about antibody-targeted thrombolytic agents consider whether the second generation of fibrin selective agents have any clinical advantage over the nonselective agents. In other words there is little disagreement that a moderate but general disruption of the clotting system is an undesiderable state.

But despite the broadly affirmed importance of haematologic assessments, also in recent times it may happen to read "It was not the practice to perform routine haematological assessment, the patients being managed purely on clinical grounds"[2].

A particular kind of complication is represented by the so called transgraft hemorrhage. This problem represent a particular chapter in the field of complications if contraindication are carefully evaluated, and more in details if the graft has been positioned more than 3 months before the beginning of thrombolysis. First report about this kind of complications are of 1982[39], and were referred to Dacron Knitted graft. This complication was attributed to the capacity of the lytic substances to solve also the old fibrin coat occluding graft porosity[33]. It has been recorded also transgraft hemorrhage in case of gore-tex graft[5,41]. In these cases it is more difficult to find the reason of hemorrhage. Rosner et al.[41] postulate that lesions generated by surgical manipulation are the causes of blood extravasation. Also sepsis even if asymptomatic and local trauma must be considered, if indication and contraindications were carefully evaluated before the institution of this therapy.

CONCLUSIONS

In conclusion we want to stress that the inability of thrombectomy to achieve uniform success in the restoration of circulation is frequently due to failure to remove distal propagating thrombus and to the inability to recognize the thrombosis cause.

In these cases the use of "low dose" catheter directed therapy is the treatment of choice for its best results and its no significant systemic effect.

In other terms, local thrombolysis in late graft thrombosis can restore the blood flow avoiding surgical emergency therapy, it also permits the performance of minimal surgical interventions or percutaneous angioplasty.

The effectiveness of intra-arterial thrombolytic therapy in the management of the late graft thrombosis is impressive. However over half of the patients of our series were normally considered out of any time limit for starting an effective thrombolysis, and in some cases they have been successfully treated. The indications for thrombolytic therapy must be wider also because this kind of treatment didn't preclude, if ineffective, any surgical procedure in any time it become necessary.

Close involvement between surgery and thrombolytic therapy is essential. We recommend a more wider use of thrombolysis also because the prospect of selective clot lysis instead of, or preceding, reconstruction is attractive.

The condition of the affected limb, and the patient should be carefully monitored. Any deterioration, particularly resulting in neurological impairment, should be considered an indication for alternative treatment to thrombolysis.

The use of new lytic drugs may contribute to achieve more lysis. Preliminary results with new drugs or association of lytic agents and/or adjuvant drugs are encouraging, with a durable complete lysis in 93% of the cases, not only in distal arterial occlusions but also in late graft thrombosis. In conclusion, we might expect more limb salvages.

REFERENCES

1. Ascer, E., Collier, P., Gupta, S.K., Veith, F.J., (1987) Reoperation for polytetrafluoroethylene bypass failure; the importance of distal outflow site and operative technique in determining outcome. *J Vasc Surg,* 5: 298-310.
2. Barr, H., Lancashire, M. J. R., Torrie, E.P.H., Galland, R.B., (1991) Intra-arterial thrombolytic therapy in the management of acute and chronic limb ischemia. *Br J Surg,* 78: 284-287.
3. Bartlett, S.T., Olinde, A.J., Flinn, W.R., McCarthy, W.J., Fahey, V.A., Bergan, J.J., Yao, J.S.T., (1987) The reoperative potential of infrainguinal bypass: Long-term limb and patient survival. *J Vasc Surg,* 5: 170-179.

4. Becker, R.C., (1991) Seminars in Thrombosis, Thrombolysis and Vascular Biology. *Cardiology*, 78:13-22.
5. Becker, G.J., Holden, R.W., Rabe, F.E., (1984) Contrast extravasation from a Gore-tex graft: a complication of thrombolytic therapy. *A J R*, 142: 573-4.
6. Berridge, D.C., Gregson, R.H.S., Makin, G.S., Hopkinson, B.R., (1990) Tissue plasminogen activator in perpheral arterial thrombolysis. *Br J Surg*, 77: 179-182.
7. Berridge, D.C., Gregson, R.H.S., Hopkinson, B.R., Makin, G.S., (1991) Randomized trial of intra- arterial recombinant tissue plasminogen activator, intravenous recombinant tissue plasminogen activator and intra-arterial streptokinase in peripheral arterial thrombolysis. *Br J Surg*, 78: 988-995.
8. Brewster, D.C., Lasalle, A.J., Robinson, J.G., (1983) Femoropopliteal graft failures: clinical conse- quences and success of secondary reconstructions. *Arch Surg*, 118: 1043-7.
9. Cohen, L.H., Kaplan, M., Bernhard, V.M., (1986) Intraoperative streptokinase: an adjunct to mechanical thrombectomy in the management of acute ischemia. *Arch Surg*, 121: 708-715.
10. Cragg, A., Smith, T., Corson, J., (1991) Two urokinase dose regimes in native arterial and graft occlu-sions: initial results of a prospective, randomized clinical trial. *Radiology*, 178: 681-686.
11. D'Addato, M., (1986) Intra-arterial thrombolysis with urokinase in acute arterial thrombosis of limbs. In: Progress in angiology, edited by Balas, P., pp. 557 561, Minerva Medica, Torino.
12. Durham, J.D., Geller, S.C., Abbott, W.M., Shapiro, H., Waltman A.C., Walker, T.G., Brewster, D.C., Athanasoulis, C.A., (1989) Regional infusion of urokinas into occluded lower-extremity bypass grafts: long term clinical results. *Radiology*, 172: 83-87.
13. Early, G.L., Hannah, H.III, (1985)A technique for postembolectomy streptokinase infusion. *Arch Surg*, 120: 1395-1397.
14. Earnshaw, J.J., Gregson, R.T.H.S., Makin, G.S., Hopkinson, B.R., (1987) Early results of low dose intra-arterial streptokinase therapy in acute and subacute lower limb arterial is-chemia. *Br J Surg*, 74:504-507.
15. Earnshaw, J.J., (1991) Thrombolytic therapy in the management of acute limb ischemia. *Br J Surg*, 78:261-269.
16. Eskridge, J.M., Becker, G.J., Rabe, F.E., Richmond, B.D., Holden, R.W., Yune, H.Y., Klatte, E.D., (1983) Catheter-related thrombosis and fibrinolytic therapy. *Radiology*, 149: 429-434.
17. Fennerty, A.G., Levine, M.N., Hirsh, H J., (1989) Hemorrhagic complications of throm-bolytic thera-py in the treatment of myocardial infarction and venous thromboembolism. *Chest*, 95 (2): 88-97.
18. Flinn, W.R., Harris, J.P., Rudo, N.D., (1981) Atheroembolism as cause of graft failure in femoro-distal reconstruction. *Surgery*, 90: 698-706.
19. Fiessinger, J.N., Vitoux, J.F., Pernes, J.M., Roncato, M., Aiach, M., Gaux,J.C., (1986) Complica- tions of intraarterial Urokinase-Lys-Plasminogen infusion therapy in arterial is-chemia of lower limbs. *A J R*, 146: 157-159.
20. Gaston, J.G., Sensarma, P.K., Sadiq, S., (1991) Urokinase infusion in total occlusion of periphal vascular disease. *Kans Med*, 3: 73-75.
21. Graor, R.A., Risius, B., Young, J.R., Geisinger, M.A., Zelch, M.G., Smith, J.A.M., Ruschhaupt, W.F., (1984) Low-dose streptokinase for selective thrombolysis: systemic ef-fects and complications. *Radiology*, 152: 35-9.
22. Graor, R.A., Risius, B., Young, J.R., Lucas, F.V., Beven, E.G., Hertzer, N.R., Krajewski, L.P., O'Hara, P.J., Olin, J., Ruschhupt, W.F., (1988) Thrombolysis of peripheral arterial bypass grafts: surgical thrombectomy compared with thrombolysis. A preliminary report. *J Vasc Surg*, 7: 347-355.
23. Haber, E., Quertermous, M.D., Matsueda, G.R., Runge, M.S., Bode, C., (1990) Antibody-targeted thrombolytic agents. *Jpn Circ J*, 54: 345-353.
24. Hargrove, W.C., Berkowitz, H.D., Freiman, D.B., McLean, G., Ring, E.J., Roberts, B., (1982Recanalization of totally occluded femoropopliteal vein graft with low-dose strep-tokinase infusion. *Surgery*, 92: 890-5.
25. Katzen, B.T., Edwards, K.C., Albert, A.S., Van Breda, A., (1984) Low-dose direct fibrinolysis in peripheral vascular disease. *J Vasc Surg*, 1: 718.
26. Katzen, B.T., Van Breda, A., (1988) The current status of catheter directed fibrinolysis in the treatment of arterial and graft occlusions. In: Arterial surgery: new diagnostic and operative techniques, edited by Bergan, J.J., Yao, J.S.T., pp 119-134. Grune & Stratton, Orlando.

27. McNamara, T.O., Fischer, J.R., (1985) Thrombolysis of peripheral arterial and graft occlusions: improved results using high-dose urokinase. *A J R,* 144: 769-75.
28. Meyerovitz, M.F., Goldhaber, S.Z., Reagan, K., Polak, J.F., Kandarpa, K., Grassi, C., Donovan, B.C., Bettman, M.A., Harringon, D.P., (1990) Recombinant tissue-tipe plasminogen activator versus urokinase in periferal arterial and graft occlusions: a randomizzed trial. *Radiology,* 175: 75-78.
29. Minar, E., Ahmadi, R.A., Ehringer, H., Marosi, L., Scholf, R., Czembirek, M., Czembirek, H., (1986) Local low-dose thrombolytic therapy of peripheral arterial occlusive disease. In: Conservative therapy of arterial occlusive disease,edited by Trubestein, G., pp 42-50. George Thieme Verlag. Stuttgart, NewYork.
30. Mori, K.W., Bookstein, J.J., Heeney, D.J., Bardin, J.A., Donnelly, K.J., Rhodes, G.A., Dilley, R.B., Warmath, M.A., Bernstein, E.F., (1983) Selective streptokinase infusion: clinical and laboratory correlates. *Radiology,* 148: 677-682.
31. Parent, F.N.III, Bernhard, V.M., Pabst, T.S.III, McIntyre, K.E., Hunter, G.C., Malone, J.M., (1989) Fibrinolytic treatment of residual thrombus after catheter embolectomy for severe lower limb ischemia. *J Vasc Surg,* 9: 153-160.
32. Perler, B.A., White, R.I.Jr., Ernst, C.B., Williams, G.M., (1985) Low-dose thrombolytic therapy for infrainguinal graft occlusions: an idea whose time has passed? *J Vasc Surg,* 2: 799-805.
33. Perler, B.A., Kinnison, M., Halden, W.J., (1986) Transgraft hemorrhage: a serious complication of low-dose thrombolytic therapy. *J Vasc Surg,* 3: 936-938.
34. Pernes, J.M., Vitoux, J.F., Brendit, P., Raynaud, A., Parola, J.L., Roth, J.P., Angel, C.Y., Fiessinger, J.N., Roncato, M., Gaux, J.C., (1986) Acute peripheral arterial and graft occlusion: treatment with selective infusion of urokinase and lysil-plasminogen. *Radiology,* 158, 481-5.
35. Pernes, J.M., De Almeida, A.M.C., Vitoux J.F., Fiessinger, J.N., Brenot, Ph., Gaux, J.C., (1988) Thrombolyse locale dans le oblitrations artrielles aigus des membres inferiurs et des pontages. *Arteres et Veines,* 7: 87-92.
36. Quinones-Baldrich, W.J., Zirler, E.R., Hiatt, J.C., (1985) Intraoperative fibrinolytic therapy: an adjunct to catheter thromboembolectomy. *J Vasc Surg,* 2: 319-322.
37. Quinones-Baldrich, W.J., Ziomek, S., Henderson, T.C., Moore, W.S., (1986) Intraoperative fibrinolytic therapy: experimental evaluation. *J Vasc Surg,* 4: 229-32.
38. Quinones-Baldrich, W.J., Baker, J.D., Busuttil, R.W., Machleder, H.I., Moore, W.S., (1989) Intraoperative infusion of lytic drugs for thrombotic complications of revascularization. *J Vasc Surg,* 10: 408-417.
39. Rabe, F.E., Becker, G.J., Richmond, B.D., Yune, H.Y., Holden, R.W., Dilley, R.S., Klatte, E.C., (1982) Contrast extravasation trough Dacron grafts: a sequela of low-dose streptokinase therapy. *A J R.,* 138: 917-920.
40. Risius, B., Zelch, M.G., Graor, R.A., Geisinger, M.A., Smith, J.A.M., Piraino, D.W., (1984) Catheter directed low-dose streptokinase infusion: a preliminary experience. *Radiology,* 150: 349-355.
41. Rosner, N.H., Doris, P.E., (1984) Contrast extravasation trough a Gore-tex graft: a sequela of low-dose streptokinase therapy. *A J R,* 143: 633-34.
42. Rush, D.S., Gewertz, B.L., Chien-Tai, L., Neely, S.M., Ball, D.G., Beasley, B., Zarins, C.K., (1983) Selective infusion of streptokinase for arteial thrombosis. *Surgery,* 93: 828-833.
43. Sautot, J., Demerciere, J.F., Sautot, M.D., (1976) Traitement thrombolytique isole', ou completant le traitement chirurgical, des ischemies aigues gravissimes des membes inferieurs. *Lyon Chirurgical,* 2: 92-96.
44. Seabrook, G.R., Mewissen, M.W., Schmitt, D.D., Reifsyder, T., Brandyk, D.F., (1991) Percutaneous intraarterial thrombolysis in the treatment of thrombosis of lower extremity arterial reconstructions. *J Vasc Surg,* 13: 646-651.
45. Sicard, G.A., Schier, J.J., Totty, W.G., Gilula, L.A., Walker, W.B., Etheredge, E.E., Anderson, C.B., (1985) Thrombolytic therapy for acute arterial occlusion. *J Vasc Surg,* 2: 65-78.
46. Sullivan, K.L., Gardiner, G.A., Kandarpa, K., Bonn, J., Shapiro, M.J., (1991) Efficacy of thrombo-lysis in infrainguinal bypass grafts. *Circulation,* 83: 99-105.
47. Van Breda, A., Robinson, J.C., Feldman, L., Waltman, A.C., Brewster, D.C., Abbott, W.M., Athanasoulis, C.A., (1984) Local thrombolysis in the treatment of arterial graft occlusions. *J Vasc Surg,* 1: 103-107.
48. Van Der Wall, E.E., Van Dijkman, P.R.M., De Roos, A., Doornbos, J., Van der Laarse, A., Manger Cats, V., Van Voorthuisen, A.E., Matheijssen, N.A.A., Bruschke, A.V.G., (1990) Diagnostic signifi-cance of gadolinium-DTPA (diethylenetriamine penta-acetic acid) en-

hanced magnetic resonance imaging in thrombolytic treatment for acute myocardial infarction: its potential in assessing reperfusion. *Eur J Radiol,* 11: 1-9.
49. Veith, F.J., Ascer, E., Gupta, S.K., White-Flores, S., Srayregen, S., Scher, L.A., Samson, R.H., (1985) Tibiotibial vein bypass grafts: a new operation for limbs salvage. *J Vasc Surg,* 2: 552-557.
50. Verstraete, M., Hess, H., Mahler, F., Mietaschk, A., Roth, F., Schneider, E., Baert, A., Verhaeghe, R., (1988) Femoro-popliteal artery thrombolysis with intra-arterial infusion of rt-PA report of a pilot trial. *Eur J Vasc Surg,* 2: 155-159.

Re-Operative Surgery For Aortoiliac Vascular Disease With Reference to Atherosclerotic Progression and Complications of Artificial Prosthetics

G.J. Eckholdt and L.H. Hollier

Department of Surgery, Ochsner Clinic and Alton Ochsner Medical Foundation, Louisiana State University Medical Center and Tulane University Medical Center, New Orleans, Louisiana, U.S.A.

INTRODUCTION

Surgery of the aorta and its immediate branches is performed with acceptable morbidity and mortality. Advances in preoperative evaluation, intraoperative management, and postoperative care have allowed patients to recover quickly from major aortic surgery and derive long-term benefit from surgical intervention. Nevertheless, as atherosclerosis is a progressive disease in most advanced cases, bypass grafts or endarterectomized aortic segments may experience failure in a small percentage of patients, not necessarily related to the prosthetic material itself nor the native aorta. Often, atherosclerotic occlusive disease progresses in the superficial femoral and profunda femoris arteries, causing failure of the aortic graft and recurrent symptoms of claudication or frank ischemia of the lower extremity.

In addition, artificial prosthetics themselves are subject to disease progression in the form of neointimal hyperplasia occurring over a period of months to years, a process usually confined to anastomotic areas, but most pronounced at distal anastomoses and often causing graft attrition in the first few years after placement[18]. A second complication related to suture lines is anastomotic pseudoaneurysm, most often seen at femoral anastomoses. This complication demands evaluation of the entire prosthesis and its incorporation into host tissues.

Besides anastomotic aneurysm, in patients subjected to surgery originally for aneurysmal disease of the infrarenal aorta, true aneurysm can develop above the proximal anastomotic line involving the mesenteric circulation and even the thoracic aorta, making re-operative surgery in these cases difficult and complex. These cases demand careful and precise preoperative studies and planning prior to surgical intervention.

Another infrequent complication of prior aortic surgery, again taxing the most proficient vascular surgeon, is graft infection, probably the most serious threat to a patient's life and limb. The morbidity and mortality of this complication remains high in these patients despite prompt graft excision and extra-anatomical bypass. In selected patients, in situ graft replacement may be an alternative if bleeding from an anastomotic disruption and not intraabdominal sepsis is the pathologic finding.

Finally, technical errors made at the initial operation can result in immediate postoperative complications often requiring immediate or delayed re-operative surgery. These problems include colonic ischemia due to interruption of either the hypogastric arteries or the inferior mesenteric artery or collaterals, including the "meandering mesenteric" artery.

Preoperative planning based on angiographic findings should address the internal iliac arteries which are essential to pelvic perfusion and often provide important colonic and lower extremity collaterals. Vasculogenic impotence and colonic or even spinal cord ischemia can result from excluding the hypogastrics from direct grafting or indirect perfusion following aortofemoral bypass.

This paper will address complications necessitating re-operative surgery on the aorta or its prosthetic replacement and discuss preventive measures to avoid redo surgery.

Preventive Measures

Although intuitively simple, patients should be strongly discouraged from smoking prior to primary or secondary surgery. It is well known that smoking is a major risk factor in the progression of atherosclerosis in both coronary and peripheral vascular beds, and studies show poorer patency among grafts placed in patients who continue to smoke[25,42]. In addition to attempting to control extraneous negative determinants of graft survival, the vascular surgeon should thoroughly evaluate the patient preoperatively for other unrecognized vascular disease which could prohibit success of the planned re-operative intervention. Clinical history is extremely important in uncovering any overt coronary disease. In addition, the coronary angiographic data reported by Hertzer et al. [27] who studied patients undergoing peripheral vascular surgery, are impressive. Severe correctable coronary artery disease was identified in 250 patients among a group of 1000, many of whom required coronary artery bypass grafting prior to their peripheral vascular procedures.

Despite the prevalence of coronary disease among vascular patients, it is unnecessary to perform coronary angiography in all vascular patients since, in selected patients, noninvasive studies of coronary perfusion and ventricular function have become effective in identifying patients at risk for coronary events[15,20,23,34,39]. Recently, dipyridamole-thallium imaging has been proven effective in selecting patients who may benefit from coronary angiography and revascularization, either via bypass grafting or balloon angioplasty, prior to peripheral vascular surgery. With judicious use of the noninvasive tests of coronary disease, effective management of the peripheral vascular patient can be achieved with minimal cardiac morbidity and mortality[20]. In particular, in cases of re-operative surgery which may be more involved and difficult both for the surgeon and patient, cardiac morbidity may be increased and should be addressed prior to the re-operative procedure.

Preoperative Planning

Prior to any redo surgery on the aorta or its immediate branches, the patient's primary disease process and original operative procedure should be studied thoroughly with the original history and presentation kept in mind along with the original angiograms or CT scans and operative notes.

Whether the patient underwent surgery for aneurysmal or occlusive disease of the aorta is important to document. The level of the proximal anastomoses should be known in cases both of occlusive and aneurysmal disease as well as whether any reimplantations of the renal arteries or inferior mesenteric artery was performed. Whether the proximal anastomosis was performed in an end-to-end or end-to-side fashion should be obtained from the operative note. If a thromboendarterectomy of the aorta was performed, the level at which the endarterectomy began and ended along with the management of the iliac and femoral vessels should be noted. In cases of aorto-bifemoral bypass, the level at which the femoral anastomoses were performed and the handling of the profunda femoris should be known. If a pseudoaneurysm of the aortic prosthesis has developed, the entire graft needs evaluation to rule out an infectious cause and to determine whether any other pseudoaneurysms or aneurysms have developed. Prior to reoperation, all data related to the original disease and operation and current presentation should be gathered and incorporated into a systematic approach to management.

In order to complete this historical data, angiography in cases of occlusive disease and CT scanning complemented by angiographic studies for aneurysmal disease are essential to planning re-operative aortic surgery. In cases of occlusive disease, multi-plane arteriography more precisely delineates occlusive disease of the common, external and internal iliac vessels than does traditional anterior-posterior projections[47]. Posterior iliac or hypogastric plaques are well visualized with this approach. Important mesenteric collaterals, whether based on an inferior mesenteric artery, a meandering mesenteric artery or a hypogastric collateral, will be appreciated on angiograms and thus may be incorporated into the revascularization.

In order to avoid colonic ischemia, another infrequent but morbid complication after aortic surgery, consideration should be given to reimplantation of the inferior mesenteric artery under certain circumstances. Criteria including severe superior mesenteric artery disease, exclusion of hypogastric circulation, an inferior mesenteric artery stump pressure less than 40 mmHg, or a history of prior colon resection may each necessitate inferior mesenteric artery reimplantation[6]. Interruption of collaterals to the bowel may be more frequent in a difficult case involving dissection around vessels and other structures in a re-operative field.

In addition, if aorto-bifemoral bypass is contemplated, pelvic perfusion must be maintained to one and, if possible, both hypogastric arteries. Iliopoulos et al.[31,32] have studied both clinically and experimentally the "critical" hypogastric circulation and detailed the catastrophic effects of inadequate pelvic perfusion after surgery and displayed the importance of maintaining bilateral hypogastric perfusion when considering a procedure which may not provide direct or indirect blood flow to the hypogastric arteries. Both Cronenwett et al.[13] and Seagraves and Rutherford[46] discuss methods to ensure pelvic perfusion from limbs of a bifurcated aortic graft with improvement of symptoms in patients with buttock claudication and/or impotence.

Patients who have had prior aortic replacement for aneurysmal disease require both an abdominal and thoracic CT scan to evaluate the entire aorta. All anastomotic lines should be visualized in cases of both anastomotic pseudoaneurysm and true aneurysm.

In a large group of over 130 patients who have undergone repair of a thoracoabdominal aneurysm, approximately 21% have had prior infrarenal aortic replacement (Figs. 1, 2). The importance of continued surveillance of patients with aortic aneurysmal disease cannot be overemphasized.

Surgical Techniques - Extra-abdominal

Although aorto-bi-iliac and aorto-bifemoral bypass for occlusive and aneurysmal disease is durable[11], complications related to both re-occlusive and aneurysmal phenomena as well as complications of the prosthesis itself can occur and may demand management to prevent limb loss and mortality.

In cases where a single limb of an aorto-bifemoral bypass becomes occluded, a femoral approach to the occlusion may be feasible, especially if the occlusion occurs acutely within hours or a few weeks[4,8,30,36]. This involves a groin exploration with exposure of the femoral anastomosis and control of the other adjacent vessels followed by passage of a balloon catheter and removal of thrombus and re-establishment of flow.

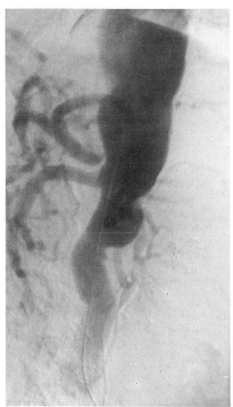

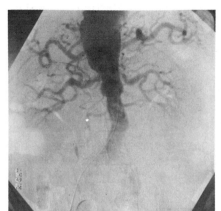

Figs. 1-2. This transfemoral aortogram displays a large thoracoabdominal aneurysm above an infrarenal aortic graft placed for aneurysmal disease.

In cases where the occlusion is more chronic, an endarterectomy loop stripper may be inserted into the graft limb with removal of the adherent occlusive debris while maintaining proximal balloon occlusion of the limb.

Angioscopy may play a valuable role in this instance[51], evaluating the results of both balloon thrombectomy and mechanical thrombo-endarterectomy. Other methods which have more limited roles in these instances are thrombolytic therapy and balloon angioplasty. Thrombolysis with urokinase often serves as only a temporizing measure in these cases where a more definitive distal reconstruction of the profunda femoris is often necessary. Similarly, balloon angioplasty may allow recanalization of an occluded bypass limb and serve to delineate the more distal problem which needs to be corrected.

Many studies have stressed the importance of the profunda femoris artery in maintaining the patency of aorto-bifemoral bypass graft limbs. In cases where extra-abdominal reconstruction is necessary, a profundoplasty may be helpful to ensure the longevity of the graft limb[38,40]. The profundoplasty can be performed with autogenous vein or adjacent, transposed endarterectomized superficial femoral artery. More distal exposure for extended profundoplasty can be obtained for more extensive disease threatening limb viability.

In patients with an occluded aortic limb, extra-anatomical femoral-femoral bypass may be an alternative[17]. Again, with biplane aortography, disease of the patent limb of the bypass graft and its immediate branches should be excluded. This technique avoids re-operative abdominal surgery and can be performed under local anesthesia in patients who are prohibitive risks for major aortic reconstruction.

Abdominal Approaches

When an entire aorto-iliac or aorto-femoral bypass fails or a proximal stenosis is recognized within a graft limb or a pseudoaneurysm or true aneurysm develops at the level of the abdominal aorta, an abdominal approach to the aorta may be required. In large studies[12,22,26], successful re-exploration of the graft has been performed with revision or replacement of the aortic graft. Complications and mortality have been acceptable. Often in patients with occlusive disease, the proximal graft itself can be left in place and used as the takeoff of the new aortic bifurcated graft, minimizing extensive dissection at the level of the left renal vein and avoiding juxta- or supra-renal aortic crossclamping. If, however, a situation mandates supra-renal or supra-celiac crossclamping, this can be achieved successfully with acceptable mortality and a low incidence of acute renal failure[48].

If transperitoneal exposure of the aorta will be extremely difficult due to multiple prior operations or if definite supra-renal aortic crossclamping will be required, two approaches to avoid the original operative field may be employed. Medial visceral rotation has been used very successfully in cases where supra-celiac crossclamping has been necessary for mesenteric ischemia[14]. Both extensive trans-aortic endarterectomy and anterograde mesenteric bypasses have been performed with acceptable morbidity and mortality via medial visceral rotation for aortic exposure. Another approach, extraperitoneal, has been used very effectively in cases of redo surgery. It involves an oblique left flank incision through which access is provided to the retroperitoneum and a posterior approach to the aorta which obviates dissection in a re-operative field[48].

Although very similar to the approach to thoracoabdominal aneurysms, this incision need not extend into the pleural space, but it does give access to the subdiaphragmatic aorta and its mesenteric branches. This exposure is excellent for recurrent aneurysmal disease above a prior infrarenal aortic graft. With both of these approaches, bleeding from major aortic branches is well controlled with balloon occluding catheters placed within the aorta, another advantage of this posterior approach. Less dissection and fewer clamps are necessary for distal control.

Another useful maneuver which can be performed from both of these approaches is endarterectomy of the supra-renal aorta, the extent of which dictated by the severity of the disease[10].

Extra-anatomical

Extra-anatomical bypass is particularly useful when infection of an aortic prosthesis is highly suspected or confirmed. Although the incidence of aortic graft infection is low[2], it can provide extremely difficult and challenging management problems.

Most commonly, axillo-bifemoral bypass with ring-enforced PTFE is employed before or after excision of an infected aortic prosthesis. Most recent studies[24,41], indicate that the extra-anatomical bypass should be placed prior to excision of the aortic graft to improve blood flow to the lower extremities and pelvis before aortic crossclamping, negating ischemic time and overall operative and general anesthetic time as the axillo-bifemoral bypass can be done under local anesthesia.

If the groins are involved with the septic process, remote distal bypass can be performed to either the distal profunda femoris arteries using a more distal anterior approach or virgin lateral approach, adjacent to the sartorius muscle, again avoiding the infected groins. Other extra-anatomical bypasses may employ the obturator foramen[49] to direct a graft away from an infected groin or limb of an aortic prosthetic. Other less frequently used extra-anatomical bypasses in very selected patients include ascending aortic to femoral bypass[9] and thoracic aortic-to-aortic or femoral bypass[45]. These procedures are very infrequently used or needed, but may be a viable alternative in patients who have undergone multiple prior abdominal operations for vascular disease or other reasons or have aortic graft infection limited to the abdomen.

SPECIFIC SURGICAL PROBLEMS

An Occluded Aorto-Iliac or Aorto-Femoral Graft Limb

Early after aortic surgery an extra-abdominal approach with thrombectomy and/or endarterectomy can be performed successfully[30]. These may need to be combined with revision of the distal anastomosis or profundoplasty, preferably with autogenous vein or adjacent superficial femoral artery. Late occlusion of a graft limb may require revision of the graft limb or complete graft replacement depending on angiographic findings. An extraperitoneal approach can be used to replace or revise a single graft limb. If the patient cannot tolerate major abdominal surgery, femoral-femoral bypass is a durable alternative if biplane angiography shows that the donor femoral artery has minimal proximal external or common iliac occlusive disease. Anastomotic revision with profundoplasty may occasionally need to be combined with more distal bypass for improved runoff and patency of the graft[1,7,43,50].

A Completely Occluded Aortic Graft. In additional to progression of proximal disease, technical problems should be considered as a possible cause in cases of an occluded aorto-iliac or aorto-femoral bypass. Angiograms are very helpful in deciding the operative approach to these patients. Technical problems may include a proximal anastomosis too distal on the aorta[5] or limbs of the bifurcated graft sewn into diseased iliac arteries. A peculiar finding in women which may cause graft failure is hypoplastic aortic syndrome[33]. These women, who are often smokers, have small aortas and should have grafts tailored obliquely at the proximal anastomosis, otherwise one is tempted to use a graft that may be too small. Thromboendarterectomy with vein patch is an alternative in this group.

In the group of patients with aortic graft failure or thrombosis of an aortic endarterectomy, an aortic replacement with a bifurcated aorto-bifemoral bypass is the treatment of choice. A repeat aorto-iliac bypass probably should not be done here, although we do not necessarily consider primary aorto-bifemoral bypass as the initial procedure of choice for aorto-iliac occlusive disease[1]. The procedure can be performed through a retroperitoneal approach or transperitoneally with medial visceral rotation, two maneuvers to avoid difficult re-operative abdominal exposures. Depending again on angiographic data, supra-renal crossclamping with more involved revascularization may be necessary. An endarterectomized proximal juxtarenal aorta can serve as the origin of the synthetic graft.

Aneurysm and Pseudoaneurysm. Aneurysmal dilatation of the aorta at or above the proximal anastomosis requires replacement of the aneurysmal segment. The approach may be direct through a transperitoneal route, but a safer, more strategic exposure is retroperitoneal. The aneurysm likely involves the renals and may entail supra-celiac or thoracic aortic crossclamping, which can easily be performed with the retroperitoneal exposure. These patients, in addition to renal failure, are subject to spinal cord ischemia and paraplegia which can be reduced to a minimum with appropriate measures[29].

Pseudoaneurysm of the proximal aortic or distal anastomoses requires graft revision or replacement at the site of disruption (Figs. 3-4). Recent evidence[3] also indicates that late pseudoaneurysm may result from bacterial colonization with coagulase negative Staphylococcus. With proper culture techniques, Kaebnick et al. have isolated a slime-producing Staphylococcus from 87% of their pseudoaneurysms[35]. In another study, Downs et al. have found bacteria by electron microscopy in twenty of twenty-six cases of anas-

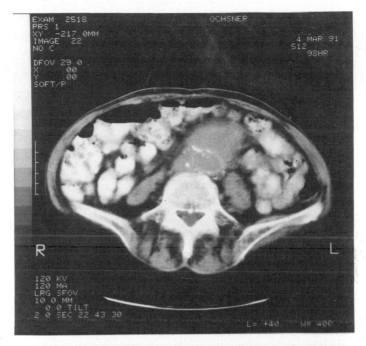

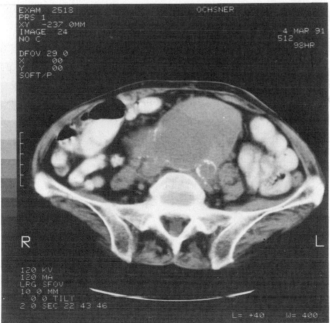

Figs. 3-4. A CT scan demonstrates a large pseudoaneurysm which developed at the level of the aortic bifurcation.

tomotic pseudoaneurysm[19]. Given this knowledge, the incorporation of the entire prosthesis in cases of pseudoaneurysm should be evaluated. Often, replacement of the graft or involved limb will be necessary. In these cases, PTFE may be the conduit of choice. Compared to Dacron grafts, PTFE grafts have reduced bacterial adherence[44] and may therefore be an advantage in the presence of coagulase negative Staphylococcus.

Infected Aortic Graft. One of the most dreaded complications of aortic surgery is graft infection and its sequelae. Most recent large series support the use of extra-anatomical bypass, prior to aortic graft excision[24,41]. Three of the immediate complications of this procedure are persistent abdominal sepsis, infection of the new bypass and aortic stump blowout, which is usually fatal. The difficulty with the aortic stump arises after debridement and the inability to provide adequate tissue coverage of the oversewn aorta. The major long-term morbidity of remote extra-anatomical bypass are poor long-term patency and the need for amputation[41]. To avoid these complica-tions which exact a high morbidity and mortality, in situ graft replacement has been successful in selected patients[16,21,28,52]. However, selection is essential. It requires making a distinction between infection and simple aorto-enteric erosion[28]. This distinction has clinical applications which strongly influence the management of these patients. Graft excision followed by PTFE graft replacement may be feasible in patients with minimal signs of infection, but if the patient has obvious signs of infection, he is best served by extra-anatomical reconstruction followed by aortic graft excision. All patients who undergo in situ replacement or oversewing of the aortic stump need tissue coverage, usually greater omentum. These patients also require long-term antibiotic therapy, usually for life.

REFERENCES

1. Baird RJ, Feldman P, Miller JT, et al (1977). Subsequent downstream repair after aorta-iliac andaortafemoral bypass operations. *Surgery* 82:785-793.
2. Bandyk DF (1990). Aortic graft infection. In: Seminars in Vascular Surgery, edited by Bandyk DF, pp. 122-132, W. B. Saunders Co., Philadelphia, PA.
3. Bergamini TM (1990). Vascular prostheses infection caused by bacterial biofilms. In: Seminars in Vascular Surgery, edited by Bandyk DF and Rutherford RB, pp. 101-109, W. B. Saunders, Co., Philadelphia, PA.
4. Bernhard VM, Ray LI, Towne JB (1977). The reoperation of choice for aortofemoral graft occlusion. *Surgery* 82:867-874.
5. Bernhard VM (1985). Late vascular graft thrombosis. In: Complications in Vascular Surgery, edited by Bernhard VM and Towne JB, pp. 187-204, Grune and Stratton, Inc., Orlando, FL.
6. Brewster DC, Franklin DP, Cambria RP, et al (1990). Intestinal ischemia complicating abdominal aortic surgery. *Surgery* 109:447-454.
7. Brewster DC, Perler BA, Robison JG, et al (1982). Aortofemoral graft for multilevel occlusive disease. Predictors of success and need for distal bypass. *Arch Surg* 117:1593-1600.
8. Cohn LH, Moore WS, Hall AD (1969). Extra-abdominal management of late aortofemoral graft thrombosis. *Surgery* 67:775-779.
9. Cooley DA, Wukasck DC (1979). Aortoiliac occlusive disease. In: Techniques in Vascular Surgery, pp. 130-146, W. B. Saunders Co., Philadelphia, PA.

10. Cowgill LD (1987). Endarterectomy of the suprarenal abdominal aorta. In: Cardiac Surgery: State of the Art Reviews, edited by Cowgill LD, pp. 515-520, Hanley and Belfus, Inc., Philadelphia, PA.
11. Crawford ES, Bomberger RA, Glaeser DH, et al (1981). Aortoiliac occlusive disease: Factors influencing survival and function following reconstructive operation over a twenty-five year period. *Surgery* 90:1055-1067.
12. Crawford ES, Manning LG, Kelly TF (1976). "Redo" surgery after operation for aneurysm and occlusion of the abdominal aorta. *Surgery* 81:41-52.
13. Cronenwett JL, Gooch JB, Garrett E (1982). Internal iliac revascularization during aortofemoral bypass. *Arch Surg* 117:838-839.
14. Cunningham CG, Reilly LM, Rapp JH, et al (1991). Chronic visceral ischemia. Three decades of progress. *Ann Surg* 214:276-288.
15. Cutter BS (1991). Interpretation and results of intravenous dipyridamole-thallium scintigraphy. In: Seminars in Vascular Surgery, edited by Rutherford RB, pp. 83-89, W. B. Saunders Co., Philadelphia, PA.
16. Daugherty M, Shearer GR, Ernst CG (1979). Primary aorto-duodenal fistula: Extra-anatomic vascular reconstruction not required for successful management. *Surgery* 86:399-401.
17. DePalma RG (1987). Reoperation for occluded aortic grafts. In: Re-operative Vascular Surgery, edited by Trout HH, Giordano JM, and DePalma RG, pp. 95-112, Marcel Decker, Inc., New York, NY.
18. DeWeese JA (1985). Anastomotic neointimal fibrous hyperplasia. In: Complications in Vascular Surgery, edited by Bernhard VM and Towne JB, pp. 157-170, Grune and Stratton, Inc., Orlando, FL.
19. Downs AR, Guzman R, Formichi M, et al (1991). Etiology of prosthetic anastomotic false aneurysms: Pathologic and structural evaluation in 26 cases. *C J Surg* 34:53-58.
20. Eagle KA, Coley CM (1991). Cost-effective use of dipyridamole-thallium imaging for cardiac risk stratification. In: Seminars in Vascular Surgery, edited by Rutherford RB, pp. 100-105, W. B. Saunders Co., Philadelphia, PA.
21. Elliot JP, Smith RF, Szilagyi DE (1973). Aorto-enteric and paraprosthetic-enteric fistulas. *Arch Surg* 108:479-490.
22. Fulenwider JT, Smith RBIII, Johnson RW, et al (1982). Re-operative abdominal arterial surgery - a ten- year experience. *Surgery* 93:20-27.
23. Goldman L (1988). Assessment of the patient with known or suspected ischemic heart disease for non-cardiac surgery. *Br J Anaesth* 61:38-43.
24. Goldstone J (1987). The infected infra-renal aortic graft. *Acta Chir Scand* 538:72-86.
25. Greenhalgh RM, Laing SP, Cole PV, and Taylor GW (1981). Smoking and arterial reconstruction. *Br J Surg* 68:605-607.
26. Haiart DC, Callam MJ, Murie JA, et al (1991). Re-operations for late complications following abdominal aortic re-operations. *Br J Surg* 78:204-206.
27. Hertzer NR, Beven EG, Young JR, et al (1983). Coronary artery disease in peripheral vascular patients. A classification of 1000 angiograms and results of surgical management. *Ann Surg* 199:223-233.
28. Higgins RSD, Steed DL, Julian JB, et al (1990). The management of aorto-enteric and paraprosthetic fistulae. *J Cardiovasc Surg* 31:81-86.
29. Hollier LH, Moore WMJr (1990). Avoidance of renal and neurologic complications following thoracoabdominal aortic aneurysm repair. *Acta Chir Scand Suppl* 555:129-135.
30. Hyde GL, McCready RA, Schwartz RW, et al (1983). Durability of thrombectomy of occluded aortofemoral graft limbs. *Surgery* 94:748-751.
31. Iliopoulos JI, Howanity PE, Pierce GE, et al (1987). The critical hypogastric circulation. *Am J Surg* 154:671-675.
32. Iliopoulos JI, Hermreck AS, Thomas JH, et al (1988). Hemodynamics of the hypogastric arterial circulation. *J Vasc Surg* 9:637-642.
33. Jernigan WR, Fallat ME, Hatfield DR (1983). Hypoplastic aortoiliac syndrome: An entity peculiar to women. *Surgery* 94:752-757.
34. Johnson GJr, Nishikimi N (1991). Identifying cardiac risk in major vascular operations. In: Seminars in Vascular Surgery, edited by Rutherford RB, pp. 63-66, W. B. Saunders Co., Philadelphia, PA.
35. Kaebnick HW, Bandyk DF, Bergamini TM, et al (1987). The microbiology of explanted vascular prostheses. *Surgery* 102:756-762.
36. LeGrand DR, Vermilion BD, Hayes JP (1982). Management of the occluded aortofemoral graft limb. *Surgery* 93:818-821.

37. Lorentzen JE, Nielsen OM (1987). Treatment of the paninfected aorto-bi-femoral pros-thesis. An alternative method using autogenous great saphenous vein. *Acta Chir Scand* 538:87-89.
38. Malone JM, Moore WS, Goldstone J (1975). The natural history of bilateral aortofemoral bypass grafts for ischemia of the lower extremities. *Arch Surg* 110:1300-1306.
39. Miller DD (1991). Clinical risk factor analysis and electrocardiographic evaluation modalities. In: Seminars in Vascular Surgery, edited by Rutherford RB, pp. 67-76, W. B. Saunders Co., Philadelphia, PA.
40. Nevelsteen A, Suy R, Daenen W, et al (1980). Aortofemoral grafting: Factors influencing late results. *Surgery* 88:642-653.
41. O'Hara PJ, Hertzer NR, Beven EG, et al (1986). Surgical management of infected ab-dominal aortic grafts: Review of a 25-year experience. *J Vasc Surg* 3:725-731.
42. Robicsek F, Daugherty HK, Mullen DC, et al (1975). The effect of continued cigarette smoking on the patency of synthetic vascular grafts in Leriche syndrome. *J Thorac Car-diovasc Surg* 70:107-112.
43. Rutherford RB (1987). The value of perioperative assessment at the time of the original revascularization in subsequent reoperation. *Acta Chir Scand* 538:46-49.
44. Schmitt DD, Bandyk DF, Pequet AJ, et al (1986). Bacterial adherence to vascular pros-theses. A determinant of graft infectivity. *J Vasc Surg* 3:732-740.
45. Schultz RD, Sterpetti AV (1987). Descending thoracic aorta to femoral artery bypass. In: Cardiac Surgery: State of the Art Reviews, edited by Cowgill LD, pp. 503-513, Hanley and Belfus, Inc., Philadelphia, PA.
46. Seagraves A, Rutherford RB (1987). Isolated hypogastric artery revascularization after previous bypass for aortoiliac occlusive disease. *J Vasc Surg* 5:472-474.
47. Sethi GK, Scott SM, Takaro J (1975). Multiple-plane angiography for more precise evalua-tion of aortoiliac disease. *Surgery* 78:154-159.
48. Shepherd AD, Tollefson DFJ, Reddy DJ, et al (1991). Left flank retroperitoneal exposure: A technical aid to complex aortic reconstruction. *J Vasc Surg* 14:283-291.
49. Sottiurai VS, Smith B, Dial P (1990). Aorto-bi-popliteal bypass via the obturator foramina. *J Cardiovasc Surg* 31:121-123.
50. Sterpetti AV, Feldhaus RJ, Schultz RD (1988). Combined aortofemoral and extended deep femoral artery reconstruction. *Arch Surg* 123:1269-1273.
51. Towne JB, Bernhard V (1979). Technique of intraoperative endoscopic evaluation of oc-cluded aortofemoral grafts following thrombectomy. *Surg Gynecol Obstet* 148:87-89.
52. Walker WE, Cooley DA, Duncan JM, et al (1986). The management of aorto-duodenal fis-tula by in situ replacement of the infected abdominal aortic graft. *Ann Surg* 205:727-732.

Anastomotic Aneurysms of The Aorta and Iliac Arteries

T.K. Ramos, J. Goldstone

Division of Vascular Surgery, UCSF San Francisco, California, U.S.A.

Although rare, anastomotic aneurysms continue to mar the success of abdominal aortic surgery. They are, in fact, the second most common late complication, of these procedures (thrombosis being the most common)[16,43]. In spite of an ever increasing number of patients who have undergone aorto-iliac reconstructive procedures and considerable improvement in both prosthetic graft and suture materials, the incidence of anastomotic aneurysms has not declined, as noted in a recent review by Gaylis and Dewar[14]. The reasons for this include the general improvements in patient management, which have allowed patients to survive long enough following their operations to develop late complications, as well as better methods of their detection.

DEFINITION

Anastomotic aneurysms are those that occur at an anastomosis between two vascular structures or at the site of an arterial repair (suture line). Although the majority of anastomotic aneurysms occur at sites of connection between an artery and a synthetic graft, any vascular anastomosis is at risk for becoming aneurysmal, including those which involve entirely autogenous tissue (endarterectomy, artery-to-artery, and/or artery-to-vein anastomoses). Most anastomotic aneurysms are false or pseudoaneurysms, meaning the walls of these pulsatile masses do not contain the discrete layers of normal vessel wall morphology, but instead are composed of organizing fibrous tissue and thrombus, in effect a pulsatile hematoma. Another type of anastomotic aneurysm is the recurrent true aortic aneurysm caused by aneurysmal degeneration of the aorta at the anastomotic site. Most of these, however, involve the adjacent aorta and are really para-anastomotic aneurysms, similar to the aneurysmal degeneration of arterialized vein grafts.

INCIDENCE

The overall incidence of anastomotic aneurysm formation in reported series ranges from about 1.4 to 4.0%. However, the incidence varies substantially with the method of reporting. Some authors have reported incidence rates according to number of patients or operations; others have used a ratio that includes the number of anastomoses at risk. Since every anastomosis and suture line constitute a potential site of aneurysm formation, it is more accurate to express incidence in terms of number of anastomoses. For example, Szilagyi et al.[41] reported a 3.9% incidence (by patient) of anastomotic aneurysms after 4.214 arterial reconstructive operations. Alternatively, when computed on a per anastomosis basis, the incidence was 1.7% (205 of 9.561 anastomoses). Additionally, up to 40% of patients affected have multiple anastomotic aneurysms, which also emphasizes the importance of expressing incidence rates based on anastomoses at risk rather than on patients or operations.

Other factors affecting the incidence include the indication for and type of original vascular reconstruction, the anatomic location of the anastomosis, and the intensity and length of follow-up by the vascular surgeon. By far, the most common location for anastomotic aneurysm formation is at the femoral anastomoses of aorto-femoral bypass grafts. These usually are identified between five and ten years following vascular reconstruction, are frequently asymptomatic, and are usually diagnosed by physical examination. On the other hand, aortic and iliac anastomotic aneurysms usually produce symptoms unexpectedly ten years or more after the primary vascular reconstruction, and require special imaging modalities for their diagnosis. As Table 1 demonstrates, aorta and iliac artery anastomotic aneurysms account for only a small percentage (11.0% and 12.0%, respectively) of reported anastomotic aneurysms. Nevertheless, they represent a significant life-threatening complication, one that is probably more frequent than current reports in the literature suggest.

Most cases of aortic and iliac anastomotic aneurysms have been reported and discussed in conjunction with larger series of femoral anastomotic aneurysms, and therefore, specific details regarding their etiology, presentation, evaluation and treatment are limited. Nevertheless, sufficient information is available from which to make etiologic inferences, diagnostic and therapeutic recommendations.

Table 1 - Anatomic Locations of Anastomotic Aneurysms

Author	Aortic	Iliac	Femoral	Extremities	Carotid	Other	Total
Knox[20]	8	2	22	3	-	1	36
Szilagyi et al.[41]	4	19	129	9	2	-	163
Nichols et al.[27]	3	3	36	-	-	1	43
Satiani et al.[34]	2	1	22	2	1	1	29
Briggs et al.[5]	5	1	27	-	-	-	33
Mehigan et al.[23]	1	3	19	-	-	-	23
Sedwitz et al.[35]	12	-	61	8	-	-	81
Wandschneider and Denck[49]	6	-	99	3	2	9	119
van den Akker et al.[48]	21	53	27	1	-	-	102
Gaylis and Dewar[14]	17	7	66	3	-	-	93
Downs et al.[102]	3	1	20	2	-	-	26
Total	82 (11%)	90 (12%)	528 (70.6%)	31 (4.1%)	5 (0.7%)	12 (1.6%)	748 (100%)

CLINICAL DATA - UCSF SERIES

We reviewed the records of all secondary and tertiary arterial reconstructions involving the abdominal aorta and its branches performed at the Medical Center of the University of California, San Francisco, (Moffitt-Long Hospitals) from July 1987 to December 1991. There were 164 procedures performed on 141 patients. Seventeen (12%) of these patients were operated upon for 21 anastomotic aneurysms involving the abdominal aorta and/or iliac arteries. During this same time interval, 10 additional patients were treated for recurrent abdominal aortic aneurysms, some of which involved the suture line of the primary procedure. Also, there were 8 other patients with aorto-enteric fistula involving the suture line, but without false aneurysm formation. These latter two groups of patients are not included in this clinical analysis because anastomotic aneurysms were not there their primary pathologic entity.

The 17 patients included in this review consisted of 13 men and 4 women, ranging in age from 38 to 85 years (mean age 70 years) at the time of presentation. Thirteen of them (76%) had hypertension, and all but one were being treated with antihypertensive medications. The original aorto-iliac reconstruction was performed for occlusive disease in 9 patients, and for aneurysmal disease in 8 patients. Synthetic prosthetic grafts were used for these procedures in 16 patients including 13 bifurcated grafts, 2 tube grafts, and 1 patch aortoplasty. One patient developed an anastomotic aneurysm at an iliac-arteriotomy closure site following aorto-iliac thromboendarterectomy. Interestingly, this patient had previously been treated for a recurrent anastomotic aneurysm at the contralateral iliac arteriotomy site.

The interval from the original operation to diagnosis of the anastomotic aneurysm ranged from 2 months to 20 years with a mean interval of 11 years. Abdominal, back or flank pain was the presenting symptom in 7 patients. In 4 of these patients, the aneurysm had ruptured, two into the free peritoneal cavity, and two into the retroperitoneum (contained). One of these was an iliac artery anastomotic aneurysm that occurred in a patient who had synchronous anastomotic aneurysms involving all three arterial anastomoses (Fig. 1). Five patients presented with significant gastrointestinal bleeding associated with hypotension due to anastomotic aorto-enteric fistula. Two patients with iliac artery anastomotic aneurysms presented with intermittent claudication which was felt to be due to embolic events in one, and near thrombosis of the anastomotic aneurysm and its outflow track in the other. Two patients were found to have asymptomatic aortic anastomotic aneurysms during their evaluation for femoral anastomotic aneurysms while another aortic anastomotic aneurysm was discovered in a patient who had undergone a cardiac transplant and repair of a nonanastomotic false aneurysm of his abdominal aorta secondary to an intra-aortic balloon pump injury. Only one patient in this series had a pulsatile abdominal mass as the only manifestation of an anastomotic aneurysm. The diagnosis of retroperitoneal anastomotic aneurysm was made preoperatively in 13 of the 17 patients, 6 by CT scan, 5 by angiography, and 2 by esophago-gastroduodeno-

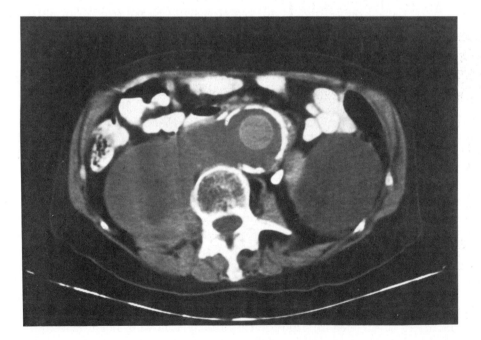

Fig. 1. CT Scan revealing retroperitoneal rupture of large right iliac artery anastomotic aneurysm. The homogeneous structure on the left represents a renal cyst.

scopy. Actually, endoscopy was diagnostic in 1 patient, and highly suggestive in the other who had the findings confirmed by abdominal computed tomography (CT) and angiography. In 4 patients, the diagnosis was only made during surgery.

Two of these were found at the time of infected graft removal following a staged extra-anatomic bypass. In another patient the proximal aortic anastomotic aneurysm ruptured in the hospital prior to the second stage procedure for removal of an infected aortic graft. The final patient underwent emergency laparotomy for uncontrollable massive gastrointestinal hemorrhage due to rupture of a proximal aortic anastomotic aneurysm into the small intestine.

As noted above, there were 21 retroperitoneal anastomotic aneurysms in these 17 patients. Fourteen were aortic, and 7 iliac in location. Two patients each had three synchronous anastomotic aneurysms involving all three of their anastomoses at risk (Fig. 2). In addition, 3 patients had synchronous femoral artery anastomotic aneurisms.

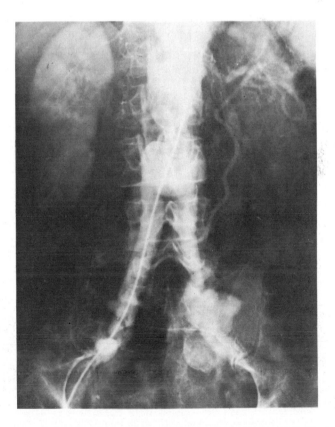

Fig. 2. Angiogram demonstrating an aortic and bilateral iliac artery anastomotic aneurysms. In addition there is aneurysmal dilatation of the aorta above the proximal anastomosis.

Thus, there were a total of 24 anastomotic aneurysms. In some instances, the anastomotic aneurysms during the interval of this study were metachronous lesions, therefore if one includes previous lesions there were a total of 33 anastomotic aneurysms of which 26 involved the abdominal aorta and iliac arteries in these 17 patients.

The anastomotic configuration of the 21 aortic and iliac anastomotic aneurysms was able to be determined in 18. At the aortic level, there were 5 end-to-end and 6 end-to-side anastomoses with one patch angioplasty. At the iliac level, there were 5 end-to-end anastomoses and one endarterectomy closure site.

The anastomotic aneurysms in this series were associated with five aorto-enteric fistulae, and with 7 clinical prosthetic graft infections. Of note, only 3 of the 7 patients with clinical evidence of prosthetic graft infection had positive intraoperative tissue or graft cultures. Two of these clinically and culture-positive prosthetic graft infections were associated with aorto-enteric fistulae.

It was possible to determine with reasonable certainty the etiology of the anastomotic aneurysms in 13 of the 17 patients in this series. Host arterial wall degeneration was incriminated whenever sutures were noted to have pulled away from the host artery but remained intact in the prosthesis (Fig. 3). This was found in 6 patients. When the former finding was not documented, and there was evidence of clinical infection, such as lack of

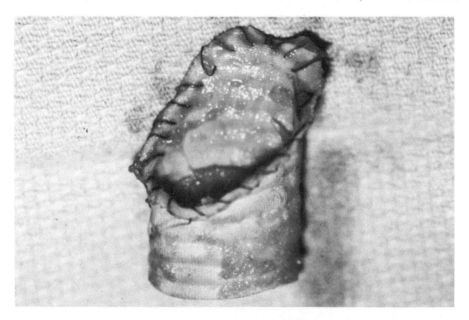

Fig. 3. Graft specimen from abdominal aortic anastomotic aneurysm showing intact suture line on prosthesis. In this case the sutures were pulled through a degenerated but not infected aortic wall. (Reproduced with permission from Goldstone J, Anastomotic Aneurysms. In: Complications in Vascular Surgery, Ed. Bernhard VM, Towne JB, pp 91. Quality Medical Publishing, Inc., St. Louis, Missouri, 1991.)

fibrous tissue incorporation of the prosthesis, periprosthetic fluid or frank pus, prosthetic graft infection was considered to be the etiology of the anastomotic aneurysm (7 patients). In the remaining 4 patients, there was not enough information available from the records to make a meaningful determination of cause.

In all cases, operative treatment consisted of resection of the retroperitoneal anastomotic aneurysm and reestablishment of distal perfusion by either anatomic interposition or extraanatomic bypass grafting. All 5 patients who underwent extra-anatomic bypass grafting did so for clinical prosthetic graft infection associated with a proximal aortic anastomotic aneurysm. However, 1 patient with a ruptured aortic anastomotic aneurysm died in the operating room before resection and bypass grafting could be performed.

There were 2 in-hospital deaths among the 17 patients, both occurring in patients who presented with complications of their anastomotic aneurysm. Both died of rupture, one due to multi-system organ failure on the 12th postoperative day, and the second occurred in the previously mentioned patient who ruptured her aortic anastomotic aneurysm while waiting for the second stage of treatment of her aortic prosthetic graft infection. Overall, 15 patients survived surgical treatment and were discharged from the hospital.

PATHOGENESIS

Most anastomotic aneurysms are anastomotic false aneurysms. These occur when there is a break in the suture line holding two vascular conduits together. This allows blood to extravasate into the peri-anastomotic space where it is frequency limited by scarring and fibrosis from the previous surgery and results in hematoma formation. Because there is continuity between the hematoma and flow of blood two things occur: remodeling and expansion. Lysis of various amounts of the thrombus results in cavity formation while connective tissue ingrowth results in formation of a fibrous capsule. The constant arterial perfusion pressure within this cavity is responsible for it's expansion.

Many factors have been implicated in the pathogenesis of anastomotic false aneurysms (Table 2). Since the existence of an anastomotic false aneurysm implies disruption in the integrity of the involved anastomosis, one or more of three things must occur for such a lesion to develop: suture failure, prosthetic failure or arterial wall failure. Hemodynamic factors frequently play a contributory role.

Suture Failure

It is well known that the strength of any arterial anastomosis involving a prosthesis is forever dependent on the stability of the suture line because permanent healing (i.e. a complete fibrous union) of the prosthetic-arterial junction never occurs. Historically, weakening, dissolution and breakage of silk suture was one of the earliest recognized factors leading to anastomotic aneurysm formation. This was felt to be responsible for many of the reported cases in the 1960's and 1970's[13,25,38,50]. With the introduction of synthetic poly- and mono-filament suture material, suture failure has been implicated less frequently as an etiologic factor. There were no cases of suture failure identified in our series of retroperitoneal anastomotic aneurysms.

However, Treinnan et al.[45] implicated suture failure in 7 of 12 cases involving the aorta and iliac arteries where synthetic suture material had been used. Early monofilament sutures such as polyethylene became brittle over time and fractured, leading to loss of anastomotic integrity, but this does not appear to be true for polypropylene which has had extensive world-wide use. Manycases of suture failure are likely due to surgical technique. For example, polypropylene suture is vulnerable to damage by inappropriate handling with surgical instruments and improper knotting results in slipping of this monofilament suture. Tissue ingrowth occurs with braided polyester suture and has a theoretical advantage of strengthening the anastomotic fibrous union[7]. However, none of the commonly used suture material today are associated with a higher incidence of anastomotic aneurysm formation than the others. Despite the universal use of permanent synthetic sutures, the incidence of anastomotic aneurysms has not significantly decreased, making other causative factors more important.

Table 2. Pathogenesis of Anastomotic Aneurysm Formation

Operational Factors	Anastomotic Components		
	Suture	Prosthesis	Artery
Defective Materials	Fracture Dissolution	Fraying Disruption Degradation Dilation	Multiple Operations Progressive Atherosclerosis Infection
Defective Technique	Improper handling Knol slippage	Angle of anastomosis Size of bevel Graft-to-artery ratio Tension	Endarterectomy Wound complications Suture depth
Hemodynamic-mechanical Stresses	Disruption	Dilatation Nondistensibility Compliance mismatch	Hypertension

Prosthetic Failure

Structural deterioration of the prosthetic graft can contribute to anastomotic aneurysm formation in a number of ways. Fraying occurs most commonly with woven Dacron grafts and allows suture material to pull through the cut edge of the graft. Disruption of individual graft fibers can also occur, and may lead to significant graft dilatation. This may be due to manufacturing defects in yarn filaments or in the design of the prosthesis. Berger and Sauvage[3] found that fiber disruption is more likely to occur with crimped, compared to non-crimped Dacron prostheses, implying that the crimping process (heat) somehow damages the fabric.

Actual chemical degradation of graft material has also been found to occur and may be related to the extent of lipid infiltration into the interstices of the prosthetic material. Although diffuse aneurysmal dilatation of a prosthesis with rupture is rare, graft dilatation is a well recognized phenomenon which occurs with all synthetic graft materials including PTFE[6]. Nunn, Freeman and Hudgins[28] performed ultrasonic evaluation of ninety-five patients with Dacron prostheses who were followed for an average of thirty-three months after implantation and found an average dilatation of 15% and 21%, in normotensive and hypertensive patients, respectively. This early graft dilatation probably represents yarn slippage with loss of compactness of the knit rather than intrinsic fiber deterioration. Nevertheless, the resulting luminal enlargement that occurs with prosthetic dilatation leads to hydrodynamic stresses on the anastomosis in accordance with Laplace's Law.

In addition to dilatation, tissue ingrowth occurs with implanted vascular prostheses making them less compliant when compared to the native arteries which have a diameter change of about 10% with each pulse wave. Mehigan et al[23]. postulated that the resulting compliance mismatch between prosthesis and artery wall, which increases axial, hoop and shearing stress, is one of the most important factors in anastomotic false aneurysm formation.

Artery Failure

The most common finding at the time of redo-surgery for an anastomotic aneurysm is partial or complete disruption of the anastomosis with intact suture within the prosthesis (Fig. 3). This is due to failure of the native artery wall and may occur if a poor quality artery is used to construct the anastomosis. The concomitant performance of endarterectomy has been mentioned by some authors as an important causative factor, but has been disputed by others, including Szilagyi and associates[41], who reported an incidence of anastomotic aneurysm formation following endarterectomy repairs of only 0.4%. Out of 21 retroperitoneal anastomotic aneurysms in our analysis only one occurred at a site where endarterectomy had been the original technique of reconstruction. It seems reasonable, however, if one considers the additional hemodynamic-mechanical stresses that occur at a graft-artery anastomosis, compared to an arteriotomy, that an improperly performed endarterectomy may be a predisposing factor for anastomotic aneurysm formation. Multiple operations resulting in perivascular fibrosis or excessive mobilization of an artery may interrupt the vasa vasorum and lead to artery wall weakness by necrosis. Satiani, Kazmer and Evans[34] found that 46% of their patients had had multiple operations at the site of anastomotic aneurysm formation and implicated this as an important factor in their development.

Progressive atherosclerosis resulting in aneurysmal dilation or obstructive lesion formation with resultant weakening of the artery wall probably contributes to anastomotic aneurysm formation in most cases. Van den Akker and associates[48] found the extent of atherosclerotic lesion formation (single- vs. multi-level disease) to be a significant risk factor. In reviewing late complications of aortic reconstructions Haiait et al.[16] found that anastomotic aneurysms and aortoenteric fistula were more common in patients with aneurysmal disease whereas graft thrombosis was a more common complication in patients with occlusive disease. However, Mehigan and associates[23] reported a 1.5% and 5.2% incidence of anastomotic aneurysms following aortic reconstructions, for aneurysmal and occlusive disease, respectively. Nineteen of the 23 anastomotic aneurysms in their series occurred at femoral anastomoses. The higher incidence of anastomotic aneurysm in association with occlusive disease was felt to be due to more extensive atherosclerotic lesions in the femoral arteries in occlusive disease, compared to aneurysmal disease. It has been suggested that occlusive atherosclerotic lesions alter the compliance of the native arterial wall producing increased stress at the anastomosis. This concept is supported by a recent report specifically addressing aortic and iliac anastomotic aneurysms where occlusive disease was the most common indication for surgery and the reconstructions involved both end-to-end and end-to-side anastomoses[45].

Hypertension is felt to contribute to anastomotic aneurysm formation by weakening the arterial wall both directly and indirectly. By predisposing to graft dilatation, hypertension weakens the artery wall through compliance mismatch. Seventy-six percent of our patients with retroperitoneal anastomotic aneurysms had hypertension and this compares similarly to reports of others[14,45]. However, some authors have pointed out that this is not significantly different from the incidence of hypertension found in control populations.

It is well known that the arterial wall can be weakened by infection and anastomotic aneurysms are a well recognized complication of prosthetic graft infection. The bacteria do not affect the integrity of the prosthesis but instead produce weakening and destruction of the adjacent arterial wall. Sedwitz, Hye and Stabile[35] found that the epidemiology of anastomotic aneurysms is changing in that over the last decade infection has become a much more important predisposing factor. In our series anastomotic aneurysms were associated with 7 clinical graft infections, but as pointed out earlier, only 3 of these patients had positive tissue cultures taken at the time of surgery. The significance of culture-negative graft infections remains controversial. One patient without evidence of clinical infection had a positive tissue culture for Staphylococcus epidermidis. Kaebneck et al[19], using ultrasonication to disrupt the graft surface biofilm and dislodge micro-colonies, recovered microorganisms from 19 of 21 clinically uninfected femoral anastomotic aneurysms. Slime producing Staphylococcus epidermidis was isolated from most of these aneurysms. A pathologic and structural analysis of twenty-six anastomotic aneurysms using gross morphologic examination along with light and scanning electron microscopy found the presence of bacteria in 20 of 26 patients[10]. Scanning electron microscopy identified microorganisms in 15 of 18 specimens where Gram's stain had been negative. None of the 26 patients in this study had clinical evidence of graft infection. We speculate that subclinical prosthetic infection or colonization, which may be manifested only by lack of prosthetic healing, and diagnosed only by special culturing techniques or histologic examination may play an important role in anastomotic aneurysm formation.

The incidence of anastomotic aneurysm is increased when wound healing problems occur after the primary arterial reconstruction. Among these are perigraft serum, lymph or blood collections. Such fluid collections impair fibrous tissue ingrowth into the prosthesis and may result in subclinical or clinical prosthetic graft infection which leads to eventual anastomotic dehiscence.

Other Factors

There are several technical factors in constructing a graft-artery anastomosis which may also contribute to anastomotic false aneurysm formation. Many authors have found an increased incidence of anastomotic aneurysm at end-to-side anastomoses when compared to end-to-end anastomoses. In an end-to-side anastomosis the radius of the anastomosis itself is larger than the artery or graft being anastomosed and therefore the suture line is subjected to increased tangential wall tension. In addition, an angle between the artery and graft in an end-to-side anastomosis which is too large leads to turbulent blood flow with eddy current formation. This results in vibration of the vessel wall and increased shear stress at the anastomosis. A graft which is cut too short, such as may occur in misjudging the spring in a crimped prosthesis, contributes to suture line tension. Similarly, if the beveled end of the prosthesis is made too small, tension at the suture line is dispersed unequally and in this situation the "toe" of the anastomosis is particularly susceptible to disruption. Finally, in an end-to-end anastomosis, if the graft diameter to host artery diameter ratio is greater than the recommended 1.4

to 1.5:1, impedance mismatch occurs resulting in additional stresses at the suture line. Most discussions pertaining to the increased risk of anastomotic aneurysm formation at end-to-side anastomoses have been in reference to the distal anastomoses of an aorto-femoral bypass graft. Recently however, van den Akker et al[48]., using life-table analysis, reported a significantly increased chance of developing an aortic anastomotic aneurysm with an end-to-side anastomosis up to fifteen years following surgery. In this study there was not a significantly increased risk of anastomotic aneurysm formation in iliac or femoral artery end-to-side anastomoses at the same follow-up period. In our series there were 10 end-to-end and 6 end-to-side anastomoses, a distribution similar to that found by Treiman et al.[45], in their series of twenty-two anastomotic aneurysms involving the aorta and iliac arteries. The difference in our findings and Treiman's et al. findings compared to those reported by van den Akker et al. may be related to the underlying arterial pathology and indication for surgery. In van den Akker's et al. study all the aortic reconstructions were performed for occlusive disease while in the other two series reconstructions for aneurysmal disease were included.

CLINICAL MANIFESTATIONS

Presentation

The clinical manifestations of anastomotic aneurysms are determined in part by their location. Those involving the femoral artery are usually asymptomatic and diagnosed by routine follow-up physical examination. Aortic and iliac artery anastomotic aneurysms are obscure and usually go unnoticed until they become large enough to produce discomfort by pressure on adjacent organs or structures or until they develop symptoms as a result of complications. Their diagnosis, which usually requires special imaging modalities, will be discussed later.

Massive lower gastrointestinal bleeding may occur if an iliac artery anastomotic aneurysm erodes into the distal small bowel, appendix, cecum or sigmoid colon. A less common complication is an iliac artery-ureteral fistula which can result in massive hematuria[2]. Ureteral compression can also occur and cause hydronephrosis. An attempt to stent a ureteral obstruction in one case report resulted in rupture of a large iliac artery anastomotic aneurysm[18]. Upper gastrointestinal bleeding is a well recognized manifestation of proximal aortic anastomotic aneurysms which have eroded into the duodenum or proximal small intestine. There were five patients with this complication in our series and all but one presented with massive upper gastrointestinal hemorrhage and hypotension. Severe back pain can occur with erosion of the vertebral bodies due to prolonged pressure of a large

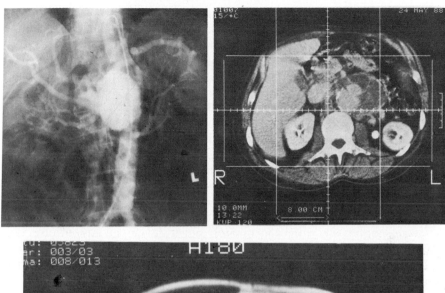

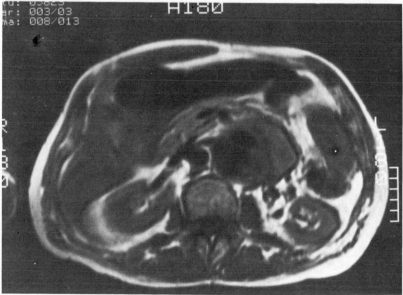

Fig. 4 A - C. Angiogram (A), CT (B) and MRI (C) of an aortic anastomotic aneurysm occurring at the site of a visceral artery Carrel patch following thoraco-abdominal aneurysm repair.

pulsatile mass[47]; but more often severe abdominal or back pain is due to rupture of the aneurysm with irritation of the parietes. Four of the seven patients in our series with rupture presented with pain (Fig. 1). One patient had a several month history of post-prandial pain associated with weight loss which evolved into a more intense, constant upper abdominal pain several days before admission to the hospital. She was found to have a false aneurysm of a visceral artery Carrel patch following repair of a thoraco-abdominal aneurysm (Fig. 4 A-C). Graft thrombosis and embolization, which occurred once each in our series, are not uncommon complications of anastomotic aneurysms.

These limb-, and life-threatening complications occur in approximately 50% of retroperitoneal anastomotic aneurysms, and may manifest several months to several years following the original vascular reconstruction. The earliest presentation in our series was a patient who ruptured a distal aortic anastomotic aneurysm two months following tube graft replacement of an abdominal aortic aneurysm. At the other end of the spectrum was a patient who presented twenty years following his original surgery with his second recurrence of an aortic anastomotic aneurysm. He also had bilateral iliac artery anastomotic aneurysms (Fig. 2). Despite having multiple metachronous and synchronous anastomotic aneurysms over an extended follow-up period, this patient fortunately never developed any serious complications.

These two patients demonstrate the difficulty in predicting when and what complications might occur with retroperitoneal anastomotic aneurysms. Since most surgeons are unwilling to take a "wait and see" approach with these lesions, what little is known about their natural history has been gained from the few patients who refused surgical treatment or who were prohibitive operative risks. Szilagyi et al.[41] reported a 3.7 year mean follow-up of patients with anastomotic aneurysms who did not undergo surgical repair. In this group there were two patients with aortic and nine with iliac anastomotic aneurysms. One patient in the former and three in the later group died of causes not related to their anastomotic aneurysms. The other aortic and four of the iliac artery aneurysms increased in size while the remaining two were stable. All three of the retroperitoneal anastomotic aneurysms which were initially observed by Treiman et al.[45] enlarged over a three to eleven month period. Enlargement resulted in fatal rupture in one of these patients.

Diagnosis

Physical examination suggests the diagnosis of aortic and iliac anastomotic aneurysms in less than 20% of patients (Table 3). Therefore additional studies are needed to detect these retroperitoneal lesions. We detected thirteen of these aneurysms preoperatively and found four of them at the time of surgery. All of the anastomotic aneurysms identified first during surgery involved the aorta and three of the patients had had angiograms in preparation for staged surgical treatment of prosthetic graft infections. None of the angiograms demonstrated the aortic anastomotic aneurysm, not an uncommon occurrence. As with true aneurysms, false anastomotic aneurysms contain thrombus which alters the angiographic appearance. We found angiography only 66% accurate in diagnosing retro-peritoneal anastomotic aneurysms and this is consistent with the finding of Treiman et al.[45] We diagnosed six retroperitoneal anastomotic aneurysms by CT scan which is currently the diagnostic modality of choice. In addition to identifying the graft-artery disruption and the proximal and distal extent of the aneurysm, CT provides useful information regarding associated complications such as hydronephrosis, prosthetic graft infection and rupture. The etiology of perivascular fluid collections can be identified by analyzing attenuation values and by using CT-guided fluid aspirations. In the case of rupture the extent and sometimes the age of hemorrhage can be assessed. Magnetic resonance imaging (MRI) which has improved resolution of perivascular structures and fluid can also demonstrate normal and abnormal blood flow patterns and may prove to be the most accurate method for diagnosing anastomotic aneurysm in the future (Fig. 4 A-C).

Table 3. Clinical Presentation of Retroperitoneal Anastomotic Aneurysms

Author	Pain	Mass	GIB	LE Isch	FAA	Asx	Total
Olsen et al. [29]	2	-	2	-	-	-	4
Treiman et al. [45]	5	4	2	4	1	2	18
Nevelsteen and Suy [26]	1	5	-	4	2	-	12
Current Series	7	1	4	2	2	1	17
Total	15 (29.4%)	10 (19.6%)	8 (15.7%)	10 (19.6%)	5 (9.8%)	3 (5.9%)	51 (100%)

GIB, gastrointestinal bleed; LE Isch, lower extremity ischemia; FAA, femoral anastomotic aneurysm; Asx, asymptomatic.

Because of the high mortality rates associated with emergency surgery for complications of retroperitoneal anastomotic aneurysms, many authors recommend annual imaging surveillance, in addition to routine office examination, for all patients who have undergone aortic reconstruction. This should certainly be performed in patients with appropriate symptoms. Ultrasonography (USG) is probably the best modality for screening because it is non-invasive, relatively inexpensive and avoids the radiation exposure associated with CT or angiography. Edwards et al.[11] reported finding asymptomatic intra-abdominal para-anastomotic aneurysms in 10%[11] of 138 patients followed with serial sonographic studies after aortic reconstruction. In eight patients the sonographic findings were confirmed by CT scan. There has been some controversy in the literature regarding the accuracy of ultrasound in diagnosing retroperitoneal aneurysmal disease, especially in reference to the iliac arteries. Therefore the results of ultrasound scans should be interpreted cautiously and confirmed when necessary with CT, MRI or angiography.

TREATMENT

Although expectant treatment has been recommended by some authors for aortic and iliac artery anastomotic aneurysms which are less than twice the diameter of the native artery, most patients should undergo prompt surgical repair as soon as the diagnosis is established. This is because there is currently no means of predicting which of these aneurysms will remain stable and asymptomatic and which will enlarge and cause limb- or life-threatening complications. In addition, as reported by Olsen, DeWeese and Fry[29], minimal trauma may result in rupture of these fragile walled false aneurysms. Most retroperitoneal anastomotic aneurysms are best treated surgically by resection and interposition prosthetic bypass grafting. However, individual cases may require alternative approaches. This is especially true when there is an associated prosthetic graft infection, and if infection is suspected based on the preoperative evaluation of the patient, surgical treatment should commence with extra-anatomic bypass grafting followed by delayed (staged) excision of the infected prosthesis[32]. On the other hand, if infection of the prosthetic graft is unexpectedly found at the time of surgery, complete prosthetic excision may be followed by patch angioplasty and/or thrombo-endarterectomy of the native system to restore flow, by in situ reconstruction with autogenous tissue or in certain cases with a new in-line synthetic Dacron or PTFE graft, or finally by extra-anatomic bypass grafting. Presently there is not enough data to favor one synthetic graft over the other for use in in situ replacement in contaminated fields. However, experimentally bacteria have been shown to adhere in smaller numbers to PTFE than to Dacron prostheses[39]. When there is infection involving the femoral anastomoses of aorto-femoral grafts, extra-anatomic bypass grafting is performed with composite synthetic and autogenous grafts: a synthetic axillo-superficial femoral artery bypass and an autogenous cross femoral bypass to avoid placing a synthetic prosthesis into an infected groin. Regardless of the clinical findings at surgery, all anastomotic aneurysms are potentially associated with prosthetic graft infection and tissue from the artery, aneurysm wall and prosthesis should be sent for bacteriologic cultures.

The basic principles of surgical technique are the same for all anastomotic aneurysms: proximal and distal control of the aneurysm's inflow and outflow vessels must be obtained by careful dissection. Until this is accomplished it is best to avoid the aneurysm itself, mobilization of which is often very difficult because of the fibrosis resulting from prior operations. Extreme care must be exercised during this dissection to avoid injuring important arterial branches, unwanted debridement of the adventitia, or disruption of the aneurysm prematurely, which can cause serious hemorrhage. Gentle handling of the aneurysm is also important to avoid dislodgement and distal embolization of mural thrombus. In emergency situations or with difficult dissections it may be easier and safer to control inflow and outflow vessels with intraluminal balloon catheters. Adequate exposure of an anastomotic aneurysm is not only important for determining it's cause, but also for enabling the surgeon to perform a secure and uncompromised repair. Since most anastomotic aneurysms are attributed to arterial wall weakness sufficient debridement of the vessel is necessary to construct a new and secure anastomosis or in the case of prosthetic graft infection sufficient debridement and mobilization are necessary to perform a secure, tension-free double layer closure of the aortic stump. Technical aids that may be useful include transcrural, supra-celiac aortic clamping for proximal control, and exposure of the aneurysm via the retroperitoneal or medial visceral rotation approaches.

Table 4. Results of Surgical Treatment of Retroperitoneal Anastomotic Aneurysms

Author	Intact		Ruptured		Total	
	Patient	Deaths	Patient	Deaths	Patient	Deaths
Olsen et al. [29]	-	-	1	1(100%)	1	1(100%)
Treiman et al. [45]	12	1(8%)	6	4(67%)	18	5(28%)
Nevelsteen and Suy [26]	10	0(0%)	-	-	10	0(0%)
Current Series	8	0(0%)	9	2(22%)	17	2(22%)
Total	30	1(3%)	16	7(44%)	46	8(17%)

Results of Treatment

Although generally excellent and durable results have been reported, the repair of anastomotic aneurysms can be difficult and significant morbidity and mortality can occur.

Satiani, Kazman and Evans[34] summarized the results of operative treatment of 411 anastomotic aneurysms in 350 patients. Overall there was an 8.5% procedure-mortality rate, an 8% amputation rate and a 7.2% recurrence rate. However, the nature and location of the lesion greatly influence the results. For example, retroperitoneal anastomotic aneurysms, particularly those presenting with complications such as graft infection, aorto-enteric fistula or free rupture, are associated with the highest mortality rate (Table 4). In our series, 12 of 17 patients presented with these grave complications. In nine patients the anastomotic aneurysm had ruptured: five into hollow viscera (aorto-enteric fistula), two into the retroperitoneum (contained), and two intraperitoneal (free). In addition there were seven clinical prosthetic graft infections. The mortality rates for patients with these complications were as follows: prosthetic graft infection, 14%; aorto-enteric fistula, 40%; and free rupture, 50%.

We advocate a very aggressive approach to the evaluation and treatment of patients with symptoms following aortic reconstruction. All patients in this series were operated on within a few hours to a few days following diagnosis or suspected diagnosis of aortic or iliac artery anastomotic aneurysm. Delay inevitably leads to further problems and risk of rupture. Little is known about recurrence rates with regard to retroperitoneal anastomotic aneurysms. Two of our patients had recurrent aneurysms. One of these presented with his second recurrent aortic anastomotic aneurysm and was found to have synchronous iliac anastomotic aneurysms bilaterally (Fig. 2). The other patient, who had a recurrent right iliac artery anastomotic aneurysm presented during our study period with an aneurysm of his left iliac artery anastomosis.

PREVENTION

Careful construction of every graft-artery anastomosis, keeping in mind the operative factors which contribute to anastomotic aneurysm formation, and meticulous surgical technique are the most important ways of preventing this complication of arterial reconstruction. Permanent synthetic sutures should be used whenever a prosthetic graft is implanted and all anastomoses should be constricted without excessive tension. Non-crimped prostheses may have an advantage in this regard but are generally available only as PTFE. An appropriately sized graft with a correctly beveled end should be attached at an acute angle for end-to-side anastomoses to limit anastomotic stresses. When an endarterectomy is required to ensure adequate luminal size, larger suture bites of the artery should be taken. One should ensure adequate hemostasis, lymphstasis and handle tissue delicately to prevent postoperative blood and lymph collections as well as tissue necrosis. This is important since wound complications are quite common in patients who subsequently develop anastomotic aneurysms.

Control of systemic factors such as hypertension as well as other risk factors for atherosclerosis (diabetes mellitus, hyperlipidemia and smoking) may retard host arterial wall degeneration as well as alter certain prosthetic changes that occur over time (dilatation, lipid infiltration). These factors are under less control by the surgeon than are those factors relating to the technical performance of the arterial reconstruction.

CONCLUSIONS

Patients who present with symptoms following aortic reconstruction which may be attributed to retroperitoneal anastomotic aneurysm (painful pulsatile mass, gastrointestinal bleeding or sepsis) should undergo aggressive evaluation with CT or MRI and angiography. In some cases endoscopy or radiolabelled blood cell (erythrocyte or leucocyte) scans may be useful. In addition, patients who present with one anastomotic aneurysm should be evaluated for other synchronous aneurysnns and followed at least annually for the development of metachronous lesions. When an aortic or iliac artery anastomotic aneurysm is diagnosed urgent surgical therapy should bc instituted where ever co-morbidity does not present a prohibitive operative risk.

GRANT ACKNOWLEDGEMENT

Supported in part by the Pacific Vascular Research Foundation and the Gladstone Foundation for Cardiovascular Disease.

REFERENCES

1. Amparo, E.G.,Higgins, C.B.,Hoddick, W., Hricak,H. Kerlan, R.K.,Ring, E.j., Kaufman, L., Hedegecock, M.W., (1984) Magnetic Resonance Imaging of Aortic Disease: Preliminary Results, *Am. J. Radiol.,* 143: 1203-1209.
2. Andreasen J.J., Fahrenkurg, L., Madsen P. V.,(1991) Massive hematuria due to iliac artery/ureteral fistula. Case report. *Eur. J. Surg.,* 157:223-224.
3. Berger, K., Sauvage, L.R., (1981) Late fiber deterioration in Dacron areterial grafts. *Ann. Surg.,* 193:447-491.
4. Blumberg, R. M.,Gelfand, M. L., Barton, E. A., Bowers, C.A., Gittleman, D.A., (1991) Clinical significance of aortic graft dilation. *J. Vasc. Surg.,* 14:175:180.
5. Briggs, R. M.,Jarstfer, B.S., Collins, G. J., (1983) Anastomotic aneurysms. *Am. J. Surg.,* 146: 770-773.
6. Campbell, C.D., Brokks, D.H., Webster, M.H., Bondi, R.P., lloyd, J.C., Hynes, M.F., Bahnson, H.T., (1976), H.T., Aneurysm formation in expanded polytetrafluoroethylene prostheses. *Surgery,* 79:491-493.
7. Conn, J., Beal, L., (1977) A study of polybutilate lubricated polyester sutures. *Surg. Gynecol. Obstet.,* 144:707-709.
8. Courbier, R., Larranaga, J., (1982) Natural history and management of anastomic aneurysms. In: Aneurysms: Diagnosis and treatment, edited by Bergan, J.J., Yao, J.A.T., pp 567-580. Grune and Stratton, New York.
9. Dennis, J.W., Littooy, J.N., Greisler, H.P., Baker, W.H.,(1986) Anastomotic pseudo-aneurysms: A continuing late complication of vascular reconstructive procedures. *Arc. Surg.,* 121: 314-317.
10. Downs, A.R.., Guzman, R., Formichi, M., Courbier, R., Jausseran, J.M., Branchereau, A., Juahn, C., Chakfe, N., King, M , Eng, P., Guidoin, R., (1991) Etiology of prosthetic anastomotic false aneurysms: Pathology and structural evaluation in 26 cases. *Can. J. Surg.,* 34:53-58.
11. Edwards, J.M., Teefey, S.A., Zierler, R.E., Kohler, T.R., (in press) Intra-abdominal para-anastomotic aneurysm after aortic bypass grafting. *J. Vasc. Surg.,* 15 (in press).
12. Ernst, C.B., (1989) Pathogenesis and management of recurrent femoral anastomotic aneurysms and aortic anastomotic aneurysms. In: Current critical problems in vascular surgery, editet by

Veith, F.J., PP 352-356. Quality Medical Publishing, Inc., St. Louis, Missouri.

13. Gardner, T.J., Brwley, R.K., Gott, V.L., (1972) Anastomotic false aneurysms. *Surgery,* 72:474-478.

14. Gaylis, H., Dewar, G., (1990) Anastomotic aneurysms: Facts and fancy. *Surg. Annual,* 22:317-341.

15. Goldstone, J., (1991) Anastomotic aneurysms. In: Complications in vascular surgery, edited by Bernhard, V.M., Towne, J.B., pp 87-99. Quality Medical Publishing, Inc., St. Louis, Missouri.

16. Haiant, D.C., Callam, M.J., Murie, J.A., Ruckley, C.V., Jenkins, A., McL, (1991) Reoperations for late complication following abdominal aortic operation. *Br. J. Surg.,* 78: 204-206.

17. Haimovici, H., (1989) Extrafemoral anastomotic aneurysms: General considerations and techniques. In: Vascular surgery principles and techniques, edited by Haimovici, H., pp 691-697. Appleton and Lange, East Norwalk, Connecticut.

18. Jaeger, H.J., Kerin, M.J., Kruegener, G.H., MacFie, J., (1991) Rupture of false aneurysms secondary to passage of ureteric stent. *Br. J. Urol.,* 68: 101-102.

19. Kaebnick, H.W., Bandyk, D.T., Bergamini, T.W., Towne, J.B., (1987) The microbiology of explanted vascular prostheses. *Surgery,* 102: 756-762.

20. Knox, W.G., (1976) Peripheral vascular anastomotic aneurysms: A fifteen-year experience. *Ann. Surg.,* 183:120-123.

21. Lee, J.K.T., Ling,D., Heiken, J.P., Glazer, N.S., Sicard, G.A., Totty, W.G., Levitt, R.G., Murphy, W.A., (1984) Magnetic Resonance Imaging of Abdominal Aortic Aneurysms. *Am. J. Radiol.,* 143: 1197-1202.

22. Mark, A.,Moss, A. A., Lusby, R., Kaiser, J.A., (1982) CT evaluation of complications of abdominal aortic surgery. *Radiology,* 145: 409-414.

23. Mehigan, P.G., Fitzpatrick, B., Browne, H.I., Bouchier-Hayes, D.J., (1985) Is copliance mismatch the major cause of anastomotic arterial aneurysms?: Analysis of 42 cases. J. Cardiovasc. *Surg.,* 26: 147-150.

24. Mikati, A., Marachi, P., Watel, A., Warembourg, jr., H., Roux, J.P., Noblet, D., Soots, G., (1990) End-to-side aortoprosthetic anastomoses: Long-term computed tomography assessment. *Ann. Vasc. Surg.,* 4: 584-591.

25. Moore, W.S., Hall, A.D., (1970) Late suture failure in the pathogenesis of anastomotic false aneurysms. *Ann. Surg.,* 172: 1064-1068.

26. Nevelsteen, A., Suy, R., (1989) Anastomotic false aneurysmsof the abdominal aorta and the iliac arteries. *J. Vasc. Surg.,* 10:595..

27. Nichols, W.K., Stanton, M.Silver, D. Kertzer, W.T., (1980) Anastomotic aneurysms following lower extremity revascularization. *Surgery,* 88: 336-374.

28. Numm, D.B., Freeman, M.H., Hudgins, P.C., (1979) Postoperative alterations in size od Dracon arterial grafts: An ultrasonic evaluation. *Ann. Surg.* 189: 741-745.

29. Olsen, W.R., DeWeese, M.S., Fry, W.J., (1966) False aneurysms of abdominal aorta: A late complication of aortic aneurysmectomy. *Arch. Surg.,* 92: 123-130.

30. Paasche, P.E., Kinley, C.E., Dolan, F.G., Gozna, E.R., (1973) Consideration of suture line stresses in the selection of synthetic grafts for implantation. *J.Biomech.,* 6:253-258.

31. Plate, G., Hollier,L.A., O'Brien, P., Pairolero, P., Cherry, K.J., Kazmier, F.J., (1985) Reccurent aneurysms and late vascular complications following repair of abdominal aortic aneurysms. *Arch. Surg.,* 120: 590-594.

32. Reilly, L.M., Stoney, R. J., Goldtstone, J., Ehrenfeld, W.K., (1987) Improved management of aortic graft infection: The influence of operation sequence and staging. *J. Vasc. Surg.,* 5: 421-431.

33. Richardson, J.V., McDowell, H.A., (1976) Anastomotic aneuwysms following arterial grafting: A 10-year experience. *Ann. Surg.,* 184: 179-182.

34. Satiani, B., Kazmers, M., Evans, W., (1980) Anastomotic arterial aneurysms: A continuing challenge. *Ann. Surg.,* 192: 674-682.

35. Sedwitz, M. M., Hye, R.J., Stabile, B.E., (1988) The changing epidemiology of pseudoaneurysm: Therapeutic implications. *Arch. Surg.,* 123: 473-476.

36. Sladen, G.J., Gerein, A.N., Miyagishima, R.T., (1987) Late rupture of prosthetic aortic grafts: Presentation and management. *Am. J, Surg.,* 153: 453-458.

37. Starr, D.S., Weatherford, S.C., Lawrie, G.M., Morris, G.C., (1979) Suture material as a factor in the occurence of anastomotic false aneurysms: An analysis of 26 cases. *Arch. Surg..,* 114: 412-415.

38. Stoney, R.J., Albo, R.J., Wylie, E.J., (1965) False aneurysms occuring after arterial grafting operations. *Am.J. Surg.,* 110: 153-161.

39. Sugarman, B., (1982) In-Vitro adherence of bacteria to prosthetic vascular grafts. *Infection,* 10: 9-12.
40. Sumner, D.S., Strandness, Jr., D. E., (1967) False aneurysms occuring in association with thrombosed prosthetic grafts. *Arch. Surg.,* 94: 360-362.
41. Szilagyi, D.E., Smith, R.T., Elliott, J.P. Hageman, J.H., Dall'Olmo, C.A., (1975) Anastomotic aneurysms after vascular reconstruction: Problems of incidence, etiology, and treatment. *Surgery,* 78: 800-816.
42. Taylor, L.M., Van Kolken, R.J., Baur, G.M., Porter, J.M., (1981) Precise diagnosis of aortic anastomotic aneurysm by computed tomographic scan. *Arch. Surg.,* 116: 1209-1211.
43. Thompson, W.M., Johnsrude, I.S., Jackson, D.C., Older, R.A., Wechsler, A.S., (1977) Late complications of abdominal aortic reconstructuve surgery: Roentgen evaluation. *Ann. Surg.,* 185: 326:334.
44. Thompson, B.W., Read, R.C., Campbell, G.S., (1979) Uninfected false aneurysms after arterial reconstruction with prosthetic grafts. *Am. J. Surgery.,* 138: 920-923.
45. Treiman, G.S., Weaver, J.A., Cossman, D.V., Toran, R.T., Cohen, J.L., Levin, P.M., Treiman, R.L., (1988) Anastomotic false aneurysms of the abdominal aorta and the iliac arteries. *J. Vasc. Surg.,* 8: 268-273.
46. Turnipseed, W.D., Acher, C.W., Detmer, D.E., Berkoff, H.A., Myerowicts, P.D., Crummy, A.B., Belzer, F.O., (1982) Digital subtraction and B-mode ultrasonography for abdominal and peripheral aneurysms. *Surgery,* 92: 619-626.
47. Usselman, J.A., Vint, V.C., Kleeman, S.A., (1979) CT diagnosis of aortic pseudoaneurysm casusing vertebral erosion. *Am. J. Radiol.,* 133: 1177-1179.
48. van den Akker, P.J., Brand, R., van Schilfgaarde, R., van Bockel, J.H., Terpstra, J.L., (1989) False aneurysms after prosthetic reconstructions for aorto-iliac obstructive disease. *Ann. Surg.,* 210: 658-666.
49. Wandschneider, W., Denck, N., (1988) Anastomotic aneurysms—an unsolvable problem. *Eur. J. Vasc. Surg.,* 2: 115-119.
50. West, J.P., Lattes, C., Knox, W.G., (1971) Anastomotic false aneurysms. *Arch. Surg.,* 103: 348-350.

Revascularization of The Lower Limbs From The Descending Thoracic Aorta After Failure of Aorto-iliac Reconstruction

A. Branchereau, P. Moracchini, P.-E. Magnan,
H. Espinoza and J.-P. Mathieu

Department of Vascular Surgery
Sainte Marguerite Hospital, University of Aix-Marseille, France

The procedure used to manage patients after failure of aorto-iliac reconstruction must meet two requirements. First because the overall condition of these patients, who usually have extensive atherosclerosis, is usually poor, it must be as uninvasive as possible; second it must restore adequate blood flow to the lower limbs.

Descending thoracic aorta to femoral artery bypass for revascularization of the lower limbs was described by both Stevenson[37] and Blaisdell[2], in 1961. A few years later Blaisdell was to describe axillo-femoral bypass (AFB)[3] which became more popular. However, in recent years, encouraging results have been obtained with descending thoracic aorta to femoral artery bypass[4,7,12,21,34,36] whereas AFB has been criticized[18,29].

In this study we present the technique of bypass from descending thoracic aorta for lower limb revascularization after failure of aorto-iliac reconstruction as well as the short and long term results we have obtained. Based on our experience and a review of the literature, we discuss the place of this technique in this particular situation.

SURGICAL TECHNIQUE

Surgical techniques and strategies used after unsuccessful aorto-iliac reconstruction must be considered for the 3 main causes of failure which are late occlusion, infection or false aneurysm.

Late Occlusion

The patient is twisted so that his shoulders are turned 60° and his pelvis 30° with respect to the table. This position allows a simultaneous approach to the thorax and both femoral arteries (Fig. 1).

Intraoperative monitoring includes central venous and direct arterial pressure measurements, continuous electrocardiography, and Swan-Ganz catheter. Selective tracheal intubation is not required.

Approach and tunnelization require five cutaneous incisions and one diaphragmatic incision (Figs. 1 and 2). A short left lateral thoracotomy in the 7th or 8th intercostal space allows access to the distal thoracic aorta.

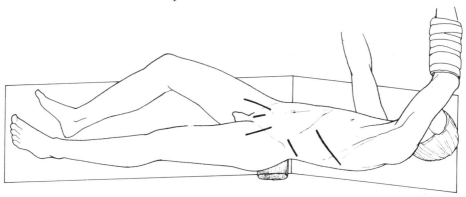

Fig.1. Patient position and skin incisions for descending thoracic aorta to femoral artery bypass.

Femoral arteries are approached as usual. A 10 to 12 cm horizontal incision, centered on the mid axillary line half-way between the iliac crest and the 12th rib, is used to tunnel the prosthetic graft behind the left kidney. A 5 cm vertical suprapubic incision allows to tunnel the right limb of the graft through the prevesical space to the right femoral triangle. The right limb is often too short and must be extended. The diaphragm is incised in the posterior phrenicostal sinus, at a point near the vertebral body, at the level of the accessory crux or the medial lumbocostal arch. This incision is made blindly using the tip of scissors introduced into the thorax. Progression is guided by the surgeon's free hand placed behind the left kidney through the lumbar incision (Fig. 2). Only the pleura is sectioned, the muscle fibers of the diaphragm being separated. After dividing the pleura we limit dissection of the aorta to the left anterior margin. A single Satinsky-type clamp allows to cross-clamp the aorta and to present the edges of the arteriotomy for suture (Fig. 3). Systemic hypotension is achieved with nitroprussiate sodium during aortic cross-clamping.

We use bifurcated albumin-coated Dacron grafts without shortening the main stem[8]. The graft is sectioned obliquely in order to implant it on the left lateral aspect of the aorta and to provide a lateral and slightly posterior

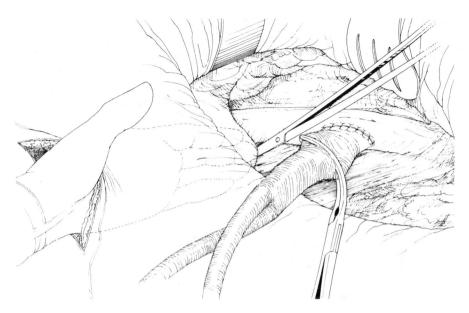

Fig. 2. Blind tunnelization, through the diaphragm, from the thorax to the retroperitoneal area

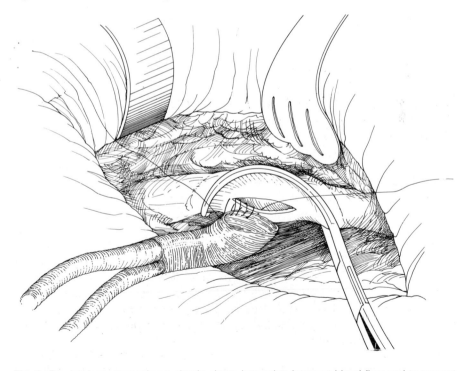

Fig. 3. Proximal anastomosis : a simple clamp is used to interrupt blood flow and to present the edges of the arteriotomy.

direction joining the diaphragmatic incision without kinking (Fig. 4). The two prosthetic limbs are placed in the sagittal plane and the graft is tunneled from the thorax to the lumbar incision through the retroperitoneal area behind the kidney (Fig. 5). The anterior limb is placed extraperitoneally, from posterior to anterior, and from left to right, to the suprapubic incision then to the right femoral triangle. The posterior limb is run directly to the left femoral triangle. The distal anastomoses are made as usual. When a patent cross-over bypass is available, a thoracic aorta to left femoral artery bypass is performed and the cross-over transposed to it.

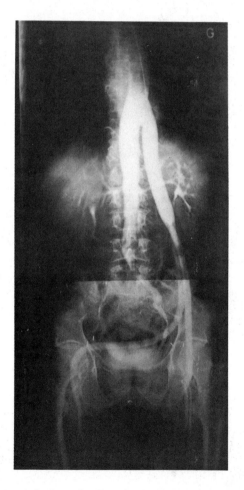

Fig. 4. Post-operative arteriogram of a thoracic aorta to femoral arteries bypass according to the basic technique.

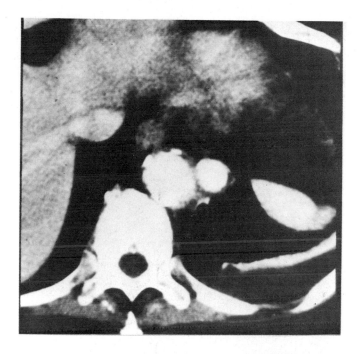

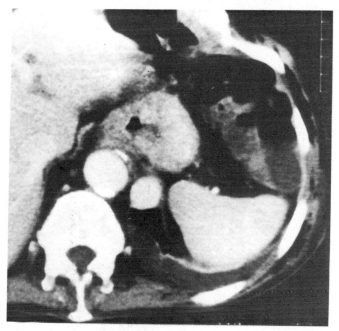

Fig. 5. CT Scan showing the course of the bypass, A: just below the proximal anastomosis, B: medial to the spleen.

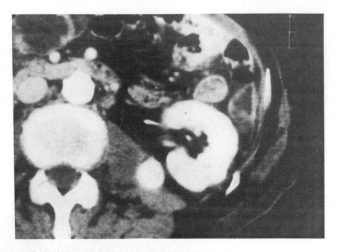

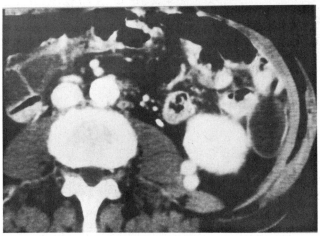

Fig. 5. (suite)C : behind the kidney, D : the two limbs are in a sagittal plane behind the kidney in front of the psoas muscle.

Post-operative Infection

Like aorto-enteric or para-prosthetic fistula, immediate or late post-operative infection pose a difficult problem. Effective management must include removal of the prosthesis, treatment of the infection and restoration of circulation to the lower limbs. Use of the thoracic aorta should be considered either if infection involves the abdominal aorta or if both femoral triangles are infected.

When the infection is limited to the abdomen, particularly in the case of an aorto-enteric fistula, the aforesaid technique can be used to make a bypass between the thoracic aorta and the femoral arteries away from the infected region. However when either of femoral triangles are infected, this technique is unfeasible because the limbs of the prosthesis would pass through the infected zone. In this situation we use a technique combining a left aorto-femoral bypass passing near the iliac spur away from the femoral triangle with femoro-femoral bypass through the perineum. Whenever possible, the femoro-femoral bypass is achieved with a vein graft[6] (Fig. 6).

The chronology of the procedure depends on the quality of the collateral circulation. When the blood supply from the iliac arteries to the lower limbs is adequate, we always perform a two-stage reconstruction. In the first stage, the infected prosthesis is removed while preserving the native aorta, leaving the patient in chronic ischaemia.

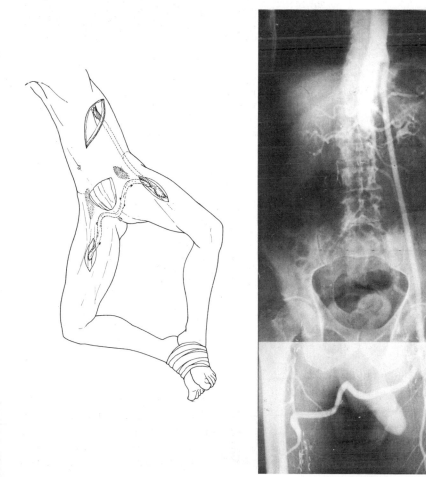

Fig. 6. Perineal bypass associated with a thoracic aorta to left femoral artery bypass. A: patient position and skin incisions. B: post-operative arteriogram.

Bypass is performed in a second stage few weeks later (3 months in one case). If collateral circulation to the lower limbs is insufficient, we perform a single procedure in which bypass is performed first, followed by removal of the prosthesis and treatment of the infected zones. This sequence avoids leaving the patient in acute ischaemia after removal of the infected prosthesis[10].

False aneurysm

A thoracophrenolaparotomy is made through the 9th intercostal space and extended extraperitoneally to the umbilicus with partial section of the diaphragm[31]. The kidney and the left renal artery are pushed forward with the viscera exposing the distal thoracic aorta, the proximal abdominal aorta and the false aneurysm. After clamping the aorta, the false aneurysm is opened, the old graft is freed, and temporarily occluded by balloon catheters. The native aorta is closed either by suture just below the renal arteries when the previous anastomosis was end-to-end, or by a prosthetic patch when the previous anastomosis was side-to-end in order to preserve flow through the internal iliac arteries. After side-to-end anastomosis on the distal thoracic aorta, revascularization of the lower limbs is achieved by end-to-end anastomosis of the new and old graft (Fig. 7).

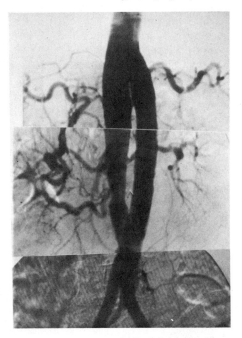

Fig. 7. Post-operative arteriogram of a thoracic aorta to bifemoral bypass in case of false aneurysm. The native aorta was closed by a prosthetic patch and after anastomosis on the thoracic aorta the new graft was anastomosed end to end with the old graft.

PATIENTS

Between November 1984 and May 1991, this technique was used to revascularize 43 lower limbs in 23 patients. Two patients had already undergone contralateral amputation and one patient was revascularized for unilateral acute ischaemia. There were 22 males and 1 female with a mean age of 58.6±8 years (range 41 to 76 years). All patients except two were heavy cigarette smokers (>20 g/day); five patients had stable coronary artery disease; four were hypertensive, and four had chronic bronchopulmonary disease.

Two patients had asymptomatic false aneurysm at the aortic anastomosis of an aorto-bifemoral bypass. Nine patients had infected prostheses: four had aorto-enteric fistula arising from an aorto-bifemoral bypass, four had infected aorto-bifemoral bypass, and one had an infected axillo-bifemoral bypass. Twelve patients had occluded prostheses causing seven chronic (4 claudication, 3 gangrene) or five acute ischaemia. All had undergone previous bypass surgery using the infrarenal aorta or axillary artery as many as four times. In the occlusion group three patients presenting bilateral thrombosis of an aorto-bifemoral bypass had undergone up to three laparotomies for various digestive disorders; two patients had undergone redo after initial aorto-bifemoral bypass; three patients suffered repeated failure of cross-over femoro-femoral bypass; two presented occlusion of an axillo-femoral or bifemoral bypass; one presented occlusion of an axillo-bifemoral bypass; one presented occlusion of an aorto-femoral bypass in association with a pre-existing occlusion of the contralateral iliac artery; and one presented occlusion of an aorto-bifemoral bypass associated with retroperitoneal fibrosis.

The basic technique, as described above, was used in 13 cases. Twelve of the grafts were diameter 14/7, and one was 16/8. A cross-over procedure was associated with a thoracic to left femoral artery bypass in six patients: a venous cross-over bypass was performed through the perineum in three cases and a subcutaneous femoro-femoral prosthetic cross-over procedure was used in three cases. Only the left lower limb was revascularized in two cases; in one the right lower limb was amputated and in the other the right lower limb was adequately vascularized and two previous cross-over procedures had failed. The throracophrenolaparotomy approach through the 9th intercostal space was used in two cases involving false aneurysm ; the new graft was implanted on the old abdominal graft: in one case on the main stem (Fig. 7) and in the other case on the origin of left limb since the right limb was already occluded associated with amputation.

Follow-up angiograms were obtained for all patients surviving more than 30 days. Late patency was established by palpation of the femoral pulses. Two patients were lost to follow-up after discharge and one was lost to follow-up after 6 months. The proximal anastomosis was controlled by CT scan in 10 patients. Thirteen patients did not undergo this investigation because of death (n=6), lost to follow-up (n=3), refusal (n=l), and follow-up of less than one year (n=3).

RESULTS

Before the 30th post-operative day or discharge, three deaths, one popliteal embolism, three prosthetic thromboses, and one paraplegia were recorded. One patient died the third postoperative day, after two successive occlusions of a cross-over bypass, with acute ischemia. Two patients died of multiple organ failure 11 and 23 days after operation. Three graft thromboses were operated on with success: in the first case, poor outflow was treated by profundoplasty: in the second the patient presented a heparin-induced thrombopenia, in the third the patient had platelet hyperaggregability potentialized by the prosthetic material; in these last two cases, thrombectomy was associated with appropriate medical treatment leading to patency. Popliteal embolism occurred in one patient, and was treated successfully on day 2. Paraplegia was observed in one patient who had undergone aortic cross-clamping associated with dissection of a large intercostal artery.

Late results were available for 18 patients (3 post-operative deaths and 2 lost to follow-up) followed for 3 to 72 months (mean: 26.7±20.8 months). Three late deaths were observed. The previously paraplegic patient died 8 months after operation due to thrombosis of the bypass. The other two patients had patent grafts and died of causes unrelated to surgery, i.e., myocardial infarction at 6 months and bladder cancer at 72 months. The cumulative life expectancy rate was 75.3± 19.3% at 5 years (Fig. 8). In addi-

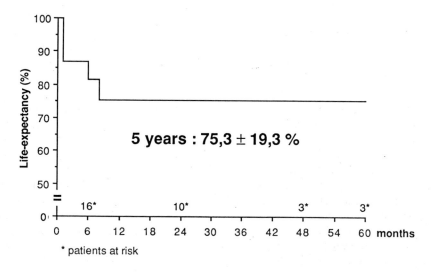

Fig. 8. *Cumulative life expectancy curve.*

tion to the patient who died with thrombosis at 8 months, two patients had late thrombosis. One patient had three episodes of thrombosis involving the right limb of the graft at 7, 16, and 21 months. The first two episodes were managed by thrombolysis and thrombectomy respectively, the last episode required amputation. The other thrombosis occurred in a thoracic aorta to left femoral artery bypass at 10 and 24 months. The first episode was successfully treated by thrombectomy but the second required amputation. The cumulative secondary patency rate was 67.4±24.9% at 5 years (Fig. 9). One patient developed a left ureteral fistula and was reoperated on 3 months later: the graft was uncrossed and an ureteral plasty was performed. This patient was without further problems at 66 months.

Ten patients have undergone CT scan at 1 year in order to detect a false aneurysm. The examination was normal in all cases.

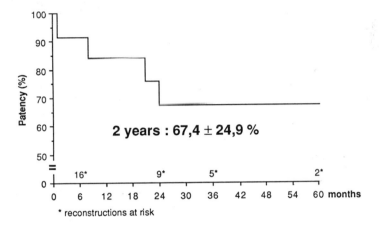

Fig. 9 - *Cumulative secondary patency curve.*

DISCUSSION

This technique of thoracic aorta to femoral bypass that we and others[4,16,20,21,25,34,36] are using seems simpler and less aggressive than the one proposed by McCarthy[12] or by Ochsner[30]: these authors divide the diaphragm and place the graft in front of the kidney. This technique is more invasive, longer to perform and more haemorrhagic.

Post-operative paraplegia did occur in one patient in this series and we are aware of other unpublished cases of medullary compromise in this setting. In our patient, a large intercostal artery had been dissected and clamped together with the aorta. In our opinion, paraplegia was due to dissection and trauma to the intercostal artery rather than to clamping of the aorta itself. Since this accident, we limit the dissection of the aorta as previously described.

The place of this technique must be discussed in relation to alternative solutions for late failure of aorto-iliofemoral bypass for revascularization of the lower limbs. AFB can be used regardless of whether the cause of failure is occlusion or infection. It is a less aggressive technique and it does not require dissection of the previous surgical field. However the risk of post-operative infection is higher than for bypass techniques using deeper routes and the risk of thrombosis is high because of poor hemodynamic conditions. In his series in which AFB was used only for failure of previous reconstruction, Oblath[29] reported a mortality rate of 41 % and a one-year patency rate of only 47%; similarly Donaldson[18] and Broome[9] also reported poor results with AFB after failure of previous reconstruction.

Table 1 - Descending thoracic aorta to femoral artery bypass : review of literature

1st Author	Year	Number of cases	Indications for late occlusion	Post-operative complications	Post-operative mortality
Stevenson [37]	1961	1	1	1 amputation	0
Blaisdell [2]	1961	1	-	0	1
Robicsek [33]	1967	1	1	0	0
Nunn [28]	1972	3	2	0	0
Froysaker [23]	1973	6	-	0	0
Finseth [22]	1974	1	-	0	0
Cevese [13]	1975	6	-	0	0
Jarrett [26]	1975	2	-	0	1
Buxton [11]	1976	1	-	1 pneumonia	0
Lakner [27]	1983	2	-	0	0
Reilly [32]	1984	5	-	0	0
Haas [24]	1985	3	-	1 hemothorax	1
Bowes [4]	1985	12	6	0	1
Feldhaus [21]	1985	18	12	1 myocardial infarction + 2 pneumonia	1
Enon [20]	1985	3	2	0	0
Rosenfeld [34]	1986	10	8	- not available	0
Schultz [36]	1986	15	15	1 thrombosis	0
Mc Carthy [12]	1986	13	5	1 hemothorax + 1 atelectasis	0
Di Marzo [17]	1987	5	-	0	1
Schellack [35]	1988	3	3	0	0
Hussain [25]	1988	8	2	0	0
Bradham [5]	1989	2	-	0	0

Late occlusion of aorto-iliac bypass is the most frequent indication for thoracic aorta to femoral artery bypass. It accounted for 12 out of 23 cases in this series and 57 out of 121 cases in the literature (Table 1). Other techniques that can be considered if thrombectomy fails or cannot be used are in situ reoperation and bypass from the coeliac aorta[1]. In situ reoperation is a long, tedious, and haemorrhagic procedure which carries a high risk of infection. Bypass from the coeliac aorta[1] by the transperitoneal route entails xyphopubic laparotomy followed by evisceration. Furthermore exposure of the coeliac aorta is difficult after previous surgery and the presence of the first graft makes passage of the second graft difficult and hazardous if a retroperitoneal route is chosen[1].

In cases involving aorto-prosthetic false aneurysm, the direct transperitoneal route is a more invasive, time consuming and haemorrhagic method. If the stump of the aorta below the renal arteries is short, the anterior approach offers only two alternatives. The first is to implant the new graft immediately below the renal arteries with a high risk of suture complication. The second is to implant the new graft on the coeliac aorta with the aforesaid disadvantages.

Table 2 - Late results of descending thoracic aorta to femoral artery bypass: review of literature

1st author	Year	N. of cases	Late patency	
Covese[13]	1975	6	30 months : PP	100 %
Feldhaus[21]	1985	18	60 months : SP	85 %
Rosenfeld[34]	1986	10	44 months : PP	90 %
Schultz[36]	1986	15	60 months : SP	80 %
Mc Carthy[12]	1986	13	22 months : PP	100 %
Hussain[25]	1988	8	36 months : SP	100 %

PP: Primary patency   SP: Secondary patency

A distinction must be made between aorto-enteric or paraprosthetic fistulas on the one hand, and infections of the prosthesis on the other. The first indication can often be treated in a single operation by in situ reconstruction with omentoplasty[14]. Lifelong antibiotics are sometimes necessary[15]. For the second indication, however, the only one-stage alternative is to remove the infected prosthesis then reconstruct with an autogenous graft (vein or endarteriectomized artery) as described by Ehrenfeld[19]; the highly invasive and haemorrhagic nature of this procedure as well as its long duration probably explain the small number of cases reported up to now. Our preference is a two-stage approach in which revasularization of the lower extremities is achieved either from the thoracic aorta as described above or by AFB with the aforesaid disadvantages.

It is difficult to evaluate the results of this technique as only 121 observations have been published, most as case reports. Only five series include 10 or more cases[4,12,21, 34,36]. Postoperative mortality was 6 out of 121 cases in the literature (Table 1) and 13% in our series. Mortality seems to be related to high risk patient status rather than the technique itself. This is illustrated by the high late mortality rate (Fig. 8). Late secondary patency was 67.4±24.9% at 2 and 5 years (Fig. 9). These figures as well those reported in the literature (Table 2) are satisfactory considering the serious nature of the indications.

Based on these results descending thoracic aorta to femoral artery bypass can be considered as an alternative to AFB. In fact it provides better haemodynamic conditions probably with better long-term results without higher morbidity or mortality particularly.

REFERENCES

1. Barral X, Youvarlakis P, Boissier G, Cavallo G: Revascularisation des membres inférieurs à partir de l'aorte supra-cœliaque. *Ann Chir Vasc* 1986; 1: 30-35.
2. Blaisdell FW, Demattei GA, Gauder PJ Extraperitoneal thoracic aorta to femoral bypass graft as replacement for an infected aortic bifurcation prosthesis. *Am J Surg* 1961 ; 102 : 583-585.
3. Blaisdell FW, Hall AD: Axillary femoral artery bypass for lower extremity ischemia. *Surgery* 1963; 54: 563-568.
4. Bowes DE, Keagy BA, Benoit CH, Pharr WF: Descending thoracic aortobifemoral bypass for occluded abdominal aorta: retroperitoneal route without an abdominal incision. *J Cardiovasc Surg* 1985; 26: 41-45.
5. Bradham RR, Locklair PR Jr, Grimball A: Descending thoracic aorta to femoral artery bypass. *JSC Med Assoc* 1989; 85: 283-286.
6. Branchereau A, Ciosi G, Bordeaux J, Laselve L, Devin R: Femorofemoral bypass through the perineum for infection complicating arterial revascularization of the lower limbs. *Ann Vasc Surg* 1988; 2: 43-49.
7. Branchereau A, Espinoza H, Rudondy P, Magnan PE, Reboul J: Descending thoracic aorta as an inflow source for late occlusive failures following aortoiliac reconstruction. *Ann Vasc Surg* 1991; 5: 8-15.
8. Branchereau A , Rudondy P, Gournier JP, Espinoza H: The albumin-coated knitted dacron aortic prosthesis : a clinical study. *Ann Vasc Surg* 1990; 4: 138-142.
9. Broome A, Christenson JT, Eklof B, Norgren L: Axillofemoral bypass reconstructions in sixty-one patients with leg ischemia. *Surgery* 1980; 88: 673-676.
10. Bunt TJ: Synthetic vascular graft infections. II Graft-enteric erosions and graft enteric fistulas. *Surgery* 1983; 94: 1-9.
11. Buxton B, Simpson L, Johnson N, Myers K: Descending thoracic aortofemoral bypass for distal aortic reconstruction after removal of an infected dacron prosthesis. *Med J Aust* 1976; 2: 133-136.
12. Mc Carthy WJ, Rubin JR, Flinn WR, Williams LR, Bergan JJ, Yao JST: Descending thoracic aorta to femoral bypass. *Arch Surg* 1986; 121: 681-688.
13. Cevese PG, Gallucci V: Thoracic aorta to femoral artery bypass. *J Cardiovasc Surg* 1975; 16: 432-438.
14. Cooley DA: Surgical treatment of aortic aneurysms. Philadelphia, Saunders, 1986, pp 193-202.
15. Crawford ES, Crawford JL: Diseases of the aorta. Baltimore, Williams & Wilkins, 1984, pp 340-376.
16. De Laurentis DA: The descending thoracic aorta in reoperative aortic surgery. In : Bergan JJ, Yao JST (eds). Reoperative Arterial Surgery, Orlando, Grune & Stratton1986; pp 195-203.
17. Di Marzo L, Feldhaus RJ, Schultz RD: Surgical treatment of infected aortofemoral grafts : a fifteen year experience. *Vasc Surg* 1987; 21: 229-236.
18. Donaldson MC, Louras JC, Bucknam CA: Axillofemoral bypass : a tool with a limited role. *J Vasc Surg* 1986; 3: 757-763.
19. Ehrenfeld WK, Wilbur BG, Olcott CN IV, Stoney RS: Autogenous tissue reconstruction in the management of infected prosthetic grafts. *Surgery* 1979; 85: 82-92.
20. Enon B, Chevalier JM, Moreau P, Lescalie F, Pillet J: Revascularisation des membres

inférieurs à patir de l'aorte thoracique descendante. *J Chir* 1985; 122: 539-543.

21. Feldhaus RJ, Sterpetti AV, Schultz RD, Peetz DJ Jr: Thoracic aorta-femoral artery bypass : indications, technique and late results. *Ann Thorac Surg* 1985; 40: 588-592.
22. Finseth F, Abbott WM: One stage operative therapy for Salmonella mycotic abdominal aortic aneurysm. *Ann Surg* 1974; 179: 8-11.
23. Froysaker T, Skagseth E, Dundas P, Hall KV: Bypass procedures in the treatment of obstructions of the abdominal aorta. *J Cardiovasc Surg* 1973; 14: 317-321.
24. Hass KL, Moulder PV, Kerstein MD: Use of thoracic aortobifemoral artery grafting as an alternative procedure for occlusive aortoiliac disease. *Ann Surg* 1985; 51: 573-576.
25. Hussain SA: Descending thoracic aorta to bifemoral bypass graft without laparotomy. *Int Surg* 1988; 73: 260-263.
26. Jarrett F, Darling RC, Mundth ED, Austen G: Experience with infected aneurysms of the abdominal aorta. *Arch Surg* 1975; 110: 1281-1286.
27. Lakner G, Lukacs L: High aortoiliac occlusion : treatment with thoracic aorta to femoral arterial bypass. *J Cardiovasc Surg* 198; 24: 532-534.
28. Nunn DB, Kai MA: Bypass grafting from the thoracic aorta to femoral arteries for high aorto-iliac occlusive disease. *Surgery* 1972; 72: 749-55.
29. Oblath RW, Green RM, De Weese JA, Rob CG: Extra-anatomic bypass of the abdominal aorta. Management of postoperative thrombosis. *Ann Surg* 1978; 187: 647-652.
30. Ochsner JL: Use of thoracic aorta in revascularization of the lower extremity. In : Bergan JJ, Yao JST (eds). Evaluation and treatment of upper and lower extremity circulatory disorders Orlando, Grune & Stratton 1984; pp 361-368.
31. O'Mara CS, Williams GM: Extended retroperitoneal approach for abdominal aortic aneurysm repair. In : Bergan JJ, Yao JST (eds). Aneurysms diagnosis and treatment, Grune & Stratton 1982; pp 237-343.
32. Reilly LM, Ehrenfeld WK, Stoney RJ: Delayed aortic prosthetic reconstruction after removal of an infected graft. *Am J Surg* 1984; 148: 234-239.
33. Robicsek F, Mc Call MM, Sanger PW, Daugherty HK: Recurrent aneurysm of the abdominal aorta. *Ann Thorac Surg* 1967; 3: 549-552.
34. Rosenfeld JC, Savarese RP, De Laurentis DA: Distal thoracic aorta to femoral artery bypass a surgical alternative. *J Vasc Surg* 1985; 2: 747-750.
35. Schellack J, Fulenwider JT, Smith RB III: Descending thoracic aortofemoral-femoral bypass a remedial alternative for the failed aortobifemoral bypass. *J Cardiovasc Surg* 1988; 29: 201-204.
36. Schultz RD, Sterpetti AV, Feldhaus RJ: Thoracic aorta as source of inflow in reoperation for occluded aortoiliac reconstruction. *Surgery* 1986; 100: 635-645.
37. Stevenson JK, Sauvage LR, Harkins HN: A bypass homograf from thoracic aorta to femoral arteries for occlusive vascular disease. *Ann Surg* 1961; 27: 632-637.

Secondary Follow-Up

G.R. Pistolese, A. Ippoliti, G.A. Giordano, E. Crispo,
S. Ronchey and A. Ascoli Marchetti

Department of Vascular Surgery, University "Tor Vergata" of Rome, Italy

The surgical treatment of occlusive aorto-iliac desease offers satisfactory results both immediate, with a death rate from operation of 2-3% and a patency of over 95%, and long term results with a patency which varies from 87% to 85% over 5 years, from 70% to 77% over 10 years, from 68% to 79% over 15 years, from 55% to 68% over 20 years, as is evident from the examinations of the principles series of the relevant literature[2,10,16,52].

These good results are to be related to the high blood flow typical of this area, to the low resistance of the vascular bed below, to the standardized operation technique and to the reliability of the prosthetic material.

The long term results have improved because of the possibility of treating the elements of risk and the eventual associated vascular deseases (coronaries, carotids, etc.), which can have a significant influence on the survival of these patients.

Thanks to the technological evolution in the field of diagnosis it has become possible to follow-up the operated patient with non-invasive methods which, as they are neither dangerous nor traumatic for the patient, can be easily repeated, are extremely reliable, and together with a clinical examination, allows a thorough check-up and bring to light possible initial pathological symptoms which are not yet completely evident. The latter may be studied later with angiography, CT Scan, MRI etc., for a more thorough diagnosis.

A high percentage of long-term successes can be, however, obtained with repeated operations. The differences in long-term patency of the principle, world-wide series, become statistically meaningful if one compares the primary patency to the secondary[10,17,20,23,28].

Possible complications occurring later are represented by bypass thrombosis (10-20%), by anastomotic false aneurysms (2-8%), and by prosthetic graft infections (0.8-3%)[2,10,16,18,22,32,33,36,46,52,54].

The most frequent complication is the thrombosis of a branch or, more rarely, of the whole aorto-bifemoral bypass. At the level of the proximal anastomosis, a later date failure is rarely due to the progression of the atherosclerotic lesion or to the deterioration in the prosthetic graft; problems at aortic level are generally of technical nature and become evident early on during the period immediately after the operation. The causes are principally due to outflow difficulties connected with the progression of atherosclerosis desease below or to the insurgence of a fibrointimal hyperplasia at the level of the distal anastomosis. Brewster, in a report on 157 reoperations for aorto-femoral bypass occlusion, recognises the cause of the complication in an inadeguate outflow in 77% of the cases[10].

In some patients it becomes necessary, at a later date, to resort to a further reoperation for a new thrombotic episode. On this subject the relative literature gives a very little data and it is difficult to evaluate because numerous Authors do not specify well the number and the characteristics of the cases which undergo multiple operation and because patients who have undergone reoperations in one center may turn to other Institutes. The most part of the series, however, record how the clinical picture at the insurgence of the complication in increasingly more serious than the initial symptoms for which the patient underwent surgery[5,27].

Darke records, in patients who were reoperated on for the first time, a long-term patency of 70%, 60% and 45% at a distance of respectively 1, 3 and 5 years. With regard to further operations the cumulative patency increased to respectively 75%, 75% and 55%[17].

The causes of a new failure are frequently to be added to those of the first thrombotic complication and the main responsibility is to be related to a limited outflow following new lesions or distal progress of the atherosclerotic desease.

It has been suggested that the cause of thrombosis may be deterioration of the prosthetic graft and, in particular, of the various type of Dacron employed in this area, but this hypotesis has been dropped. Robicsek has implanted 158 aorto-bisiliac or bifemoral grafts with one branch in Knitted and the other in Woven Dacron without finding significant differences between the two sizes regarding platelet aggregation and the patency both immediate and at distance [41].

Crawford, examining his experience in 1004 cases of aorto-iliac reconstruction, did not find any significative differences among the various symptoms which suggested the first operation and the time interval between this revascularization and the successive ones[16].

Bernhard, one of the first to work on the problem, records, in a report on his experience published in 1977 concerning 50 reoperations for prosthetic occlusion (30 TEA and 20 implants of new grafts), 3 cases (6%) of unilateral occlusion which have later developed a contralateral problem. One late occlusion among reoperation occurred in 8 cases (17.4% of revascularized limbs): 5 (62.5%) were operated on successfully in 4 cases and 3 (37.5%) were amputated without attempting further revascularization[7].

In Benhamou's experience, among 70 reoperations (8.2%) out of 850 aor-to-femoral reconstructions, no less than 21 patients (30%) needed multiple "redo surgery": 8 (11.4%) a double, 7 (10%) a triple and 6 (8.6%) a quad-ruple with an over all success rate of 85%[5].

Ameli, out of 19 patients already operated on, reports the incidence of a second surgical treatment in 31.6% (6 cases) with 2 amputations and of a further third re-operation in 17.6% (3 cases) with 1 failure. The Author reports, more over, 4 cases (14.3%) of a single branch thrombosis followed over a period of time by the occlusion of the contralateral branch in a group of 28 late complications[1].

Frisch reports a similar incidence of subsequent thrombosis of the other branch of an aorto-bifemoral bypass: 7 cases (11.3%) out of 62 episodes of prosthetic thrombosis. Among the 51 cases globally treated with a thrombec-tomy, 12 (23.5%) had a relapse and among the latter, 8 (66.6%) presented a further rethrombosis which was treated with graft substitution[22].

Nevelsteen, out of 216 patients with late complications, reports how 91 (42.1%) had shown more than one[31]. In an other article, the Author reports out of 110 reoperations for prosthetic occlusion, 33 (30%) cases of rethrom-bosis 3 (9%) of which had undergone medical treatment, 6 (18.1%) major amputations and 24 (72.7%) "redo surgery". Among the latter, 6 (25%) showed a third thrombotic episode[32].

From this data it becomes clear that a further single branch thrombotic occurrence is not so rare and that this eventuality may affect the con-tralateral branch as well.

In Brewster's experience a further reoperation was undergone by 29 (26%) of the 110 patients operated on for bypass thrombosis and, in par-ticular, 79 multiple reoperations (69%) out of a total of 157 reoperations were carried out. It concerned smokers, who had not, in the majority of the cases, suspended the use of tobacco[10]; during the first reoperation, it was necessary to install a femoro-popliteal bypass in 26% of the cases, while in following cases, this was necessary with the regard to 53%.

One gathers from this data that the cause, in the majority of the multiple reocclusion cases, is to be identified of the atherosclerotic desease at the femoro-popliteal district.

As a confirmation of this, Crawford reports how, out of 89 patients who have already undergone "redo surgery", 31 (34.8%) had required a further revascularization, aorto-femoral in 18 cases and femoro-popliteal in 17. In the latter it concerned patients with functioning aorto-femoral bypasses, but which was not sufficient to resolve the more peripheral ischemia[15].

During multiple reoperations one may be confronted with technical dif-ficulties wich requires alternative types of incision and with high surgical risk patients who require greater skill from the vascular surgeon. The surgical techniques employed may be superimposed on those employed in the primary operation even though procedures with improve out-flow are more frequently added, such as extended profundoplastic procedures or more distal femoro-popliteal bypasses. Given that the surgical risk increased by conventional revascularization, both because of general causes and local technical problems, some Authors have suggested the use of extra-anatomic bypasses to restore inflow[5,10,13,15]; others, instead, have suggested a retroperitoneal approach with whole graft substitution[29]. As an alternative, a bypass with proximal anastomosis at the level of thoracic aorta has been suggested; this should have grater haemodynamic efficiency, with lesser infection risk than the extra-anatomic model and should avoid the unfavorable local conditions connected with re-operation[9].

However, the first choice for operating should be an inguinal thrombectomy which can be undertaken under local anaesthetic with minimal surgical risk for the patients who are often in critical general conditions. This is confirmed by the high death rate from operation in those cases which required the substitution of the whole graft (5.7-9%)[15,25,27,29,52]. When an other quick in-flow is not obtained with Fogarty's catheter, before deciding on a graft substitution, it is possible to utilize the Vollmar's dissectors. In multiple operation cases the thrombectomy, even if accurately performed, does not seem to guarantee an accettable long term patency and, in these patients, it is advisable to substitute partially the prosthesis; while a total substitution or an extra-anatomic bypass are necessary in selected cases.

Also in multiple reoperation cases it is desirable to intervene as soon as possible after the acute episode in order to avoid both the adhesion of the thrombotic material to the prosthesis and distal propagation of the thrombosis.

Should the ischemic episode be recent (less than 36-48 hours), thrombolitic loco-regional treatment can be used. This permits, with selective catheterism and low doses of fibrinolithic drugs, the dissolution of the thrombosis and the re-establishment of patency. It must be taken into account, however, that, in the majority of cases, the course of the ischemic episode is not removed, but is emphasized in order to resort to its surgical solution or to a PTA[55].

Regarding particular initial occlusive lesions, endovascular surgery, which permits the solution of these high-risk situations which could cause bypass thrombosis, has been suggested[57].

The control of elements of risk and of the evolution of the atherosclerotic desease must be undertaken with great attention and assiduity in those patients who have already presented a complication, in order to pinpoint as early as possible potentially dangerous situations and resolve them without reaching the dramatic and complex clinical-anatomical picture of the thrombotic occlusion.

Early diagnosis and treatment of initial lesions with patent prostheses can esclude inadeguate inflow problems and distal thrombosis that represent a possible cause of failure of the surgical theraphy.

The formation of a false aneurysm represents a not-infrequent complication in surgery in the aorto-iliac area; the overall incidence in this pathology varies from 2 to 8% [10,14,16,18,22,46,48,50,52,54].

The pseudoaneurysms may become manifest in a very wide period of time after the first operation. The relative literature records an average of about 50-60 months[14].

Regarding the pathogenesis, among the mechanical factors, procedures capable of altering the structural characteristics of the arterial wall near the anastomosis such as an endarterectomy, favour the formation of a false aneurysm. An other problem is represented by the difference of compliance which exists between the artery and an alloplastic graft; in this way the arterial hypertension may contribute to an acceleration of the phenomenon[51].

Some Authors have suggested an ethiology connected with the fragmentation of suture material or with the prosthetic dilation[37,48].

The bacterial graft infection, mostly caused from coagulase-negative Staphilococci, has been documented in a significant number of explanted prosthesis because of false aneurysms in the absence of any factor which might give rise to the suspicion of infection[45].

Recent studies suggest how patients who run the danger of formation of false aneurysms may suffer from an aggressive form of atherosclerosis which often involves brain and coronary vessels. This factor, togheter whith those mentioned above, may promote a gradual degeneration of the anastomotic junction.

As a confirmation of this hypotesis, Schellack, by analizing his experience of 102 cases of femoral pseudoaneurysm, discovered that out of 41 patients who had undergone an aorto-bifemoral bypass, 29 (70%) had a bilateral localization and that, out of 48 patients with aorto-femoral bypass, there was a simultaneous aortic and femoral localization in 8 (17%)[44].

Among the most recent experiences, Nevelsteen, considering 869 patients operated on for aorto-femoral bypass, comfirms this fact, reporting, among 66 anastomotic false aneurysms, 10 cases (15.1%) simultaneous multiples and 5 (7.6%) consecutive multiples over a period of time[31]. Courbier describes, though with a lesser incidence, the same phenomenon in 10 patients who presented a bilateral false aneurysm out of 74 patients who have been surgically treated; he reports, moreover, how in literature Hollier & Starr report an incidence of 30% [14].

Crawford, among 30 cases of false aneurysm, in a huge group of 1287 patients who had undergone aorto-iliac surgery, brought attention to 5 patients (16.7%) who had presented an other false aneurysm at the level of an other anastomosis[15].

An early diagnosis becomes particularly important above all in consideration of the fact that, in the case of "redo surgery" the death rate percentage rises from 6-8% in the patients selected for an operative management, to 60-70% in those needing emergency operation due to aortic pscudoaneurysm rupture[18,54]. While the diagnosis of a false aneurysm of the groin may be suggested by a careful phisical examination, the same may not be invoked should the aorta or iliac arteries be involved. This eventuality is often characterized by hidden symptoms until the aneurysm rupture. According to Sieswerda, the physical examination alone may give rise to 37% false positives and 67% false negatives[46].

After the first surgical treatment, in some cases, further complications may arise such as reoccurence of false aneurysms, thrombosis and graft infection.

Szilagyi, in examining his study of 1748 operations for revascularization of aorto-iliac lesions, reports 173 cases of femoral false aneurysm, 27 of which were relapses: 23 (13.3%) represented a first recurrence and 4 (2.3%) a further pathological episode[52]. The same Author have previously reported a similar incidence of first relapse equal to 10.9% (17 out of 156 patients which had undergone surgery)[51].

Also Schellack reports, with an average interval of 73 months, 6 (7.3%) recurring pseudoaneurysms out of 82 groin cases. In particular, among 70 cases having undergone surgery, 4 (5.7%) represented a first recurrence and 2 (2.8%) a third episode. Moreover, there were 13 thromboses (18.6%) and 4 infections (5.7%)[44].

Courbier reports an incidence of 24 femoral aneurysmal relapses (22.4%) out of 107 false aneurysms operated on with an average interval of 25 months from the first reoperation compared with 41 months interval between the first operation and the surgical correction of the false anastomotic aneurysm. It concerned 4 patients with 3 relapses and 2 patients with 4 [14].

Carson, in 42 pseudoaneurysms surgically treated, analyses the various phisiopathologic aspects by comparing 22 primary cases with 20 (47.6%) relapses. There were no infection in either group, the recurrences had been repaired with the insertion of a segment of Dacron, and no technical errors were pinpointed. The differences were represented by the outcoming time which, contrary to Courbier, was longer in relapse cases (38 vs. 17 months), by the higher hypertension incidence (45 vs. 27.3%), by the greater graft dilation (16 vs. 11%) and by the type of anatomo-pathological finding (arterial and graft dilatation with separation: 85 vs. 22.7%). In particular the latter cause concerned a marked degeneration of arterial wall due to the loss of smooth muscle cells with a fragmentation of elastic lamina and elastic fibers proliferation[12].

Regarding the pseudoaneurysm, therefore, a great deal of attention should be paid to the localisation also at the level of another anastomosis, which often appears completely asymptomatic, or to its relapse. The operated patient must be followed-up using routinely echo-doppler, followed by more invasive and selective methods such as TC Scan, MRI and angiography when there is a well-founded suspicion of pseudoaneurysms, in order to evaluate more thoroughly its dimensions, its relation with contiguous structures and its evolution. Moreover, the presence of indirect tomographic signs, such as air-bubbles around the graft or peri-graft fluid collection, at least some time after the operation, may demonstrate or deny an infective etiology. In this instance, even considering the type of re-operation to be undertaken, some Authors suggest the importance of subjecting the patient to instrumental examinations capable to precociously detect a prosthetic graft infection, like leukocytes-labeled scanning[45].

Together with a precocious diagnosis, treatment is important before the insurgence of possible complications as embolism, thrombosis and hemorrage, which lead to a noteworthy increase of failures and in the death rate from operation[47].

Regarding the surgical treatment, this consists in the resection of the false aneurysm with distal revascularization, through a single re-anastomosis or by an eventual interposition of a new prosthetic segment. It is thought that, at femoral level, the termino-terminal anastomoses has a lesser relapse and thrombosis incidence compared with the latero-terminal one. Carson emphasize the importance of prosthetic branch substitution avoiding a second anastomosis between the old graft and the femoral artery, both in order to achieve greater guarantees of good-function at distance, but chiefly to avoid the risk of relapses which are always difficoult to treat[12].

Particulary attention should be reserved to thrombotic or pseudoaneurismal complications in patients already submitted to reoperations for surgical problems of a previous aorto femoral bypass. The importance of early detection of these events and the immediate surgical repair, before their clinical evolution, avoid the dramatic and severe anatomo-clinical findings represented by further relaps that lead to very poor results.

To be greatly feared, because of their high morbility and mortality rate, are the prosthetic graft infecions in the aorto-iliac area. They have an incidence, in literature, that varies from 0.7 to 2.6%.

The conventional surgical treatment, based on the infected graft removal and consequent limbs revascularization with an extra-anatomical bypass, has not generally produced satisfactory results as it has an high mortality (up to 75%) and an amputation rate ranging from 8 to 58%, according to the most important series[8,11,19,24,30, 33,38,49], even though Reilly reports, in her experience of 101 patients, an overall death rate equal to 28% in the first 6 month postoperatively, with a reinfection rate of 13% which reached 20% in high-risk patients[39]. O'Hara underlines how 40% of patients with in-fected aortic grafts had undergone more than 2 reoperation (2.1) for repairing prosthetic occlusion before the diagnosis of infection was made[33].

Studies of infections' natural history from its insurgence to its evolution, have demonstrated the importance of detecting its presence before it becomes evident. When the diagnosis is made at this stage, the necessary treatment will inevitably bring about that high incidence of complicances and death rate which relevant literature reports[35].

During the last few years, research has been orientated towards the definition of a procedure which allows precocious diagnosis in order to utilise new strategic tactics in early and therefore less aggressive stages. Encouraging results have been obtained with Indium or Tecnetium leucocytes-labeled scanning, method which has an accuracy near to 90%[43]. Some Authors suggest using the MRI; the latter permits, in fact, the pin-pointing of an inflammatory reaction and the differentiation between haemorragic and serous fluids, even if of distinguishing the differences among the characteristics of non-haemorrahic fluids[34].

The improved knowledge of the behaviour of prosthetic graft infection, of the etiologic agents and of the greater incidence in well-defined groups of patients, have led to a new post-operative management. It has been demonstrated to be necessary to carry out periodical, short term check-up especially in particular groups of patients: diabetics, patients who have undergone more than one operation, or patients with a femoral vascular anastomosis. These examinations should aim at the earliest possible detecting of symptoms and signs which may suggest the possible presence of an infection.

The surgical correction purely limited to the apparent infected area, togheter with antibiotic prophylaxis and with the correction of eventual immunological changes, has given encouraging results.

Regarding the aortic infections which have undergone conservative treatment, the documentation over the last 10 years reports an overall death rate of 19-21%. In case of aorto-enteric fistulas, in patients treated in a conservative way, a survival rate equal to 87% without complication with a follow-up of 1-5 years is recorded[21, 26, 42].

Walker, out of 23 cases treated with this technique, report an immediate success rate of 78.3% with an operatory mortality of 21.7%. In an average follow-up of 5.2 years, among the 18 survivors, there were 3 complications at the level of the proximal anastomosis with the death of 2 patients; the other 15 (83.3%) did not report other problems[56]. Bandyk, out of 19 infected prosthesis (16 aorto-femoral, 2 axillo-femoral, 1 femoro-popliteal grafts) treated by the systemic administration of antibiotics, removal of the infected graft, excision of periprosthetic material involved in inflammatory process, prosthetic substitution with PTFE graft and protective flap over sartorious muscle, did not report thrombosis or reinfection for an average period of 26 months (follow-up: 6-60 months)[3,4].

Regarding infected femoral anastomosis, many Authors tend to use a conservative treatment or, at least, a partial excision od the prosthesis immediatly above the infected area and the lenghtening of the affected branch with a PTFE graft distally anastomized under the infection. These operations seems to reduce the death rate and the incidence of major amputations. Bandyk, in his series of 17 infected graft by Gram (-) bacteria, treated by partial resection and distal bypass in PTFE, does not report cases of re-infection and records only one reoperation at a distance of 3 years because of a graft branch thrombosis[3,4].

The conservative treatment of proximal infections in more debated even though many Authors have made use of it. Quick[38] reports, in fact, the cases of 4 patients treated by drainage of infected area and local irrgation with antibiotics drugs repeated for 17 days-5 weeks: in one case infection occurred again after 3.5 years. Also Tobin report a case successfully treated means of drainage and repeated irrigation with antibiotic solutions[53]. Robinson has, moreover, suggested the possibility of in situ re-manufacturing reporting excellent results in 10 patients treated by him for graft infection at aortic level, without reinfections or deaths during a follow-up period of 10 months-9 years[42].

The correction purely limited to the apparent infected area, that sems to give encouraging results, allows operations with minor trauma and surgical risk for the patient; this is possible only with an early and accurate detection of the infection before its extention to all the prostheses.

On the contrary Ricotta, out of 32 cases of treated aortic graft infection, 12 of which with partial excision and 20 with total graft removal, records a death rate equal to 75% in the first group, while, among the patients of the second group with extra-anatomic revascularization, no reccurring infection, amputation dehiscence of aortic stump over an average period of 34 months has been reported. There was a statistically significant decrease in the postoperative complications in the group with whole graft removal, especially in those cases treated with extra-anatomic bypass[40].

The presented series are, however, still very limited and the problem of graft infection is one of the most scrious and to be feared in the field of aorto-iliac surgery.

The patient who has already undergone "redo surgery" for a graft infection must be included in a follow-up protocol with close-tined and more thorough examinations (ecography, TC scan, Tecnetium labeled leukocytes scan, etc.) because the early dia-gnosis af a relapse infection can be treated when the general conditions are still satisfactory and therefore present fewer general surgical risks with a better immunitary response from the patient, by substituting, if possible, only the infected segment of the prosthetic graft.

In conclusion, the patients who presents a complication which is either thrombotic, pseudoaneurysmatic or infective, and for this reason has undergone "redo surgery" must be followed-up with more frequent and accurate examinations which permits the identification of those situations of risk needing the earliest treatment possible before the insurgence of the often dramatic and difficult to resolve anatomo-clinical picture represented by a further relapse.

REFERENCES

1. Ameli F.M., Provan J.L., Williamson C., Keuchler P.M.: Etiology and management of aorto-femoral bypass graft failure. *J. Cardiovasc. Surg.* 1987; 28: 695-700
2. Baird R.J.: Techniques and results of arterial prosthetic bypass for aorto-iliac occlusive disease. *Can. J. Surg.* 1982; 25: 476
3. Bandyk D.F., Bergamini T.M., Kinney E.V., Seabrook G.R., Towne J.B.: In situ relacement of vascular prostheses infected by bacterial biofilms. *J. Vasc. Surg.* 1991; 13: 575-83

4. Bandyk D.F.: When can an infected prosthetic arterial graft be treated by in situ prosthetic graft replacement. 18°Annual Symp. Current Critical Problems and New Horizons in Vascular Surgery; New York, november1991
5. Benhamou A.C., Kieffer E., Tricot J.F., Maraval M., Thoai M.L., Natali J.: "Redo" surgery for late aortofemoral graft occlusive failures. *J. Cardiovasc. Surg.* 1984; 25: 118-125
6. Bergeron P., Espinoza H. Rudondy P., Ferdani M., Martin J., Jausseran J.M., Courbier R.: Fistules Aorto-duodénales secondaires: Intérèt du pontage axillo-fémoral premier. *Ann. Chir. Vasc.* 1991; 5: 4-7
7. Bernhard W.M., Ray L.I., Towne J.B.: The reoperation of choice for aorto-femoral graft occlusion. *Surgery* 1977; 82: 867-874
8. Bleyn J., Kinsbergen G.: A case against immediate revascularization after uni- or bilateral removal of infected aortobifemoral (end-to-site) prosthetic grafts. *J. Cardiovasc. Surg.* 1988; 29: 264-67
9. Branchereau A., Espinoza H., Rudondy P., Magnan P., Reboul J.: Descending thoracic aorta as an inflow source for late occlusive failures following aortoiliac reconstruction. *Ann. Vasc. Surg.* 1991; 5: 8-15
10. Brewster D.C.: Surgery of late aortic graft occlusion. In: Aortic surgery, pag. 519; J.J. Bergan, J.S.T. Yao eds.; W.B. Saunders Company, London, 1989
11. Calligaro K.D., Veith F.J., Gupta DS.K., Ascer E., Dietzek A.M., Franco C.D., Wengerter K.R.: A modified method for management of prosthetic graft infections involving an anastmosis to the common femoral artery. *J. Vasc. Surg.* 1991; 11: 485-92
12. Carson S.N., Hunter G.C., Palmaz J., Guernsey J.M.: Recurrence of femoral anastomotic aneurysms. *Am. J. Surg.* 1983; 146: 774-778
13. Charlesworth D.: The occluded aortic and aortofemoral graft. In: Reoperative arterial surgery, pag. 271; J.J. Bergan, J.S.T. Yao eds.; Grune and Stratton, Orlando, New York, 1986
14. Courbier R., Larranaga J.: Natural hystory and management of anastomotic aneurysms. In: Aneurysms: diagnosis and treatment, pag. 567; J.J. Bergan, Y.S.T. Yao eds.; Grune and Stratton, New York, 1982
15. Crawford E.S., Manning L.G., Kelly T.F.: "Redo" surgery after operations for aneurysm and occlusion of abdominal aorta. *Surgery* 1977; 81:41-52
16. Crawford E.S., Bomberger R.A., Glaeser D.H., Saleh S.A., Russel W.L.: Aorto-iliac occlusive disease: Factors influencing survival and function following reconstructive operation over a 25 year period. *Surgery* 1981; 90: 1055-1067
17. Darke S.G.: The surgical management of occluded aortobifemoral grafts. In: The maintenance of arterial reconstruction, pag. 351; R.M. Greenhalgh, L.H. Hollier eds.; W.B. Saunders Company, London, 1991
18. Dennis J.W., Littooy F.N., Greisler H.P., Baker W.H.: Anastomotic pseudoaneurysms. *Arch. Surg.* 1986; 121: 314-317
19. England D.W., Simms M.H.: Recurrent aorto-duodenal fistula: A final solution? *Eur J. Vasc. Surg.* 1990; 4: 427-29
20. Fiorani P., Spartera C., Pistolese G.R.: Indicazioni al trattamento chirurgico delle lesioni aorto- iliache: il bypass aorto-femorale. *Min. Med.* 1979; 70: 2189
21. François F., Thevenet A.: Conservative treatment of prosthetic aortic graft infection with irrigation. *Ann. Vasc. Surg.* 1991; 5: 199-201
22. Frisch N., Bour P., Berg P., Fieve G., Frisch R.: La trombectomie dans les occlusions tardives des pontages aorto-femoraux: resultats tardifs. *Ann. Chir. Vasc.* 1991; 5: 16-20
23. Hyde G.L., McCready R.A., Schwartz R.W., Mattingly S.S., Ernst C.B.: Durability of thrombectomy of occluded aortofemoral graft limbs. *Surgery* 1983; 94: 748-751
24. Jacobs M.J.H., Reul G.J., Gregoric I., Cooley D.A.: In-situ replacement and extra-anatomic bypass for the treatment of infected abdominal aortic grafts. *Eur. J. Vasc. Surg.* 1991; 5: 83-86
25. Kanaly P.J., Dilling E.W., Robinson H.B., Elkins R.C.: Discussion and management of late failures in reconstructive procedures involving the abdominal aorta. *Am. J. Surg.* 1978; 136: 709-713
26. Lorentzen J.E.,, Nielsen O.M.: Aortobifemoral bypass with autogenous saphenous vein in treatment of paninfected aortic bifurcation graft. *J. Vasc. Surg.* 1986; 3:666-8.
27. Malone J.M., Moore W.S., Goldstone J.: Life expectancy following aortofemoral arterial grafting. *Surgery* 1977; 81: 551-556
28. Malone J.M., Goldstone J., Moore W.S.: Autogenous profundoplasty: the key to long term patency in secondary repair of aorto femoral graft occlusion. *Ann. Surg.* 1978; 188: 817-823
29. Najafi H., Dye W.S., Javid H.: Late thrombosis affecting one limb of aortic biforcation graft.

Arch. Surg. 1975; 110: 409-412
30. Nevelsteen A., Suy R.: Autogenous vein reconstruction in the treatment of aortobifemoral prosthetic infection. *J. Cardiovasc. Surg.* 1988; 29: 315-317
31. Nevelsteen A., Suy R.: Occlusions tardives apres pontage aorto-femoral en dacron. *Ann. Chir. Vasc.* 1991; 5: 32-37
32. Nevelsteen A., Wouters L., Suy R.: Aortofemoral dacron reconstruction for aorto-iliac occlusive isease: a 25-year survey. *Eur. J. Vasc. Surg.* 1991; 5: 179-186
33. O'Hara P.J., Hertzer N.R., Beven E.G., Krajewski L.P.: Surgical management of infected abdominal aortic grafts: Review of a 25-year experience. *J. Vasc. Surg.* 1986; 3: 725-731
34. Olofsson P.A., Auffermann W., Higgins C.B., Rabahie G.N., Tavares N., Stoney R.J.: Diagnosis of prosthetic aortic graft infection by magnetic resonance imaging. *J. Vasc. Surg.* 1988; 8: 99 105
35. Pabst T.S., Bernhard V.M., McIntyre K.E., Malone J.M.: Gastrointestinal bleeding after aortic surgery. *J. Vasc. Surg.* 1988; 8: 280-5
36. Pistolese G.R., Ippoliti A., Ranucci A., Tozzi A., Ronchey S.: Chirurgia aorto-iliaca: Stato dell'arte. Atti II Congresso internazionale sulle protesi vascolari, pag. 221; P. Pietri ed.; Monduzzi Editore, Bologna, 1989
37. Postlethwait R.W.: Long term comparative study of nonadsorbable sutures. *Ann. Surg.* 1970; 171: 892
38. Quick C.R.G., Vassallo D.J., Colin J.F., Heddle R.M.: Conservative treatment of major aortic graft infections. *Eur. J. Vasc. Surg.* 1990; 4: 63-67
39. Reilly L.M., Stoney R.J., Goldstone J., Ehrenfeld W.K.: Improved management of aortic graft infection: The influence of operation sequence and staging. *J. Vasc. Surg.* 1987; 5: 421-31
40. Ricotta J.J.: Total excision and extra-anatomic bypass for aortic graft infection. 18° Annual Symp. Current Critical Problems and New Horizons in Vascular Surgery; New York, november 1991
41. Robicsek F., Duncan G.D., Daugherty H.K., Cook J.C., Selle J.G., Hess P.J.: "Half and half" woven and knitted dacron grafts in the aortoiliac and aortofemoral positions: Seven and one-half years follow-up. *Ann. Vasc. Surg.* 1991; 5: 315-319
42. Robinson J.A., Johansen K.: Aortic sepsis: Is there a role for in situ graft reconstruction? *J. Vasc. Surg.* 1991; 13: 677-84
43. Roddie M.E., Peters A.M., Danpure H.J., Osmann S., Handerson B.L., Lavender J.P., Carroll M.J., Neirinkcx R.D., Kelly J.D.: Inflammation: imaging with Tc-99m HMPAO-Labeled leukocytes. *Radiology* 1988; 166: 767
44. Schellack J., salam A., Abouzeid M.A., Smith R.B., Stewart M.T., Perdue G.D.: Femoral anastomotic aneurysms: a continuing challenge. *J. Vasc. Surg.* 1987; 6: 308-317
45. Seabrook G.R., Schmitt D.D., Bandyk D.F., Edmiston C.E., Krepel C.J., Towne J.B.: Anastomotic femoral pseudoaneurysms: an investigation of occult infection as an etiologic factor. *J. Vasc. Surg.* 1990; 11: 629-634
46. Sieswerda C., Skotnicki S.H., Barentsz J.O., Heystraten F.M.J.: Anastomotic aneurysms - an Underdiagnosed complication after aorto-iliac reconstructions. *Eur. J. Vasc. Surg.* 1989; 3: 233-238
47. Spartera C., Speziale F., Santoro P., Zaccaria A., Pistolese G.R.: Anastomotic aneurysms after aorto-femoral bypass. Prevention and treatment. *Surgery in Italy* 1979; 9: 79-89
48. Starr D.S., Weatherford S.C., Lawrie G.M., Morris G.C.: Suture material as a factor in the occurrence of anastomotic false aneurysms. *Arch. Surg.* 1979; 114: 412-415
49. Szilagyi D.E., Smith R.F., Elliott J.P., Vrandecic M.P.: Infection in arterial reconstruction with synthetic grafts. *Ann. Surg.* 1972; 176: 321-333
50. Szilagyi D.E., Smith R.J., Elliott J.P., Hagemann J.H., Dall'Olmo C.A.: Anastomotic aneurysms after vascular reconstruction: Problems of incidence, etiology, and treatment. *Surgery* 1976; 78: 800-816
51. Szilagyi D.E., Elliott J.P., Smith R.F., Hageman J.H., Sood R.K.: Secondary arterial repair: the management of late failures in arterial reconstructive surgery. *Arch. Surg.* 1975; 110: 485-493
52. Szilagyi D.E., Elliott J.P., Smith R.F., Reddy D.J., McPharlin M.: A thirty-year survey of the reconstructive surgical treatment of aorto-iliac occlusive disease. *J. Vasc. Surg.* 1986; 3: 421-436
53. Tobin K.D.: Aortobifemoral perigraft abscess: Treatment by percutaneous catheter drainage. *J. Vasc. Surg.* 1988; 8: 339-43
54. Treimann S., Weaver F.A., Cossman D.V., Foran R.F., Cohen J.L., Levin P.M., Treiman R.L.:

Anastomotic false aneurysms of the abdominal aorta and the iliac arteries. *J. Vasc. Surg.* 1988; 8: 268-273

55. van Breda A., Robinson J.C., Feldman L.: Local thrombolysis in the treatment of arterial graft occlusions. *J. Vasc. Surg.* 1984; 1: 103-112

56. Walker W.E., Cooley D.A., Duncan J.M., Hallman G.L., Ott D.A., Reul G.J.: The management of aortoduodenal fistula by in situ replacement of infected abdominal aortic graft. *Ann. Surg.* 1987; 205: 727-32

57. White G.H., White R.A., Kopchok G.E., Colman P.D., Wilson S.E.: Endoscopic intravascular surgery removes intraluminal flaps, dissections and thrombus. *J. Vasc. Surg.* 1990; 11: 280-288

58. Yashar J.J., Weyman A.K., Burnard R.J., Yashar J.: Survival and limb salvage in patients with infected arterial prosthese. *Am. J. Surg.* 1978; 135: 499-504

REDO SURGERY IN INFRAINGUINAL AREA

"Redo" Surgery in The Infrainguinal Area

R.M. Greenhalgh

*Department of Surgery, Charing Cross and Westminster
Medical School, Charing Cross Hospital, London, U.K.*

The chapters which are included in this section of the book range from prevention of unnecessary "redo" surgery by getting the operation right in the first case, through to follow-up after the secondary procedure. The use of intra-arterial ultrasound imaging is in its infancy. There is very much more experience with intra-vascular endoscopy and of course, electromagnetic flow probes. Doppler ultrasound and Duplex scanning have also been used as well as on-table arteriography to check that an operation has been done properly the first time. Intra-vascular ultrasound is the latest in the line of instruments used to check that the operation is as near perfect as possible. This facility may prove to be ideal or it may be better in some respects than others and the chapter in this section debates these issues.

It is not essential always to operate a second time when a bypass fails as sometimes the symptoms do not merit reoperation. Indications for redo surgery as considered next and improved strategy for secondary operations in this situation. Nowadays some surgeons are leaving their first choice conduit, saphenous vein and using a prosthetic material for bypass to the suprageniculate popliteal in the first instance. If such a bypass fails, the vein is there and can be used if necessary.

Endovascular procedures are developing rapidly and sometimes these can be used in the redo situation. The place of atherectomy, laser angioplasty and conventional angioplasty is considered in this section and these have to be considered as an alternative to a second arterial bypass. On those occasions on which an endovascular technique was used on the first occasion, the first bypass may be needed for the "redo" procedure.

Careful audit and surveillance of a reconstruction is always important but it is even more important after a failure than at any other time. During the secondary follow-up, it is necessary to monitor patients' habits and consider whether they should be taking platelet inhibitory therapy and to what extent they are listening to advice to stop smoking. One has to bear in mind that many of the patients say one thing and do another and during the secondary follow-up period, these issues become vitally important.

Is Intravascular Ultrasound Imaging Helpful in Preventing Restenosis After PTA ?

H. van Urk[1], W.J. Gussenhoven[2,4], N.A.J.J. du Bois[1],
S.H.K. The[2,4], H. Pieterman[3], C.T. Lancée[2],
F.C. van Egmond[2] and N. Bom[2]

*Departments of Vascular Surgery[1], Thoraxcenter[2] and
Radiology[3] and Intercardiology Institute[4]
University Hospital Rotterdam, The Netherlands*

INTRODUCTION

Percutaneous transluminal angioplasty, with or without the use of laser energy, is attractive as an alternative to vascular surgical reconstruction because of the simplicity of the procedure, avoiding the need of general anaesthesia, long skin incisions and associated woundhealing problems. The method appeals to both patients an intervention radiologists, whereas a majority of the vascular surgeons have either refrained from applying this technique or have frankly critisized the procedure.

One of the main reasons for this difference in opinion from two sides of the disciplines involved in the treatment of peripheral vascular disease is formed by the discrepancy between an allegedly high initial (technical) success rate and the ensuing long-term results. A major factor in determining the disappointing late patency after PTA is the relatively high incidence of recurrent stenosis[8]. Another factor is undoubtedly the absence of uniform reporting standards, as pointed out recently by Rutherford[9].

The problem of restenosis is found both in peripheral PTA and after coronary PTA. Different regimen for drug treatment aimed at preventing restenosis have not lead to improvement: clinical trials of multiple agents have been unsuccessful in altering the rate of restenosis following coronary angioplasty[2]. Moreover, the role of PTA in the management of renovascular hypertension caused by atherosclerotic disease is still debated[1] and controversy still exists about the treatment with PTA of infra-inguinal vein graft stenoses[12].

The application of endovascular ultrasound is a relatively new development in the field of vascular diagnostic procedures. The role of endovascular imaging in the armamentarium of the vascular surgeon or interventional radiologist has yet to be determined. However, from the experimental in-vitro and in-vivo experience and the preliminary observations in the clinical situation, the method appears to have several advantages over angiography and angioscopy: endovascular ultrasound provides both qualitative and quantitative information about the vessel wall and atherosclerotic lesions that cannot be obtained by any other method in comparable detail and accuracy.

It is postulated that the information obtained by intra-arterial ultrasonic imaging will lead to a better understanding of the pathophysiologic effects that are caused by balloon angioplasty. Based on this information it may be feasible to modify or adept our angioplasty policy in order to overcome or reduce the problems of re-stenosis.

In this article we describe our clinical experience up to date, which is entirely based on the close correlation between histologic and ultrasonic cross-sections of normal and diseased arteries as shown in previous in-vitro and in-vivo experiments.

INTRAVASCULAR ULTRASOUND SYSTEM

All clinical investigations were performed with a high frequency intravascular device currently under dcevelopment in our laboratory. This prototype (Du-Med™, Rotterdam, The Netherlands) consists of a 32 MHz single-element ultrasound transducer mounted in the tip of a 5.2 F catheter and covered with an acoustically transparent dome (Fig. 1).

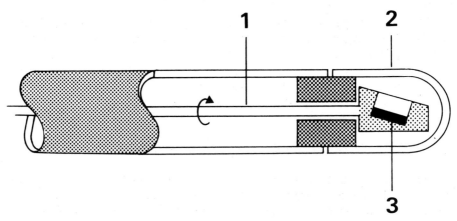

Fig. 1. Schematic drawing of ultrasound catheter tip. (1) drive shaft, (2) transparent dome, (3) ultrasound element.

The ultrasound element is motor-driven by a flexible drive-shaft, providing continuous real-time cross-section images of the vessel wall (up to 16 images per second). The ultrasonic images are displayed on a monitor by means of a video-scanned memory of 512 x 512 pixels with 256 gray levels. Axial resolution of the system is 75 micron and lateral resolution is better than 200 micron at a depth of 1 mm.

TECHNIQUE

The catheter is introduced through a 7 F introducer sheath, either percutaneously or "à vue" after surgical dissection of the artery, usually the common femoral or superficial femoral artery. Percutaneous studies are performed under local anesthesia, intraoperative studies were always performed under general anesthesia. The ultrasound catheter is advanced into the artery, either antegrade to the superficial femoral and popliteal artery or retrograde to the external and common iliac arteries. The tip of the catheter is passed beyond the stenotic segment, as known from previous angiography or under fluoroscopic control. No attempt is made to advance the catheter with force, but usually the stiffness of the catheter allows the tip to pass through soft materials like recent clot formation. The position of the tip of the catheter is monitored under fluorscopy with the help of a radiopaque ruler. If a total occlusion cannot be passed due to a rigid or calcified obstruction, a Nd-Yag laser (Medilon-2, MBB) is used to obtain a channel. While the catheter is pulled back slowly, the ultrasonic images are displayed in real-time and are also recorded on a videorecorder for off-line studies. Small amounts of heparinised saline solution are injected through the introducer sheath in order to replace the echogenic blood with a non-echogenic solution for the time of a few heart beats, in order to achieve a better outline of the lumen.

A completion angiography is always performed to compare ultrasonic and angiographic images. The procedure is repeated after balloon angioplasty has been performed.

Quantitative analysis of the stored data is performed with the help of an IBM compatible PC/AT computer equipped with a DT 2851 framegrabber and a PC mouse for manual contour tracing[10].

ULTRASONIC CHARACTERISTICS OF ARTERIAL WALL

The clinical application of endovascular ultrasound and the interpretation of the ultrasonic images is entirely based on the characteristics of echogenecity of the different layers of the arterial wall and the different components of atherosclerotic lesions as found in earlier in-vitro studies[5,6].

As iliac, femoral and popliteal arteries are histologically classified as "muscular" arteries, because the media of the vessel wall consists mainly of smooth muscle cells (in contrast to "elastic" arteries, where the media mainly contains elastin fibers), all these arteries are easily identifyable on ultrasonic interrogation because of the typically "hypoechoic" media, resulting in a characteristic three-layered appearance of the muscular artery wall. This hypoechoic media serves as a landmark in the recognition of atherosclerotic lesions, like diffuse intimal thickening. The echo-lucent zone between intima and adventitia allows computer tracing of the outer boundary of an atherosclerotic lesion. The inner boundary of a normal artery can be traced by tracking the bright echoes of the internal elastic lamina. The inner surface of a diseased artery can be outlined by flushing the artery with saline solution, thus replacing the backscatter echoes from flowing blood resulting in an echo-free lumen area.

The lesion area is defined as the region enclosed by these two contours and can be calculated by subtracting the area of the free lumen from that of the "media-bounded" area[11].

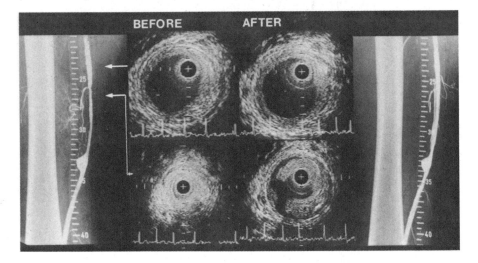

Fig. 2. Angiography and corresponding ultrasound images before (left) and after (right) balloon dilatation.
Upper level: normal artery (no dilatation).
Lower level: severe stenosis before PTA, plaque rupture and partial dissection after PTA.

The different components of atherosclerotic lesions produce different echo patterns:

lipid deposition	- hypoechoic
diffuse intimal thickening	- soft echoes
collagen-rich fibrous tissue	- bright echoes
calcified lesions	- bright echoes with shadowing behind the lesion

ENDOVASCULAR INTERVENTIONS

The most striking observation after balloon angioplasty is the frequent finding of atherosclerotic plaque rupture and dissection between plaque and remaining arterial wall (Fig. 2).

This phenomenon is sometimes displayed very obviously on angiography, but is frequently obscured and can only be suspected in other cases. This largely depends on the location of the dissection with regard to the direction of the X-ray projection. Tangential projection reveals a dissection easily, whereas a rupture in the ventral or dorsal part of the vessel wall can be obscured on A-P projection.

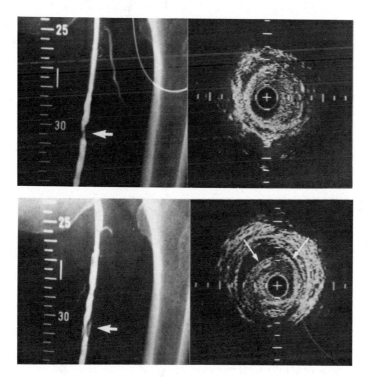

Fig. 3 A-B. A: Angiography and corresponding ultrasound image a level of severe stenosis before PTA. Remaining free lumen diameter 3 mm (calibration on ultrasound image in millimeters). B: Same vessel and same location as in fig. 3a, now after PTA. Note plaque rupture at 12 o'clock and partial dissection of flaps from 8-3 o'clock. Bloodflow in original lumen is slower than in false lumen (dissected area), as evidenced by higher echogenecity of blood arount the catheter.

Intravascular ultrasound not only recognizes this type of lesion at any sector of the circumference of the arterial wall, it actually visualizes the movements of a ruptured plaque inside the lumen as caused by the pulsatile blood flow (Fig. 3).

Computer analysis of this phenomenon has confirmed that the original concept of co-axial dilatation as described by Dotter and Judkins in 1964[3] is erroneous. Dotter theorized that the atheromatous plaque obstructing the lumen of the artery would be compressed by the co-axial catheter like fresh snow is compressed by footsteps. From computer calculations as mentioned above it has clearly been shown that the difference between pre- and post-PTA ultrasonic cross-sections with regard to increase of free lumen area, is entirely based on stretching of the media-bounded area, wheras the plaque area virtually stays the same.

Stretching of the media and adventitia occurs primarily in the sector of the vessel wall that has relatively few disease. Measuring the thickness of the atherosclerotic plaque provides one parameter for classifying the severeness of arteriosclerotic disease, measuring the thickness of the media appeared to be another reliable discriminating factor. The phenomenon of "thinning" of the media with progression of atherosclerotic disease, as described by Glagov[4] for coronary arteries was confirmed by our studies in peripheral arteries[7].

Conversely, the presence of a normal sized media behind a thickened "intimal" area consisting of soft echoes may be an indicator that this lesion consists of mural thrombus rather than an intimal lesion.

Currently no consensus exists about the potential harm or benefit of vessel wall dissections after PTA. Some authors argue that the false lumen will create an area of low bloodflow which is prone to induce thrombus formation and therefore a possible cause of acute occlusion by thrombosis. Others feel that in real tight stenoses no long-term patency may be expected unless the vessel wall is over-stretched, as manifested by intimal dissection. At present we have not sufficient arguments to take a stand about the prognostic value of creating and detecting plaque rupture and/or dissection. However, we feel that these "complications" are underestimated by angiographic control studies, as we have observed this finding in a vast majority of clinical cases and it may well be that this phenomenon is mandatory to some degree in order to establish a successful PTA with long-term patency (Fig. 4).

An important cause for failure of PTA after initial technical success is the occurrence of intimal hyperplasia causing re-stenosis and occlusion. There is little doubt that intimal hyperplasia should be regarded as "overshooting" of the normal tissue reaction to vascular trauma. The migration and multiplication of smooth muscle cells, the main components of intimal hyperplasia, is stimulated by various growth factors which in turn are triggered by different forms of trauma. PTA undoubtedly is such a trauma to the vessel wall. The key to solving this problem may be found in regulation of the "healing-response" by various (combinations of) drugs. Another factor may be modulation of the traumatic stimulus by modifying the effects: selective positioning of short stents at the entree and/or re-entree of dissections may be of potential value in a regimen to reduce the re-stenosis phenomenon.

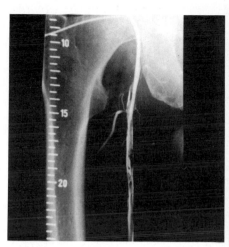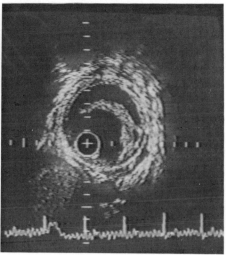

Fig. 4 A-B. A: Angiography of superficial femoral artery after PTA. Extensive dissection or thrombus formation at level 16-25 cm. B: Corresponding ultrasound image: atherosclerotic plaque with dissection, no thrombus. Plaque can be seen moving in real-time image with pulsatile bloodflow.

Endovascular ultrasound may be helpful in detecting plaque ruptures and dissections, and can be used to monitor the proper and selective placement of stents.

CONCLUSION

The place of endovascular ultrasound in the diagnosis and management of vascular disease in general and as monitoring procedure during PTA in particular, is not established yet.

From our clinical experience so far, we conclude that endovascular ultrasound has been very helpful in our understanding and knowledge about the effects of PTA. Whether the information obtained in this way will allow us to modify our policy during the procedure, resulting in an improvement of both immediate success and long-term patency, will have to be the subject of further clinical investigation. A randomized study for this purpose is now underway.

REFERENCES

1. Braun, L.A., Ramsay, L.E. (1987) Is "improvement" real with percutaneous transluminal angioplasty in the management of reno-vascular hypertension? *Lancet*, 1313-1316.
2. Dalman, R.L., Porter, J.M. (1989) Will interventional angiography replace vascular surgery? *J. Vasc. Surg.* 10: 129-134.

3. Dotter, C.T., Judkins, M.P. (1964) Transluminal treatment of arteriosclerotic obstruction; description of a new technique and a preliminary report of its application. *Circulation* 30: 654-670.
4. Glagov, S., Weisenberg, E, Zanus, C.K. et al (1987) Compensatory enlargement of human atherosclerotic coronary arteries. *N. Engl. J. Med.,* 3126: 1371-1375.
5. Gussenhoven, W.J., Essed, C.E., van Egmond, F.C. et al. (1989) Intravascular ultrasonic imaging: histologic and echographic correlation. *Eur. J. Vasc. Surg.,* 3: 571-576.
6. Gussenhoven, W.J., Essed, C.E., Frietman, P., Mastik, F. et al (1989) Intravascular echographic assessment of vessel wall characteristics; a correlation with histology. *Int. J. Card. Imaging,* 4: 105-116.
7. Gussenhoven, W.J., Pijl, P., Frietman, P., Gerritsen, G.P. et al (1990) Thinning of the media in atherosclerosis: an in vitro/in vivo intravascular echographic study. *Circulation* Suppl. III: 82.
8. Johnston, K.W., Rae, M., Hogg-Johnston, S.A. et al (1987) 5-Years results of a prospective randomized study of percutaneous transluminal angioplasty. *Ann. Surg.,* 206: 403-413.
9. Rutherford, R.B (1991) Standards for evaluating results of interventional therapy for peripheral vascular disease. *Circulation* 83 (Suppl. I): 6-11.
10. Wenguang, L., Gussenhoven, W.J., Bosch, J.G., Mastik, F. et al (1990) A computer-aided analysis system for the quantitative assessment of intravascular ultrasound images. *Computers in Cardiology:* 333-336.
11. Wenguang, L., Gussenhoven, W.J., Zhong, Y., The, S.H.K. et al. (1991) Validation of quantitative analysis of intravascular ultrasound images. *Intern. J. Card. Imaging,* 6: 247-253.
12. Whittemore, A.D., Donaldson, M.C., Polak, J.F. and Mannick, J.A. (1991) Limitations of balloon angioplasty for vein graft stenosis. *J. Vasc. Surg.,* 14: 340-345.

Indications for Infrainguinal Redo Surgery

D. Charlesworth

AMI Alexandra Hospital, London, U.K.

The expression 'Redo femoropopliteal surgery' implies two things, that some form of surgery has already been carried out and, that by definition, that surgery involved the arteries in the thigh.

The reasons why surgical treatment is preferred to medical management are referred to as the "indications" and the word is qualified by an adjective absolute or relative. These terms are widely understood, an absolute indication for operation implies that the surgeon considers operation is the only rational and ethical method of treatment.

When the indications are said to be relative surgery may be one of several alternatives or may be the only mode of treatment but not necessarily needing to be done at that time. Whatever the indications were for the original operation, it is the indications at the time 'redo' is contemplated which count. This applies particularly to femoropopliteal surgery when the original indication may have been claudication (relative) and a redo becomes imperative when the bypass fails and the patient develops pain at rest. As far as choice of operation is concerned whatever options were available originally they will inevitably be restricted when redo surgery is contemplated.

Figura 1 is a graph of cumulative patency against time, it is representative of the type of graph published to illustrate the long term patency of femoropopliteal bypasses. It has three components in which the rate of change in patency varies, initially there is a sharp drop, then a second phase, finally a third slow fall off with time.

The first two phases represent early failures, approximately half fail early, for either technical reasons or errors in selection 1 (inadequate run-in, high distal impedance, "poor run-off" or a bad conduit such as a very small bore vein). The other half fail because of the development of a stricture at the proximal or distal end of the graft, sometimes a stricture within a vein graft.

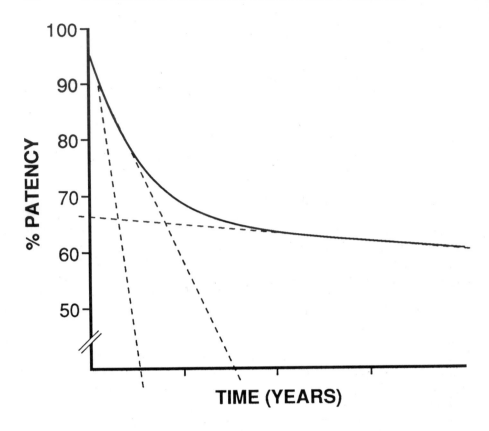

The indications for redo surgery, when we consider this group of early failures are influenced by a) the reason for the first operation, and b) the condition of the leg after the bypass occludes.

For example, if a claudicant has a femoropopliteal bypass and it occludes early, leaving the foot cold and ischaemic, then the indications for redo surgery are absolute and pressing. Alternatively, if a patient with pregangrene and who has only one patent crural artery and an in situ femorodistal bypass occludes, it is debateable whether further surgery is worthwhile.

When an arterial reconstruction fails within days further surgery should be done without delay unless there are overriding reasons to the contrary (i.e. the patient is unfit for surgery). If we assume that everything was done prior to the first operation to ensure good "run-in", redo affords an opportunity to identify technical faults, replace the conduit and improve "run-off".

EARLY FAILURE

                              CORRECT TECHNICAL ERROR
                              IMPROVE RUN IN
    UNFIT   REDO   CHANGE CONDUIT
                              IMPROVE RUN OFF

Approximately 50% of early failures occur within twelve months of operation and occlusion is preceded by a gradually increasing stenosis[2,3].

Two facts should be borne in mind:

1. The stenoses do not always give rise to symptoms
2. Redo surgery for a stenosis gives much better results than 4 redo after an occlusion.

If we assume that all stenoses will inevitably lead to occlusion it follows that by detecting stenoses and correcting them, long term patency will improve. However, we know from observation that only a quarter to a third of all stenoses will progress to complete occlusion. Hence, if the overall incidence of stenoses is between 15% for femoropopliteal bypasses and 20% for femorodistal bypasses, then only 4% to 5% of all grafts will progress to complete occlusion.

The question is, should we treat all stenoses as and when they are detected, or should we try to identify those which will progress to complete occlusion? Clinical observation to identify stenoses is totally inadequate, 65% of stenoses are asymptomatic, and pulses are palpable distal to the bypass. Measurements of ankle pressures is useful and a fall of greater than 0.2 in the ankle/brachial index is indicative of a stenosis but is not completely reliable, "a drop of A.P.1 does not predict 4 patients with impending graft failure".

Measurements of velocity, by waveform analysis of signals obtained by insonating the bypass with ultrasound, taken from within both the stenosed and unstenosed portions of the bypass provide information from which better estimates of the degree of stenosis can be made. On the basis that the increase in velocity within a stenosis is proportional to the cross sectional area of the lumen of the stenosis, various indices have been derived.

PSV1/ PEAK SYSTOLIC VELOCITY INDEX (PSV INDEX) =
PSV_1/PSV_2 (stenosed)

But we should bear in mind that the peak systolic velocity in a graft upstream from a stenosis is also influenced by the stenosis. This index produces a better discriminant than the change in peak velocity alone or the ankle to brachial pressure index.

On the basis of velocity measurements percentage stenosis can be calculated:

$$\% \text{ stenosis} = 100 \, (1 - V_1/ V_2)$$

Serial measurements of stenosis may provide information of deterioration and impending occlusion. However, stenoses of less than 50% diameter have no hydraulic consequences which means that observations of progressive deterioration are not accurate until the stenoses are severe, and the errors in the method are large.

One can calculate that when the velocity in the stenosis is four times greater than the velocity in the tube ($V_2 = 4 \times V_2$) then the error in the estimate of stenosis from V_1 / V_2 is probably in the region of 50%. This means thatitis not possible to detect with accuracy an increase in stenosis of 15% to 20%. Until we have reliable methods of detecting progressive stenoses it seems reasonable to redo all stenoses of greater than 75% (area).

When it comes to late failures the number of variables increases considerably. For example, a 65 year old claudicant has a successful bypass (saphenous vein) which occludes after five years and his syptoms recur. He will be 70 years old with an increased operative risk, there is a 25% chance that the contralateral leg will also give problems, a prosthesis will be necessary and run off may be further compromised.

The alternative would be a young patient to whom occlusion of a bypass had brought symptoms of pregangrene and, for whom every effort should be made to revascularise the leg.

LATE FAILURE

UNFIT   PREGANGRENE
CLAUDICATION ONLY

Late failure does allow for careful re-investigation of both run-in and run-off. The findings will influence the decision to operation, particularly since in most cases it will be necessary to use a prosthesis.

Redo surgery for infection complicating the initial operation is also influenced by a variety of factors. If the initial operation invoked the use of a prosthesis it will almost inevitable mean that the prosthesis will need to be removed. Whether it is necessary, even possible, to replace the bypass with another routed though some extra anatomic will vary from patient to patient and will depend principally on whether the foot becomes critically ischaemic when the original conduit is removed.

REFERENCES

1. Charlesworth D., Harris P.L., Cave F.D., TaylorL.: Undetected aorto-iliac insufficiency: a reason for early failure of saphenous vein bypass grafts for obstruction of the superficial femoral artery. *Br J Surg,* 1975; 62:567-70.
2. Moody P., Gould D.A., Harris P.L.: Vein graft surveillance improves patency in femoropopliteal bypass. *Eur J Vasc Surg,* 1990; 4:117-121.
3. Grigg M.J., Nicolaides A.N., Wolfe J.H.N.: Femorodistal vein bypass graft stenoses. *Br J Surg,* 1988; 75:737-40.
4. Berkowitz H.D., Greenstein S., Barker C.F. et coll.: The failure of reversed vein bypass grafts. *Ann Surg,* 1989; 210:782-86.
5. Barnes R.W., Tompson B.W., McDonald C.M., et al.: Serial non-invasive studies do not herald postoperative failure of femoropopliteal or femorotibial bypass grafts. *Ann Surg,* 1989; 210:486-91.

Technical Problems With Re-Do Reconstruction

P. Lewis and J.H.N. Wolfe

Department of Vascular Surgery, St Mary's Hospital,
University of London, U.K.

INTRODUCTION

Graft throbosis in an inevitable complication of infrainguinal reconstruction. Hypercoagulability States and graft surface thrombogenicity are often thought to cause graft occlusion but are rarely demostrable. In contrast, most graft occlusions are associated with detectable anatomical abnormalities. Thus re-do surgery is essential for continued limb salvage.

Early graft thrombosis, occurring within 1 month of surgery, is generally thought to represent an error in judgement or techique. Judgmental errors include incorrect selection of inflow or outflow anastomotic sites and unsatisfactory bypass conduit. The common technical errors are anastomotic stenosis, clot formation within the graft or outflow tract, proximal clamp injuries and intact valves in situ vein bypasses. Immediate re-operation and correction of the surgical error is the widely accepted method of managing early graft thrombosis and will not be considered further.

Later graft occlusion, caused by progressive disease in the graft or inflow/outflow tracts, is primarily responsible for the well recognized attrition of grafts. This process of delayed occlusion has led to the development of specific re-do surgical techniques which have significantly improved the overall results of arterial reconstruction for limb salvage. The techniques responsible for improved secondary patency rates are subject of this discussion and reflect the philosophy of our vascular unit.

THE PROBLEMS

The strategy for re-operation is determined by the clinical presentation and mechanical site of delayed graft failure and is dependent on the type of graft used in the primary procedure (Table 1).

Management of the occluded graft itself is primarily influenced by the type of conduit and clinical presentation. A conservative approach to graft occlusion is sometimes appropriate when the leg is viable and the patient has adequate mobility. Acute ischaemia, presenting with a white, anaesthetic foot, obviously demands urgent attention. With prosthetic graft this may be achieved by surgical thrombectomy and vein graft may be unblocked by thrombosis if surgery is undertaken immediately after thrombosis. Otherwise occluded vein soon becomes thrombogenic and a secondary infra-inguinal reconstruction should be considered. In chronic ischaemia, intra-arterial thrombolysis is a reliable alternative to surgical thrombectomy, particularly when a vein graft is occluded and we increasingly use Streptokinase or tPA intra-arterially to delineate the cause of the failure so that a localised procedure can be performed.

Maintenance of graft patency is usually dependent on correction of a haemodynamically significant stenosis or occlusion. If these stenosis are less than 2 cm in length then balloon dilatation is effective; longer stenoses require an extensionjump graft from the graft to patent distal vessels. Recognition of such lesions before graft occlusions occurs, by graft surveillance, is an important development that may prevent limbs being placed at risk. Stenosis and aortic/iliac to profunda bypass occasionally produces limb salvage.

Table 1

A)	Clinical presentation	Acute ischaemia Chronic ischaemia Viable limb
B)	Mechanical site	Inflow Graft Outflow
C)	Tube graft	Vein Prosthetic

Angiography

Pre-operative angiography is essential to confirm graft occlusion and identify the extent of thrombosis. The underlying stenosis/occlusion is, however, unlikely to be demonstrated. Per-operative angiography performed after graft thrombectomy and restoration of flow is imperative to display any mechanical abnormalities that may promote re-thrombosis. Doppler ultrasonography is a useful adjunct; a biphasic flow signal confirming an adequate outflow tract.

Dissection

Re-do surgery commonly necessitates re-exploration of the groin and dissection is facilitated by careful sharp dissection with a scalpel and number 10 blade. After an incision through the old scar, dissection should proceed in a lateral direction on to the fascia overlying sartorius and medially onto the femoral vessels. This approach minimises damage to lymphatics and a lymphatic fistula, which is classically associated with re-do groin exploration may be prevented. A patent profunda femoris artery may be a useful donor or recipient vessel and may be isolated medial or lateral to sartorius through and incision placed to avoid the previous scarring in the groin. Attempts to re-isolate the popliteal artery should be avoided. The combination of fibrosis from previous surgery and or acces may make surgery difficult and result in damage to the popliteal vein or nerve. Furthermore, there are satisfactory alternatives; the tibio-peroneal trunk can be isolated by dissecting through clean tissue beneath the origin of soleus or the crural arteries can be isolated in the lower calf where they lie superficially between muscle tendons. In the upper calf these vessels lie deep between muscle bellies; exposure is more limited, extensive muscle dissection is usually necessary, and the wound is more prone to haematoma formation.

Bypass Graft

The choice of bypass conduit is largely determined by circumstance. Ipsilateral autolougus long saphenous vein, the bapass of choice, is rarely available. Controlateral long saphenous vein mau also have been used for coronary or arterial reconstruction. Arm vein is short in lenght, often smaller siameter and frequently sclerosed due to previous venepuncture. However, reversed brachiocephalic vein, harvested between elbow and shoulder, is an excellent conduit for extension jump grafts[1] and veno-venous composite grafts can be manufactured from 2 lenghts of vein[2]. Of the prosthetic graft, PTFE has the best patency rates in infra-inguinal reconstruction but few find it of value to crural vessels. Compliance mismatch at the distal graft-artery anastomosis fraquently causes narrowing due to myointimal hyperplasia[3]. However, vein interposition using a venous collar or both produces patency rates approximately 25% worse than in correspoding vein grafts[4]. Anastomotic suture technique is particularly important in graft-crural vessel anastomoses. Magnification and fine microinstruments are essential pre-requisites of good suture technique. Seven/zero Prolene should be the largest gauge suture material used and needle selection is important; an 8 mm needle is the optimum size for crural reconstruction.

SPECIFIC TECHNIQUES

Surgical Thrombectomy

As a general rule successful thrombectomy requires proximal and distal arteriotomies. The distal arteriotomy enables visualization of the distal anastomosis, clearance of thrombus from the run-off vessels and flushing of the graft with blood or heparinized saline. A 4 F Fogarty catheter is used to clear the graft and a 2 F Fogarty catheter may be gently employed to extract thrombus from distal arteries. The newer "adherent clot catheters" may effect better prosthetic graft clearance than conventional balloon catheters. Flushing with heparinized saline helps dislodge adherent thrombus. When dissection of the distal extebt of the graft is technically difficult (see above) flushing should be avoided in order to prevent distal thrombo-embolism. Under these circumstances, angioscopy may be evaluable adjunct to confirm extraction of all thrombus.

Thrombolysis

Intra-arterial thrombolysis is currently regarded as the optimal method of graft recana lization providing immediate viability of the limb is not threatened[5]. Although lysis may be effective several weeks after graft occlusion, the results are best when treatment is started within days of thrombosis. Intra-arterial thrombolysis has an important application in thrombosis of vein graft and popliteal or crural vessels since mechanical thrombectomy may damage the endothelial lining leading to recurrent thrombosis.

Streptokinase is the first line thrombolytic agent principally because of expense but tPA is used for repeat thromboliysis because of the possibilitiy of the streptokinase hypersensitivity. The thrombolytic agent may either be administered by bolus or continous infusion and the catheter should be advanced until complete clot lysis is achieved.

Intra-operative thrombolytic therapy is gaining in popularity in situatios were run-off vessels remain occluded after successful mechanical thrombectomy of the graft itself. A regime of 100.000 units of Streptokinase or 5 mg of tPA infused over 30 mionutes is currently recommended although clinical trials are still awaited.

Aortic/Iliac-Profunda Bypass

Graft occlusion, precipitated by inflow obstruction, also causes thrombosis of the common femoral artery and a veritable extent of the ipsilateral iliac segment. However, the profunda femoris artery often remains patent and can be used as the recipient vessel. Proximal reconstruction from the aorto-iliac segment may be undertaken via the transperitoneal, retroperitoneal or cross over routes, depending on the distribution of disease in the aorto-iliac vessels and the general condition of patient. The aortic/iliac-profunda approach has the advantages of avoiding scar tissue in the groin and the need to perform graft thrombectomy or thrombolysis. Also the possibility that the graft or outflow tract may have contributed to the occlusive event are obviated. If the aortic/iliac-profunda bypass does not improve the circulation sufficiently to relieve rest pain then an extension femoro-distal graft may be needed. The indication for extension grafting is usually apparent after observation of the limb over a period of days.

Angioplasty

Angioplasty is an attractive alternative to re-do surgery. In practice this opportunity most commonly rises when a vein graft stenosis is discovered during a graft surveillance programme or after intra-arterial thrombolysis. Good results have been obtained for balloon dilatation of short stenoses (less than 2 cm)[6] but there is now increasing evidence that longer stenoses should be sublitted to open surgery[7].

Extension Jump Grafting

The commonest cause of failure of an infra-inguinal graft is progressive stenosis in the distal extent of the graft, the distal anastomosis or the immediate run-off vessels. Successful mechanical thrombectomy and patch angioplasty necessitate dissection of the distal graft and anastomosis. Extension jump grafting is a easier alternative which avoids difficult dissection through scar tissue. The original graft is identified in the mid or lower thigh and a jump graft is constructed to a patent crural vessel[1]. Brachiocephalic vein is particularly useful for this relatively short bypass which can be placed subcutaneously.

Secondary Infra-Inguinal Reconstruction

Long standing thrombosis of a vein graft and the popliteal trifurcation beyond a prosthetic graft are both relative contraindications to graft thrombectomy. Under these conditions a secondary infra-inguinal procedure may be indicated. Reversed controlateral long saphenous vein may be used buth adequate lengths of vein are frequently unavailable. Prosthetic femoro-distal reconstruction is then the only method of limb salvage. Limb salvage rates using prosthetic grafts alone are disappointing but PTFE with a vein collar or both provide reasonable results. Our limb salvage rates are 50% at 3 years for > 70 cm PTFE/collar femoro-distal reconstructions for patients in whom available vein as already been used and the alternative is amputation. Perioperative haemorheological enhancement with Dextran 70 and long term anti-thrombotic therapy with Warfarin are important adjuvant measures.

Fasciotomy

Successful reconstructions may fail because of raised compartment pressures in the calf. Fasciotomy should therefore be considered in the management of all ischaemic legs. If fasciotomy is undertaken all 4 compartments must be decompressed. Many approaches have been described but our preference is the double incision technique. Incisions placed over the medial and the lateral aspects of the calf proivide easy access to all 4 compartments and enables necrosed muscle to be removed when necessary.

CONCLUSION

We have an active approach to reconstruction in the critical leg and only 3% of patients receive primary amputation. Following reconstruction an aggressive surveillance programme, coupled with further intervention, means that these patients require a mean of 1.1 secondary operations over a period of 3 years. These re-do procedures improve the patency rates and limb salvage rates by 16% .

REFERENCES

1. Wolfe J.H.N., Taylor P.R.: Repair of the failing femoro-distal. In: Vascular Surgical Techniques. Eds Greenhalgh R.M., W.B. Saunders Co, London, 1989.
2. Harris R.W., Andros G., Salles-Cunha S.X., et al.: Totally autogenous veno-venous composite bypass grafts. *Arch Surg,* 1986, 121:1128-1132.
3. Imparato A.M., Bracco A., Kim G.E., et al.: Intimal and neo-intimal fibrous proliferation causing failure of arterial reconstruction. *Surg,* 1972, 72:1007-1017.
4. Wolfe J.H.N., Tyrrell M.R.: Justifying arterial reconstruction to crural vessels - even with a prosthetic graft. *Br J Surg,* 1991, 78: 897-898.
5. Van Breda A., Robinson J.C., Feldman L., et al.: Local thrombolysis in the treatment of arterial graft occlusions. *J Vasc Surg,* 1984, 1: 103-110.
6. Veith F.J., Weiser R.K., Gupta S.K., et al.: diagnosis and management of failing lower extremity arterial reconstructions. *J Cardiovasc Surg,* 1984, 25:381-386.
7. Cohen J.R., Mannick J.A., Couch N.P., et al.: Recognition and management of impending vein graft failure. *Arch Surg,* 1986, 121:758-9.

Improved Strategies for Secondary Operations on Infrainguinal Arteries

F.J. Veith

*Division of Vascular Surgery, Montefiore Medical Center
Albert Einstein College of Medicine
New York, New York, U.S.A.*

Infrainguinal arterial reconstructions for lower extremity ischemia include axillofemoral and femorofemoral procedures and bypasses to the popliteal and infrapopliteal arteries. All these operations have an intrinsic tendency to fail or become ineffective as time elapses. The proportion of such operations undergoing this fate increases with time and is greater for reconstructions terminating more distally in the arterial tree. Because a sizable minority of patients undergoing these operations will have circulatory deterioration in their lifetime and because this deterioration will often be associated with disabling or limb threatening manifestations, appropriate management of this condition has become an important aspect of vascular surgery and one to which the competent vascular surgeon must be committed to serve his patients' interests well. This article discusses the general principles and strategies of this management with a specific focus on the aspects of reoperative vascular surgery that differ from a primary approach to lower extremity ischemia.

INDICATIONS

In general arterial reconstruction should rarely be performed for intermittent claudication[1]. One reason for this attitude is the relatively high inevitable failure rate of these operations and the fact that failure may be associated with ischemia worse than that prompting the original operation.

This and the increased difficulty and complication rate associated with most secondary operations, particularly if arteries must be redissected, seem to justify a conservative attitude toward *primary* operations for intermittent claudication. This attitude, however, is by no means universal and present practice accepts "truly disabling" claudication as an indication for primary arterial reconstruction to at least the popliteal level. In contrast almost all present day vascular surgeons would tend to avoid secondary arterial operations for intermittent claudication.

Thus gangrene, a nonhealing ischemic ulcer or severe rest pain should be the indications for most *secondary* arterial reconstructions especially those below the inguinal ligament. Interestingly occasional patients with these classic limb threatening manifestations and poor noninvasive indices can be effectively managed by conservative measures for protracted periods[2] and such treatment, if possible, is particularly appropriate in patients who are faced with the need for a difficult distal reoperation. Thus, except for the special circumstances occurring with a "failing graft", most patients undergoing secondary arterial reconstruction should have as their indication for operation unquestionable immediate limb salvage.

ETIOLOGY

Early Reoperations (Within 30 Days). The need to reintervene soon after a primary arterial reconstruction can be generated by several situations[3]. First, the original operation can *thrombose or fail* in the early postoperative period, i. e., within 30 days. Generally this is due to a *technical flaw* in the operation or to the poor choice of inflow or outflow sites. In addition, thrombosis may occur for no apparent reason presumably due to the inherent thrombogenicity of the graft in a low flow setting. Usually this occurs only with PTFE and other prosthetic grafts, but rarely it can occur with a vein graft also. A transient *fall in cardiac output, hypotension or increased coagulability* can contribute to such unexplained thrombosis. Second, the original operation although technically satisfactory and associated with a patent bypass graft can *fail to provide hemodynamic improvement* sufficient to relieve the patient's symptoms. This in turn can be due to the choice of the *wrong operation*, e. g., the performance of an aortofemoral bypass in a patient whose femoral artery pressure was normal and who actually needed a femoro-popliteal bypass. Alternatively such hemodynamic failure could also occur in the presence of *multisegment disease* and extensive foot gangrene or infection. In this setting uninterrupted arterial circulation to the foot may be required and a primary or secondary sequential bypass may be indicated[1,4,5].

Late Reoperations (After 30 Days). Failure with graft thrombosis can occur at any time after the first postoperative month. This can be due to some of the factors already mentioned. However, it is usually due to the development of some flow reducing lesion within the bypass graft or its inflow or outflow tract. *Intimal hyperplasia* is a prominent cause of failure and graft thrombosis. This can occur with all kinds of grafts in all positions. The etiology of this process is poorly understood, and fortunately it does not affect most arterial reconstructions. When intimal hyperplasia does occur, it usually produces infrainguinal graft failure between 2 and 18 months after operation[3,6,7]. It can involve any portion of a vein graft in a focal or diffuse manner and either anastomosis of vein or prosthetic grafts. Because the lumen of the distal artery is smaller, this site is most vulnerable to flow reduction by this process. After 18 months *progression of the atherosclerotic disease* process involving the inflow or outflow tract of the arterial reconstruction becomes the predominant cause of failure and graft thrombosis. After 3-4 years a variety of other *degenerative lesions* can also afflict autogenous vein grafts and umbilical vein grafts[6,8,9]. These processes which are rare in autogenous vein grafts but extremely common in umbilical vein grafts can lead to wall changes and aneurysm formation with thrombosis or embolization.

FAILING GRAFT CONCEPT

Intimal hyperplasia, progression of proximal or distal disease, or lesions within the graft itself can produce signs and symptoms of hemodynamic deterioration in patients with a prior arterial reconstruction without producing concomitant thrombosis of the bypass graft[10,14]. We have referred to this condition as a "failing graft" because, if the lesion is not corrected, graft thrombosis will almost certainly occur[10]. The importance of this failing graft concept lies in the fact that many difficult lower extremity revascularizations can be salvaged for protracted periods by relatively simple interventions if the lesion responsible for the circulatory deterioration and diminished graft blood flow can be detected before graft thrombosis occurs.

We have now been able to detect more than 145 failing grafts and to correct the lesion before graft thrombosis has occurred[10,14]. The majority of these grafts were vein grafts but approximately 1/3 were polytetrafluoroethylene (PTFE) or Dacron grafts. Invariably the corrective procedur is simpler than the secondary operation that would be required if the bypass went on to thrombose. Many lesions responsible for the failing state could be remedied by percutaneous transluminal angioplasty (PTA), although some required a vein patch angioplasty, a short bypass of a graft lesion or a proximal or distal graft extension[10,14]. Some of the transluminal angioplasties of these lesions have failed and required a second reintervention; others have remained effective in correcting the responsible lesion as documented by arteriography more than 2-5 years later. If the failing graft is a vein bypass, detection of the failing state permits accurate localization and definition of the responsible lesion by arteriography and salvage of any undiseased vein. In contrast, if the graft is permitted to thrombose, the responsible lesion may be difficult to identify, the vein may be difficult or impossible to thrombectomize, and the patient's best graft, the ipsilateral greater saphenous vein, may have to be sacrificed rendering the secondary operation even more difficult and more likely to fail with associated limb loss. Most importantly the results of reinterventions for failing grafts, both in terms of continued cumulative patency and limb salvage rates have been far superior to the results of reinterventions for grafts that have thrombosed and failed[7,10,12,14].

This difference in results together with the ease of reintervention for failing grafts mandate that surgeons performing infrainguinal bypass operations follow their patients closely in the postoperative period and indefinitely thereafter. Ideally noninvasive laboratory tests should be performed with similar frequency. If the patient has any recurrence of symptoms or the surgeon detects *any* change in peripheral pulse examination or other manifestations of ischemia, the circulatory deterioration is confirmed by noninvasive parameters and *urgent arteriography*. If a lesion is detected as a cause of the failing state, it is corrected urgently by PTA or operation.

MANAGEMENT STRATEGIES FOR PATIENTS WITH PRESUMED INFRAINGUINAL GRAFT FAILURE

Patients with circulatory deterioration after an infrainguinal arterial reconstruction present with recurrent symptoms, a decrease in pulses in the involved limb, other changes on physical examination or a decrease in noninvasive vascular laboratory values.

These manifestations may occur at any time after operation and are presumptive evidence that the arterial reconstruction has thrombosed although they could also occur in the absence of graft thrombosis when some lesion is present in, proximal or distal to the bypass graft, i.e., with a failing graft.

Presumed Early Failure (Within 30 Days of Operation)

If the primary operation was originally justified, a secondary procedure is also mandated. If the primary operation was for limb salvage indications, early graft failure or thrombosis will always be associated with a renewed threat or even a worse threat to the limb. If the original preoperative arteriogram was satisfactory, repeat arteriography is not performed. The patient is given intravenous heparin and returned to the operating room as expeditiously as possible. Since vein grafts can be injured by the ischemia associated with intraluminal clot and since it may be more difficult to remove solid thrombotic material from vein grafts, there is greater urgency to reoperate on a patient with a failed autogenous vein graft than one with a PTFE graft. In any event reoperation should be undertaken within less than 12 hours of the detection of failure. Even greater urgency is required if calf muscle tenderness or neurological changes are associated with graft failure.

Vein Grafts. The distal incision of the arterial reconstruction is reopened. The graft thrombosis is confirmed by palpation. Control of the artery proximal and distal to the distal anastomosis is obtained and a full anticoagulating dose of intravenous heparin (7500 IU) is given. A linear incision is made in the hood of the graft (Fig. 1) so as to visualize the interior of the distal anastomosis. Balloon catheters are gently passed retrograde in

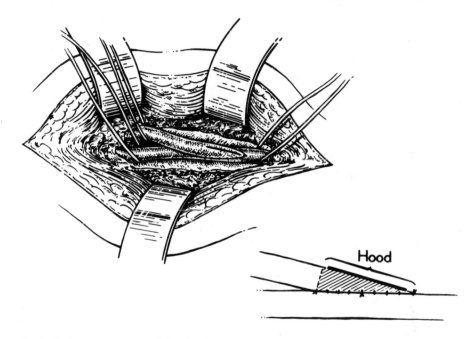

Fig. 1. Operative exposure of the distal anastomosis. The incision in the hood of the graft is made to within 1 mm of the distal end of the graft. This provides optimal exposure of the distal anastomosis and facilitates thrombectomy. (Reproduced from Collier et al.[19] with permission)

the graft to remove clot (Fig. 2). If necessary, any clot is similarly removed from the proximal and distal adjacent host artery and any visualized anastomotic defect is repaired. Valves in the vein graft may prevent retrograde passage of the catheter or it may be impossible to restore adequate, normal prograde arterial flow through the graft. In either event the proximal incision is opened and the same procedures performed at the proximal anastomosis. With flow restored and all openings in the graft closed with fine running monofilament sutures, an intraoperative arteriogram is performed to visualize the graft and the outflow tract. If no defect is seen, adequacy of the reconstruction and the inflow tract is demonstrated by direct arterial pressure measurements which should reveal no gradient in excess of 15-20 mm Hg between the distal end of the graft and the brachial or radial artery. Any gradient in excess of 25 mm Hg should be localized to the inflow tract

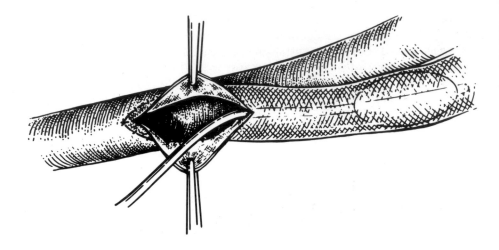

Fig. 2. Thrombectomy alone is performed through the distal graft incision when no cause for graft failure is identified. Clot is removed from the graft and, if needed, from the artery both proximally and distally. (Reproduced from Collier et al.[19] with permission)

or the graft by appropriate needle placement. If there is a gradient in the vein graft, it should be eliminated by revision. If this is impossible, the graft should be replaced by a prosthetic (PTFE) graft. Often such unexplained gradients can be due to recanalized, thrombophlebitic segments of vein. Unless removed, such segments will cause recurrent failure. If an inflow gradient is present, it should be eliminated by a suitable inflow bypass (aortofemoral, femorofemoral or axillofemoral) or occasionally by an intraoperative or postoperative balloon angioplasty.

If disease in the outflow tract is detected and is the presumed cause of graft failure, this generally is best treated by an extension to a more distal less diseased segment of the same or another outflow artery (Fig. 3).

If no defect is detected by arteriography or pressure measurements, the procedure is terminated. Despite older evidence to the contrary[15], an occasional vein graft will undergo early failure for no apparent reason and will remain patent indefinitely after simple thrombectomy. Perhaps the unexplained thrombosis was due to undetected decreased cardiac output with hypotension and decreased arterial flow.

With increasing ability to perform distal bypasses to disadvantaged outflow tracts[1,16,17], we have had some patients whose distal grafts failed early for no apparent reason other than high outflow resistance. In some of these instances thrombectomy and extension of the graft to another outflow vessel as a sequential graft has resulted in long-term graft patency and limb salvage[18].

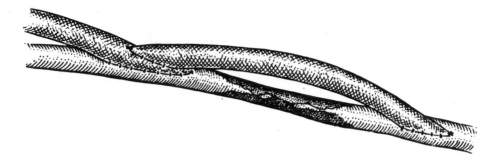

Fig. 3. If disease in the outflow tract is detected, a graft extension is performed. (Reproduced from Ascer et al.[14] with permission)

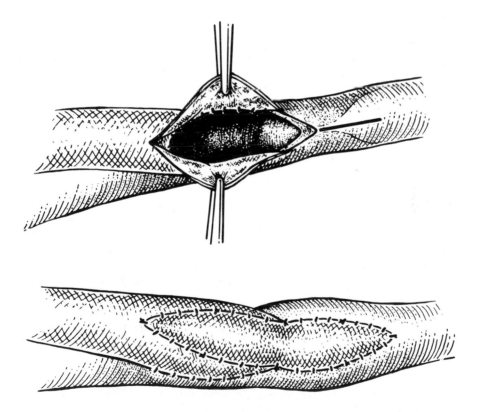

Fig. 4. Stenosis just distal to the anastomosis can be caused by an unrecognized atherosclerotic lesion. This can be corrected by extending the graft incision distally across its apex and down the recipient artery until its lumen in no longer narrowed. A patch of PTFE or vein is then inserted across the stenosis to widen the lumen. Similar treatment is appropriate for intimal hyperplasia which causes late graft occlusion. (Reproduced from Ascer et al.[14] with permission)

PTFE and Other Prosthetic Grafts. Early thrombosis of PTFE grafts is managed in essentially the same fashion as already described for early failure of vein grafts[3,14]. Differences include the almost complete freedom from graft defects as a cause of failure although occasionally a PTFE graft will be compressed, kinked or twisted because of poor tunneling technique and malposition around or through some of the tendinous structures in the region of the knee. In addition, graft thrombosis for no apparent reason is more common with PTFE grafts than vein grafts and occured in 38 of our 61 early failures in a series of 822 infrainguinal PTFE grafts[19]. Simple thrombectomy of the graft by the techniques already described resulted in patency rates in excess of 50% after 3 years, if no other defect was found and if the distal end of the graft was above the knee joint[3,14]. The secondary operative treatment in the remaining 23 cases was designed to correct the cause of early failure. In one case it consisted of a patch angioplasty for outflow stenosis (Fig. 4), and in 22 cases it was a graft extension for inflow or outflow disease[19].

Presumed Late Failure (1 Month or More After Operation)

All patients with presumed late graft failure should undergo a standard transfemoral or translumbar arteriogram with visualization of all arteries from the renals to the forefoot[1]. If a failing graft is found, it is urgently treated by a reintervention as already discussed. If a failed or thrombosed graft is present, the patient is not subjected to reinterventional treatment unless the limb is unequivocally threatened. Surprisingly, even though the original operation was performed for limb salvage with critical ischemia[20], the limb may not be rethreatened when the original arterial reconstruction occludes[3]. Ten to 25 percent of patients will be able to tolerate occlusion of a limb salvage bypass and function effectively indefinitely. This proportion seems to increase as the interval between the primary operation and its failure increases. Presumably this phenomenon occurs because the original limb threatening lesion has healed by virtue of the bypass and does not recur with the renewed ischemia. Alternatively, improved collaterals maintain the limb better after some graft failures than before the operation for reasons that remain obscure.

When graft thrombosis is associated with renewed critical ischemia and an imminently endangered lower extremity, aggressive reintervention is indicated and is very important in achieving optimal limb salvage results[1]. Management strategies differ depending on the type of graft and its location.

Axillofemoral and Femorofemoral Grafts. When failure of one of these grafts occurs, the inflow tract of the graft should be examined angiographically. With axillofemoral grafts it is possible to perform an aortic arch arteriogram by the translumbar route*. Similar examination should evaluate

---

* Personal Communication. S. Sprayregen, C.Bakal, J. Cynamon, 1988.

the inflow or donor iliac system with failed femorofemoral grafts. If significant inflow disease is found, it may be corrected by PTA or a new bypass from an alternate site must be performed. If, for example, inflow iliac disease has caused failure of a femorofemoral graft, it can be corrected by PTA or an aortobifemoral bypass, or an aortic limb can be brought to the thrombectomized femorofemoral graft.

The same arteriogram should also seek evidence of progression of outflow disease and should define patent distal segments that can be used to bypass such outflow disease if necessary. An example of this would be progression of deep femoral artery disease in a patient for whom that vessel was providing outflow for an axillofemoral or femorofemoral bypass. In this circumstance the poplitel artery should be evaluated angiographically and thrombectomy of the graft should be followed by a profundaplasty or graft extension to the undiseased deep femoral or popliteal artery.

After suitable arteriographic examination, the patient is subjected to a secondary operation. The graft is opened over the hood or hoods of the distal anastomoses so the interior of the distal anastomosis can be inspected. With axillofemoral grafts this is facilitated if the original femorofemoral limb is placed over the distal end of the axillary limb. In this way a single opening in the graft permits thrombectomy of all prosthetic grafts, thrombectomy of arteries in one groin, and diagnosis and correction of anastomotic problems at one distal anastomosis. Although occasionally successful, the practice of blind balloon catheter thrombectomy of any distal anastomosis via an opening in the graft remote from the anastomosis is to be condemned. The chance of damage to the anastomosis, intimal injury or plaque disruption in the adjacent artery is too great. While it is true that the anastomosis and its adjacent arteries must be dissected free and controlled and that this procedure may be difficult because of scar, it is clearly worth the effort. If distal anastomotic intimal hyperplasia is detected as the cause of graft failure, it is treated by a graft extension or by incising across the hyperplastic lesion and inserting a patch graft (Fig. 4). In the latter circumstance the incision and patch are usually placed across the origin of the deep femoral artery.

If no cause of failure is found on preoperative arteriography or intraoperative inspection, an intraoperative arteriogram is performed. If no defects or partially obstructing lesions are found, as is often the case with failed axillofemoral grafts, the reoperative procedure is terminated and good results can be expected. The value of these reoperations for failed extraanatomic bypasses is substantially increased late patency rates[21] with a three year *additional* patency rate, calculated from the time of reoperation, of 75%[14].

An alternative approach, which is particularly useful if multiple failures have occurred, is to perfom a totally new bypass using undissected arteries. In this regard the ascending or descending thoracic aorta, the retroperitoneally approached aorta or iliac arteries are useful options to provide inflow. The distal portions of the deep femoral artery and the laterally approached popliteal artery are good options to provide outflow.

Generalities Applying to Reoperations or Secondary Operations After Late Failure of Femoropopliteal or Infrapopliteal Bypasses

In the circumstances, if the graft is confirmed to be thrombosed by arteriography, reintervention is only undertaken if the limb is in immediate jeopardy. If this is the case, *Complete Contrast Arteriography* must precede any secondary operation to provide some information, albeit perhaps incomplete, as to why the graft failed and to define possible therapeutic options by demonstrating remaining patent distal arterial segments and the quality of undissected proximal arteries which may be used for bypass origin such as the mid or distal portions of the deep femoral artery[22,23].

Bilateral *Contrast Venography* should also precede reoperation to define the lenght and quality of the remaining superficial veins[24]. This can be helpful in patients with failed vein grafts by revealing unused accessory greater saphenous veins, short saphenous veins, arm veins and occasionally an unused main saphenous trunk. Duplex ultrasonography can also be helpful in predicting the lenght and diameter of useable upper or lower extremity venous segments. Venography is also indicated preoperatively in patients who have previously had a prosthetic bypass. Often the greather saphenous vein in such cases has been damaged at the first operation or by scarring.

The standard surgical approaches to arteries in patients who have undergone previous failed bypasses are often rendered more difficult or even impossible to use of surgical scarring and/or infection. For that reason a variety of *Unusual Approaches* to all the infrainguinal arteries whit allow these vessels to be approached through virginal tissue planes have been developed[22]. These approaches can be helpful in avoiding scarred standard access routes and can be essential if a previous operation was complicated by infection. These unusual approaches include direct access routes to the second and third portions of the deep femoral artery medial or lateral to the sartorius muscle[22,23]. These routes obviate the need to use a scarred or infected groin to trace the deep femoral down from its origin. They also permit the distal portions of the artery to be used to provide inflow for a distal shorter vein graft. We have now used these direct distal approaches to the deep femoral artery in more than 70 secondary cases. Another set of unusual approaches provides lateral access to the above knee or below knee popliteal artery[25]. These are particularly useful in the presence of medial incision sepsis and permit the popliteal artery to be used for bypass inflow or outflow even in the presence of groin and medial thigh infection[25]. In addition all 3 leg arteries can be approached medially or laterally and adequate exposure obtained to perform an anastomosis. The lateral approach, which involves fibula resection, allows access to all parts of the tibial and peroneal arteries[25-27].

We have devised a method for exposing the lower third of the peroneal artery well from a medial approach. This technique involves division of the long flexor muscles and tendons to the toes and foot and is particularly suited if an in situ bypass to the distal third of the peroneal artery is to be performed. Finally, we have developed surgical approaches to the terminal branches of the posterior tibial artery and the dorsalis pedis artery[22,28]. Any of these branches which include the medial and lateral plantar branches of the posterior tibial artery and the lateral tarsal and deep metatarsal arch branches of the dorsalis pedis artery can be used for secondary bypass operations[16]. The deep metatarsal arch is accessed via a dorsal incision with removal of portions of the shaft of the second and perhaps third metatarsal bones[28].

Another principle that is particularly useful for secondary procedures is the *Short Vein Graft or Distal Origin Bypass* concept. Every bypass to the popliteal or infrapopliteal vessels need not originate from the common femoral artery[1,29]. Grafts to these distal arteries may originate from the superficial femoral, popliteal or even tibial arteries without compromising late patency results provided no important inflow disease is present[16,29]. Such short vein grafts are particularly useful in secondary bypass operations since they allow the surgeon to avoid previously scarred or infected areas and they facilitate the use of the limited remaining superficial veins as bypass conduits. Certainly they are better than prosthetic grafts[30]. Moreover it has recently been show that short vein grafts probably have better patency rates than long vein grafts, particularly when they are used as bypasses to disadvantaged outflow tracts[16,17].

Two *types of secondary arterial reconstruction* are available to the vascular surgeon who is planning a reintervention for a failed infrainguinal bypass. The first, which is termed a *"Reoperation"*, employs some form of graft thrombectomy and revision or extension in an effort to save all or as much of the original graft as possible. The other type of secondary operation involves placement of a *Totally New Secondary Bypass Graft* preferably but not necessarily using previously undissected patent arteries for the origin and insertion of the bypass. The choice of which type of secondary bypass to employ is dependent on a number of variables including the type of primary bypass (PTFE or autogenous vein), the nature and location of the lesion responsible for the failure of the primary operation, the surgeon's training and experience, the residual arterial and superficial venous anatomy, and most importantly the location of the primary bypass. Because of the importance of the latter factor, the management of different kinds of failed primary operations that require reintervention will be considered separately.

Failed Femoropopliteal or Infrapopliteal Autogenous Vein Grafts. In this setting thrombectomy of the occluded vein graft is not attempted unless the graft is only partially thrombosed or the thrombosis has been present for less than 36 hours. Occasionally a vein graft can be salvaged in the latter two circumstances. Otherwise a totally new bypass is perfomed. If a patent isolated popliteal artery segment is present, a bypass to that segment will be attempted. An effort to perfom this with a vein graft from the ipsilateral extremity will be made using a remnant of the greater saphenous or the lesser saphenous vein. This will be facilitated by using the distal deep femoral or superficial femoral artery for inflow, if possible, and keeping the vein graft short. If no ipsilateral lower extremity vein of adequate lenght is available, a PTFE graft will have good prospects of remaining patent and providing long-term limb salvage particularly if inserted above the knee[30]. In this setting, it would be appropriate to use a PTFE graft in preference to vein from the opposite leg or upper extremities. If foot necrosis or infection is extensive in this setting, a sequential femoro-to-poplitel-to-tibial bypass should be performed with a short distal vein graft obtained from any extremity of the patient. If no patent popliteal segment is present, as short a vein graft as possible should be performed extending from the distal most artery with unobstructed proximal flow (i.e. deep or superficial femoral, popliteal or tibial artery) to the most proximal patent infrapopliteal artery which courses without significant obstruction to its terminal end. For such procedures autogenous vein from any extremity is used even if it is only 2-3 mm in diameter when distended[16,31]. PTFE grafts should only be used for bypasses to infrapopliteal arteries if absolutely no autogenous vein is available. However a secondary arterial reconstruction with such a prosthetic graft has some chance of remaining patent for several years and a moderate chance of saving the involved limb[30]. Furthermore, more recent work suggests that late patency rates for such grafts can be improved by postoperative anticoagulation[32]. Accordingly use of such a graft, though not ideal, is a better option than an amputation.

Failed Femoro-to-Above-Knee Popliteal PTFE Bypass. When failure of such a bypass results in a threatened limb and a secondary intervention is required, it is our present belief that a reoperation with an attempt at graft salvage is justified and indicated[3,14]. If the preoperative arteriogram indicates an inflow problem, this is treated appropriately by PTA or a proximal graft extension. The distal end of the graft is redissected along with its adjacent arteries (Fig. 1) and, after administration of 7500 IU of heparin, a vertical incision is made in the distal hood of the graft to permit balloon catheter thrombectomy of the graft and the popliteal artery proximally and distally (Figs. 1 and 2). Great care is exercised and minimal balloon inflation is used when passing the catheter in arteries to avoid intimal injury. Only if necessary is a proximal incision made. If the presence of a distal lesion is detected on inspection of the anastomosis or preoperative arteriography, it is treated. We still believe an incision across the lesion and patch angioplasty is best for intimal hyperplasia (Fig. 4), and a graft extension to a distal patent artery with a PTFE or vein graft (Fig. 3) is best for distal disease progression. Although this approach requires a difficult redissection of the distal anastomosis (which may be more technically demanding than performing a totally new bypass), it is justified and indicated in view of the acceptable 3 year patency results and the fact that it preserves the maximal amount of undissected patent distal arterial tree should further problems develop[14].

On the other hand, if excessive scarring or infection are present or the surgeon's preference dictates, a new bypass to patent unused arterial segments may be the best operation in this setting.

Failed Femoro-to-Below-Knee Popliteal or Infrapopliteal PTFE Bypass. When failure of such a procedure results in the need for a secondary arterial reconstruction, the best treatment is an *entirely new secondary bypass* preferably employing an autogenous vein graft using some of the strategies already discussed to minimize graft length and permit use of previously unused segments of arteries or segments approached through virginal tissue planes. The primary reason for departing from our previous strategy[3] of performing a reoperation with an attempt at graft salvage is the poorer additional patency that can be obtained with reoperations on these below knee grafts as compared to better results (over 40% 2 year patency) when a totally new secondary bypass is employed[14]. A second reason for not using the reoperation strategy is the high infection rate of 6% with such procedures, while the infection rate for a new secondary bypass is less than 1%[14].

Failure of Secondary Arterial Reconstructions. Although some vascular surgeons are reluctant to undertake multiple attempts at arterial reconstruction to salvage a threatened limb in the belief that the risks of infection and knee loss outweigh the potential benefits, we and others disagree. The results show that many patients can benefit from multiple limb salvage operations and that the benefits outweigh the risks and disadvantages, if the principles and strategies already advocated are employed[1,3,7,14,33].

GRANT ACKNOWLEDGEMENT

This work was supported by the Maming Foundation and the New York Institute for Vascular Studies.

REFERENCES

1. Veith FJ, Gupta SK, Samson RH, et al: Progress in limb salvage by reconstructive arterial surgery combined with new or improved adjunctive procedures. *Ann Surg,* 1981; 194:386-401.
2. Riverse SP, Veith FJ, Ascer E, Gupta SK: Successful conservative therapy of the severe limb-threatening ischemia: The value of nonsympatectomy. *Surgery,* 1986; 99:759-62.
3. Veith FJ, Gupta SK, Daly V: Management of early and late thrombosis of expanded polytetrafluoro-ethylene (PTFE) femoropopliteal bypass grafts: Favorable prognosis with appropriate reoperation. *Surgery,* 1980; 87:581-7.

4. Veith FJ, Gupta SK, Daly V: Femoropopliteal bypass to the isolated popliteal segment: Is polytetrafluoroethilene graft acceptable? *Surgery,* 1981; 89:296- 303.
5. Flinn WR, Flanigan DP, Verta MJ, et al: Sequential femoral-tibial bypass for severe limb ischemia. *Surgery,* 1980; 88:357-65.
6. Szilagyi DE, Smith RF, Elliot JP, Ageman JH: The biologic fate of autogenous vein implants as arterial substitutes clinical angiographic and histopathologic observations in femoropopliteal operations for atherosclerosis. *Ann Surg,* 1983; 178:232-44.
7. Witthemore AD, Clowes W, Couch NP, Mannick JA: Secondary femoropopliteal reconstruction. *Ann Surg,* 1981; 193:35-42.
8. Karkow WS, Cranley JJ, Cranley RD, et al: Extended study of aneurysm formation in umbilical grafts. *J Vasc Surg,* 1986; 4:486-92.
9. Hasson JE, Newton WD, Waltan AC, et al: Mural degeneration in the glutaraldehyde tanned umbilical vein graft: Incidence and implications: *J Vasc Surg,* 1986; 4:243-50.
10. Veith FJ, Weiser RK, Gupta SK, et al: Diagnosis and management of failing lower extremity arterial reconstructions. *J Cardiovasc Surg,* 1984; 25:381-4.
11. O'Mara CS, Flinn WR Johnson ND, et al: Recognition and surgical management of patent but hemodynamically failed arterial grafts. *Ann Surg,* 1981; 193:467-76.
12. Smith CR, Green RM, DeWeese JA: Psdeudocclusion of femoropopliteal bypass grafts. *Circulaton,* 1983; 68 (Suppl II) 88-93.
13. Berkowitz HD, Hobbs CL, Roberts B, et al: Value of routine vascular laboratory studies to identify vein graft stenosis. *Surgery,* 1981; 90:971-79.
14. Ascer E, Collier P, Gupta SK, Veith FJ: Reoperation for PTFE bypass failure: The importance of distal outflow site and operative technique in determinining outcome. *J Vasc Surg,* 1987; 5:298-310.
15. Craver JM, Ottinger LW, Darling C, et al: Hemorrhage and trhombosis as early complications of femoropopliteal bypass grafts: Causes, treatment, and prognostic implications. *Surgery,* 1973; 74:839-48.
16. Veith FJ, Ascer E, Gupta Sk, et al: Tibiotibial vein bypass grafts: A new operation for limb salvage. *J Vasc Surg,* 1985; 2:552-7.
17. Ascer E, Veith FJ, Gupta SK, et al: Short vein garfts: A superior option for arterial reconstruction to poor or compromised outflow tracts. *J Vasc Surg,* 1988; 17:370-78.
18. Ascer E, Veith FJ, Morin L, et al: Components of outflow resistance and their correlation with graft patency in lower extremity arterial reconstructions. *J Vasc Surg,* 1984; 1:817-28.
19. Collier P, Ascer E, Veith FJ, et al: Acute thrombosis of arterial grafts. In Bergan JJ, Yao JST (eds): Vascular Surgical Emergencies, New York, Grune and Stratton Inc., 1987 , pp 517-528.
20. Working Party of the International Vascular Symposium. The definition of critical ischaemia of a limb. *Br J Surg,* 1982; 69 (Suppl):S2.
21. Ascer E, Veith FJ, Gupta SK, et al: Comparison of axillo-unifemoral and axillobifemoral bypass operations. *Surgery,* 1985; 97:169-77.
22. Veith FJ, Ascer E, Nunez A, et al: Unusual approaches to infrainguinal arteries. *J Cardiovasc Surg,* 1987; 28: 58.
23. Nunez A, Veith FJ, Collier P, et al: Direct approach to the distal portions of the deep femoral artery for limb salvage bypasses. *J Vasc Surg,* 1988; 8:576-81.
24. Veith FJ, Moss CM, Sprayregen S, Montefusco C: Preoperative saphenous venograpy in arterial recontructive surgery of the lower extremity. *Surgery,* 1979; 85:253-9.
25. Veith FJ, Ascer E, Gupta Sk, Wengerter KR: Lateral approach to the popliteal artery. *J Vasc Surg,* 1987; 6:119-23.
26. Veith FJ, Gupta SK: Femoro-distal artery bypasses. In Bergan JJ, Yao JST (eds): Operative Techniques in Vascular Surgery. New York, Grune & Stratton, 1980, pp 141-150.
27. Dardik H, Dardik I, Veith FJ: Exposure of the tibial-peroneal arteries by a single lateral approach. *Surgery,* 1974; 75:372-82.
28. Ascer E, Veith FJ, Gupta SK: Bypasses to plantar arteries and other tibial branches: An extended approach to limb salvage. *J Vasc Surg,* 1988; 8:434-41.
29. Veith FJ, Gupta Sk, Samson RH, et al: Superficial femoral and popliteal arteries a inflow sites for distal bypasses. *Surgery,* 1981; 90:980-90.
30. Veith FJ, Gupta SK, Ascer E, White-Flores S, Samson RH, Scher LA, Towne JB, Bernhard VM, Bonier P, Flinn WR, Astelford P, Yao JST: Six-year prospective multicenter randomized comparison of autologous saphenous vein and expanded polytetrafluoroethylene grafts in infrainguinal arterial reconstructions. *J Vasc Surg,* 1986; 3:104-14.
31. Wengerter KR, Gupta Sk, Veith FJ, et al: Critical vein diameter for infrainguinal arterial reconstructions. *J Cardiovasc Surg,* 1987; 28:109.

32. Flinn WR, Rohrer MJ, Yao JST, et al: Improved long-term patency of infragenicular polytetrafluoroethylene grafts. *J Vasc Surg,* 1988; 7:685-90.
33. Bartlett ST, Olinde AJ, Flinn WR, et al: The reoperative potential of infrainguinal bypass: Long-term limb and patient survival. *J Vasc Surg,* 1987; 5:170-79.

Role of Endovascular Procedures in Reoperations in Infrainguinal Area

G. Agrifoglio, G. Lorenzi, M. Domanin

Department of Vascular Surgery and Angiology, University of Milan, Italy

INTRODUCTION

Direct surgical revascularization procedures and endovascular interventional techniques permit to treat successfully the occlusive disease of the lower limbs in different clinical situations.

In a variable number of patients, however, early or late treatment failure may result in disabling claudication or limb threatening ischemia. Restenosis and thrombosis may occur as a consequence of several biological, haemodinamical or mechanical factors.

Graft obstruction usually evolves from intimal hyperplasia occurring at the anastomotic sites. Neointimal overgrowth and new atherosclerotic lesions can lead to occlusion after thromboendoarterectomy (TEA). Residual parietal irregularities, elastic recoil and hyperplasia may compromise the results of percutaneous transluminal angioplasty (PTA).

Secondary surgical reconstructions has been reported to achieve good patency rates but in some cases may present considerable difficulty when the lesion occurs at an anastomosis or is located in a graft surrounded by dense scar tissue.

Percutaneous transluminal angioplasty, new endovascular procedures (Laser-PTA, atherectomy, intravascular stenting) and intra-arterial thrombolysis may provide other options in order to treat restenosis and open occluded arteries and grafts, obviating the necessity of surgical revascularization or reducing the complexity of the operation.

Despite initial enthusiasm, however, reports of several Authors show conflicting data that may suggest a more accurate patients selection.

Our experience with endovascular procedures in reoperations for recurrent lesions demonstrate a clear difference both in immediate and late patency rate between aorto-iliac and infrainguinal districts.

METHODS

This series consists of twenty four patients (23 men, 1 woman) aged thirty-five to seventy-one (average: fifty-five) presented with recurrent symptoms of claudication (5 or 20,9%), rest pain (8 or 33,3%) and tissue necrosis (11 or 45,8%) after direct arterial reconstruction or PTA.

We performed 24 endovascular recanalization procedures as reoperations a mean of 5 months after the initial operative treatment. Patients were divided in two groups according to the involved area: 1) aorto-iliac (11 Pts.); 2) infrainguinal (13 Pts.). The two groups were comparable for age, risk factors and clinical stage.

In **the aorto-iliac group** (Table 1) the original reconstruction consisted of 4 iliac PTA, 4 iliac TEA, 1 aortobiiliac TEA, 2 ilio-femoral PTFE bypass graft. Arteriography demonstrated a new stenosis in all patients previously managed with PTA and TEA (mean length: 3 cm.), whereas in the two patients with failed bypass graft angiographic investigation identified a complete occlusion proximal to the graft in one case and a narrow stenosis at the distal anastomosis in the other.

Table 1. Endovascular procedures in reoperations of the aorto-iliac group

Case	Original intervention	Redoendovascular procedures
1)	Iliac PTA	Iliac PTA
2)	Iliac PTA	Iliac PTA
3)	Iliac PTA	Iliac PTA
4)	Iliac PTA	Iliac PTA
5)	Iliac-femoral TEA	Iliac PTA + STENT
6)	Aorto-bisiliac TEA	Iliac PTA + Fem-fem crossover
7)	Iliac-femoral TEA	Iliac PTA
8)	Common iliac TEA	Iliac PTA + STENT
9)	Common iliac TEA	Iliac PTA
10)	Iliac-femoral BYPASS	Common iliac LAPTA
11)	Iliac-femoral BYPASS	Iliac PTA

PTA = Percutaneous Transluminal Angioplasty; LAPTA = Laser Assisted PTA; TEA = Thromboendoarterectomy.

As shown in Table 1, a conventional percutaneous transluminal angioplasty was carried out for concentric, smooth arterial stenosis in 7 patients and in the patient with distal graft stenosis: in one of these patients PTA was associated to a femoro-femoral bypass graft. In presence of irregular, eccentric or hardly calcific lesions PTA was completed by insertion of a Palmaz stent (2 patients).

The occluded PTFE graft was managed with thrombectomy and laser-assisted balloon angioplasty. The approach was percutaneous in seven patients and surgical in four. The lesions were dilated using a 8 or 9 mm balloon catheter. The laser thermal angioplasty was performed passing a 2.5 mm Nd:YAG powered probe activated at 14 watts. All patients underwent operation under local anesthesia with the exception of one case.

In **the infrainguinal group** (Table 2) the primary revascularization procedure consisted of 2 femoro-popliteal TEA, 3 below-knee saphenous bypass grafts with the in situ technique, 2 below knee composite grafts, one below-knee umbilical vein bypass graft, 3 above-knee femoro-popliteal PTFE bypass grafts, one PTA and one laser assisted PTA of the superficial femoral artery.

Table 2. Endovascular procedures in reoperations of the infra-inguinal group

Case	Original intervention	Redoendovascular procedures
1)	Sup. Femoral LAPTA	Sup. Femoral PTA
2)	Sup. Femoral PTA	Sup. Femoral LAPTA + STENT
3)	Femoro-popliteal TEA	Thrombectomy + Popliteal PTA
4)	Femoro-popliteal TEA	Sup.Fem.LAPTA + Profundoplasty
5)	Femoro-ant. tibial BYPASS (DARDIK)	Thrombolysis
6)	Femoro-popliteal BYPASS (PTFE)	Thrombolysis
7)	Femoro-post. tibial BYPASS (ISSV)	Thrombolysis
8)	Femoro-peroneal BYPASS (ISSV)	Thrombectomy + Thrombolysis
9)	Femoro-peroneal BYPASS (ISSV)	Thrombolysis
10)	Femoro-tibioperoneal BYPASS (ISSV)	Thrombectomy + Peroneal PTA
11)	Femoro post-tibial BYPASS (ISSV)	Thrombectomy+Tibioperoneal PTA
12)	Femoro-popliteal BYPASS (PTFE)	Distal anastomosis PTA
13)	Iliac-femoral + Fem-pop BYPASS (PTFE)	Thrombolysis

PTA = Percutaneous Transluminal Angioplasty; LAPTA = Laser Assisted PTA; TEA = Thromboendoarterectomy; ISSV = In Situ Saphenous Vein;

At the time of repeat angiography all the previously inserted grafts were occluded. As summarized in Table 2, low-dose intra-arterial thrombolitic therapy as an adjunct to conventional thrombectomy was used to restore graft patency in 6 patients. As thrombolitic agent we administered urokinase (UK) at a dosage of 50.000 to 100.000 units in thirty minutes.

After graft thrombectomy with Fogarty catheter, intraoperative control angiography revealed in three patients a distal anastomotic high grade stenosis. A percutaneous transluminal angioplasty with small caliber balloon catheters was carried out in the operating room under fluoroscopic control.

In the patient primarily treated with laser assisted PTA, a stenotic lesion developped in the femoral artery distally to the dilated site. The lesion was managed by means of a conventional transluminal angioplasty with a 5 mm balloon catheter.

The obliteration of the superficial femoral artery previously submitted to conventional PTA was recanalized by means of a laser assisted balloon angioplasty and insertion of a 5 mm diameter Strecker stent.

RESULTS

No deaths occurred within 30 days in both groups.

Operative morbidity consisted of a single case of inguinal haemorrhage after UK infusion in the infrainguinal group (7.6%), in whom no transfusion was required.

Significant differences both in initial and long-term patency rates were observed between the aorto-iliac and infra-inguinal areas (Fig. 1). In the **infrainguinal group** endovascular procedures were successful in only 5 patients (38,4%). Amputation was required in 4 patients (30,7%), whereas in two cases (15,3%) a femoro-distal bypass was performed for impending limb loss. Within three months recurrent thrombosis was observed in two patients. Thus, the cumulative long-term patency rate at 18 months, analyzed by life-table method, was only 15.3%.

Subjects who underwent endovascular procedures in **the aorto-iliac area** fared significantly better (Fig. 1). Treatment was successful in all patients with an initial patency rate of 100%. At follow-up, only one recurrent obliteration was observed. Cumulative patency rate at 6, 12 and 18 months was 90.1%.

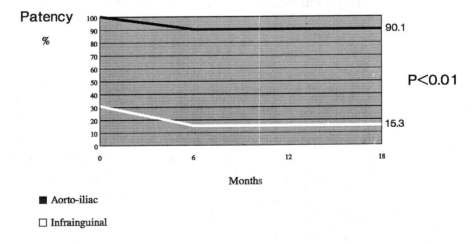

■ Aorto-iliac

☐ Infrainguinal

Fig. 1. Endovascular procedures: Comparative actuarial analysis of patency in reoperations in the aorto-iliac and infrainguinal areas.

DISCUSSION

It has been reported in the literature that a substantial number of arterial reconstructions can fail. Endovascular procedures has been considered as an alternative to redo surgery after proper patients selection. Some Authors reported encouraging results with balloon angioplasty, intra-arterial thrombolysis and, more recently, laser-assisted angioplasty. In contrast, others reports have provided less favorable early and long-term results, above all in infrainguinal reoperations.

Our experience shows that the use of endovascular techniques may obviate the need for surgery in the aortoiliac area in presence of limited lesions, but fail to restore patency in most of the cases of femoro-popliteal and femoro-distal reocclusions.

These variable results may be the consequence of differences in treated lesions, vessels caliber and distal run-off. In 81.8% of patients (9/11) of the aortoiliac group we used PTA, LPTA and stents to restore patency after failure of previous ballon angioplasty or endarterectomy. Restenoses after these revascularization procedures usually presented as smooth, concentric, prevalently fibrotic and therefore suitable for interventional procedures. Moreover, the good run-off and the large vessel caliber were conditions favoring the treatment durability.

In the infrainguinal area we managed prevalently occluded grafts (9/13 or 69.2%). Late graft obstruction generally evolves from intimal hyperplasia that leads to organized thrombus. These lesions in our experience have proven to be recalcitrant to dilation and thrombolitic therapy following thrombectomy, producing a high rate of rethrombosis. The data suggest that more favorable results may be obtained with conventional redo surgery. Interventional technologies may be of benefit in presence of limited arterial or vein graft stenosis. Perhaps the development of other laser systems that produce less thermal injury will improve the results. The potential of intravascular stenting in reoperations needs further investigations.

REFERENCES

1. Agrifoglio G, Lorenzi G. (1987): PTA e chirurgia nel trattamento della malattia aterosclerotica. In: Patologia Vascolare '87, Atti IX Congresso Nazionale Società Italiana di Patologia Vascolare, Coppanello, Giugno 1987, Monduzzi, Bologna, 467.
2. Belkin M., Donaldson M.C., Whittemore A.D. et al. (1990): Observation on the use of thrombolytic agents for thrombotic occlusion of infrainguinal vein grafts. *J. Vasc. Surg.* 11: 289.
3. Brewster D.C., La Salle A.J., Robison J.G., Strayhorn E.C., Darling R.C. (1983): Femoropopliteal graft failures: clinical consequences and success of secondary reconstructions. *Arch. Surg.* 118: 1043.
4. Dietrich E.B., Santiago O., Bahadir I. (1991): Laser-assisted angioplasty in the treatment of prosthetic graft stenosis. *Angiology*, 42: 576.
5. Harris E.J., Porter J.M. (1989): Thrombolytic therapy and modern vascular surgery: an overview. In: Goldstone J.: "Perspectives in vascular surgery" Q.M.P. St. Louis, 40.

6. Lorenzi G., Domanin M., Costantini A. (1991): PTA and laser assisted PTA combined with simultaneous surgical revascularization. *J.Cardiovasc. Surg.* 32, 456.
7. Perler B.A., Osterman F.A., Mitchelle S.E., Burdick J.F., Williams G.M. (1990): Balloon dilatation versus surgical revision of infrainguinal autogenous vein graft stenoses: long-term follow-up. *J. Cardiovasc. Surg.* 31: 656.
8. Quinones-Baldrich W.J., Baker J.D., Bussutil R.W. et al. (1988): Intraoperative infusion of lytic drugs for thrombotic complications of revascularization. *J. Vasc. Surg.* 7: 347.
9. Whittemore A.D., Donaldson M.C., Polak J.F., Mannick J.A. (1991): Limitations of balloon angioplasty for vein graft stenosis. *J. Vasc. Surg.* 14: 340.

New Technology and Reoperations: Cause or Solution in The Infrainguinal Area

E.B. Diethrich

Department of Cardiovascular Surgery, Arizona Heart Institute & Foundation and The Cardiovascular Center of Excellence at Human Hospital-Phoenix Phoenix, Arizona, U.S.A.

INTRODUCTION

For more than four decades, bypass grafting has been the primary surgical means of revascularizing lower limbs whose arterial supply is threatened by atherosclerotic occlusive disease. Endarterectomy of the limb vessels is today commonly employed only as an ancillary procedure to treat very localized disease in the common and profunda femoris arteries and in the distal runoff circulation.

Peripheral atherosclerotic lesions arise more frequently in the femoropopliteal segment than in any other area of the lower extremities, making the femoropopliteal bypass the most commonly performed surgical revascularization procedure in the peripheral circulation[16,30]. Autogenous veins remain the preferred conduit, either excised and reversed or in situ[3-5,8,14-17,19,21,25,27,29-31].

When sufficient vein material is not available or has been reserved for future coronary bypasses, synthetic substitutes can be used. Currently, the polytetrafluoroethylene (PTFE) is somewhat favored over the velour knit Dacron conduits[2,5,6]. Though initial (up to two-year) results sometimes parallel those of the autogenous vein grafts[3], synthetic grafts have only a 65% or lower patency rate at five years and even more disappointing results when used below the knee joint[7,8,18,24,29,31].

Historically, vascular reconstructions in the trifurcation arteries have not been particularly successful, primarily due to the severity of the disease (threatened limb loss and/or critical ischemia) required to justify this intervention. Typically, such advanced distal disease is not an isolated pathology but attendant to multisegment atherosclerosis, often complicated by diabetes mellitus[7,16,19,30,33].

CAUSES OF LATE FAILURE

Since most repeat vascular procedures below the inguinal ligament will involve a previously placed bypass graft, an understanding of the causes of graft failure is important to selecting new technologies for revascularization.

Vascular grafts perform well when placed in high flow, low resistance locations, such as the aortoiliac or iliofemoral segments; femorodistal reconstructions routinely fare less well due to inherently unfavorable hemodynamics associated with poor runoff[5,7]. However, graft failure is a multifactorial problem[5,7,28,30,33].

No graft is immune to the ramifications of progressive atherosclerotic disease in the native artery. Whether lesions develop proximally or distally to the graft or both, the disruption in normal flow dynamics compromises the viability of the bypass, leading to mural layering and thrombosis[7,33].

Graft failure may also occur from changes in the conduit over time[33]. Among the earlier prosthetics, fabric fatigue resulted in dilatation and elongation with kinking; failure of the fabric also produced fragmentation, fraying and disruption of strands. Newer synthetic grafts usually are resistant to atherosclerosis, but they can develop mural thrombus.

Vein grafts exhibit pressure-induced histologic changes such as intimal thickening, progressive diminution of smooth muscle in the media with a buildup in collagen tissue, and increased vascularity extending from the adventitia[18,33]. They also suffer atheromatous degeneration and fibrosis of retained valve cusps. Pseudoaneurysms as well may arise at the anastomotic sites[7].

Another cause for failure common to all graft conduits and even endarterectomized arteries is intimal hyperplasia[2,5,13,33]. This condition produces a proliferative lesion composed largely of smooth muscle cells at the anastomotic border, primarily in the graft's neointima, but sometimes extending into the intima of the recipient artery. The distal anastomosis of a femoropopliteal or femorotibial bypass is affected more often than the proximal junction[28,33].

The occurrence of this suture line reaction has been linked to a number of influencing factors: arterial pressure and flow patterns, shear stress forces, operative handling of the anastomosis, thrombogenicity of the graft, and mechanical mismatch between the graft and host artery[2,28,33].

Although the above causes singly or in combination probably account for the majority of failed grafts, there are several other factors that are contributory. Notable among these are the conditions which impact hemodynamics, namely graft length, native vessel caliber and the graft-to-vessel diameter ratio, and the status of the distal circulation[33].

As a general rule, the longer an interposed graft, the greater the resistance to flow and the poorer the long-term results; hence, one of the reasons aortofemoro-popliteal reconstructions do not fare well[16]. Small diameter recipient arteries do not presage a good result either[5]. They cannot comply with the blood volume and so contribute to turbulence in the oversized graft.

Small vein grafts may produce similar problems of incompatibility with the native vasculature, in which flow from a large caliber host artery hastens pressure-induced damage and disintegration of the vein[5].

Poor runoff has a notoriously fatal influence on grafts[2,7,28,33]. In the presence of femoropopliteal occlusive disease, the outflow tract is often compromised. Frequently, one or more of the tibioperoneal vessels will be involved, thereby reducing graft flow and setting the stage for thrombosis.

In addition to flow considerations, several systemic factors may contribute to graft failure[7,33]. The presence of diabetes mellitus has widespread vascular consequences. In the lower limbs, diabetics have an altered pattern of atherosclerotic disease presentation, with the preponderance of their lesions appearing in the infrainguinal and distal areas. Not only do they tend to have more multisegmental lesions, but atherosclerosis progresses at a faster pace in diabetics. Furthermore, they have tendencies toward infection and diffuse microangiopathy that contributes to low flow in the distal circulation.

A wealth of hypercoagulopathies can impact graft patency[18,33]. Most common are the abnormalities in platelet function associated with myeloproliferative disorders, hyperlipidemias, diabetes, smoking, and heparin-induced thrombocyto penia. Among the primary hypercoagulable conditions that can precipitate graft failure are deficiencies of antithrombin III, protein C, and protein S, along with the variety of fibrinolytic disorders and dysfibrinogenemia. Hyperviscosity syndromes, such as the polycythemias, may also play a role in early graft failure.

Other forms of cardiovascular disease, such as coronary artery disease, are commonly found in patients with failed grafts. Hypertension accelerates atherosclerosis and may hasten pressure-related alterations in graft conduits.

RESULTS OF FAILURE

The timing of graft failure may influence the various opportunities to reestablish flow using new technologies. Late graft failure can present as an acute event, with a rapid, often limb-threatening change in vascular status. This late graft occlusion generally disrupts the native artery as well as collateral flow down the first patent collateral vessel below the distal anastomosis. Patients are generally much more symptomatically aware of this occlusive process than they were before their original bypass procedure.

The other presentation of graft failure is a chronic progression of stenosis with gradual return of symptoms. Depending on the etiology of the recurrence, this symptomatology may be or may not be similar to the pre-graft claudication pattern.

The classical treatment for occlusion of an infrainguinal graft has been extirpation of the old conduit and insertion of a new graft usually distal to the original anastomosis[2,23]. Unfortunately, mobilization and removal of an old thrombosed graft is often extremely difficult because of its firm attachment to its tunnel[2]. Most grafts, especially prosthetic ones, undergo a graft-host tissue response that results not only in the formation of a pseudointima inside the graft but also a perigraft capsule of fibrous tissue.

NEW TECHNOLOGY

Today, infrainguinal graft occlusion can be approached from a new direction in many cases. An array of interventional techniques offers viable alternatives for revascularization, sparing the original conduit while attacking the suture line response and atherosclerosis at the root of the failure.

The current interventional armamentarium includes a variety of devices and techniques: thrombolytic therapy, aspiration thrombectomy, hyperplastic tissue extraction, laser recanalization, balloon dilation, atherectomy, and intravascular stents. In addition, two important assessment and guidance modalities - intravascular ultrasound and angioscopy - are enhancing the performance of these techniques and their outcome in cases of late primary graft failure.

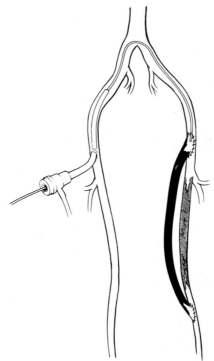

Fig. 1. For graft thrombolysis via contralateral access, the catheter is delivered to the clot site across the aortic bifurcation from the percutaneous entry site in the contralateral common femoral artery.

Thrombolysis. Catheter-directed thrombolysis is extremely valuable as a primary treatment tool in bypass graft occlusion. Because graft thrombosis is usually a manifestation of an underlying pathology, thrombolysis can offer both diagnostic and therapeutic benefits. If the graft occlusion is relatively recent (4-6 weeks), lytic infusion is almost universally effective.

The initial decision to use thrombolysis is dictated to some extent by the potential to gain satisfactory access to the origin of the occluded graft. Two approaches are commonly employed: contralateral or ipsilateral. In the former technique, an infusion catheter is delivered from a contralateral per-cutaneous access across the aortic bifurcation and placed in the common femoral artery (CFA) at the origin of the graft (Fig. 1).

Occasionally, it is possible to place a wire into the occluded graft and follow with advancement of the catheter to assure that a high concentration of lytic agent is delivered directly to the thrombosis (Fig. 2). However, if the graft origin cannot be cannulated, the catheter is positioned at the suspected origin and lysis started.

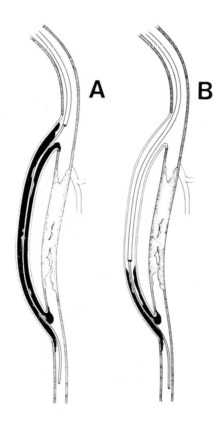

Fig. 2. It is advisable to attempt wire passage in the contralateral approach to guide the advancement of the catheter through the thrombus.

Alternately, the ipsilateral common femoral artery can be approached directly, attempting to pass a wire into the graft. This technique is almost always successful in recent occlusions.

In our standard lytic protocol, intraarterial infusion of 250.000 units of urokinase is followed by drip infusion at 40.000-80.000 units per hour for up to 48 hours. The partial thromboplastin time is maintained in the 40-90 second range with a concomitant heparin drip (800-1200 units per hour after a 1000-3000 bolus).

In the Intensive Care Unit, the lytic protocol calls for serial bedside arteriography using either a portable C-arm or a standard chest x-ray unit to monitor progress of the thrombolysis. The delivery catheter is advanced progressively into the thrombus until lysis is achieved.

Aspiration Thrombectomy. An alternative or adjunctive treatment for thrombosis involves the insertion of an 8F catheter (Renal Superflow, Schneider, Minneapolis, MN) either percutaneously or directly through an arteriotomy. The catheter is guided to the clot and strong suction applied with a 50 cc syringe. As the catheter is withdrawn (under suction), the thrombus is extracted. The technique can be used to remove residual clot that has failed to lyse after urokinase infusion.

Hyperplastic Tissue Removal. If the thrombosis is old and resistant to extraction, or if there is residual pseudointima or neointima partially across an anastomotic site, a new device, the 6F Fogarty Adherent Clot Catheter (Baxter-Edwards, Irvine, CA) (Fig. 3), is highly effective in removing the material.

Again, it is possible to use this device either percutaneously or with an open arteriotomy; however, delivery of the material through a sheath can be troublesome. An expandable sheath (Applied Vascular Devices, Laguna Hills, CA) is useful if large quantities of material are to be extracted. The orifice of the sheath incorporates an expandable ring that allows for a wide operating lumen.

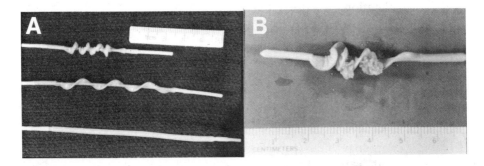

Fig. 3. The Fogarty Adherent Clot Catheter (A) is particularly helpful in removing resistant thrombus and excess neointima (B) that has contributed to the graft stenosis.

The major problem or limitation to successful graft recanalization following thrombolysis or clot extraction is the residual stenosis responsible for the occlusion. This almost always occurs at the distal anastomosis which, under most circumstances, will open at least partially after lytic therapy. If the anastomotic site does not open or a wire cannot be passed across to the artery distally, the laser is highly effective in recanalizing the occlusion.

Laser Angioplasty. Today, the most versatile vascular laser for opening distal prosthetic graft occlusions is the pulsed, near-infrared holmium:YAG system (Trimedyne, Inc., Tustin, CA), which achieves a maximum temperature of only 85°C when operated within recommended limits (3.6 J/pulse at 10 Hz). PTFE and many synthetic graft materials have satisfactorily tolerated laser therapies even with older, high-temperature models [11,20,22,26].

The holmium cool laser is coupled with a newly marketed hybrid probe design, the 2.5 mm Spectraprobe-Max. This delivery system, with its conically-shaped metal tip fitted to a 600 micron fiber, has a 0.9 mm aperture that emits approximately 50% of the laser energy. With a maximum energy density of 4000 mJ/mm[2], the Spectraprobe is highly effective in crossing occlusions resistant to standard guidewire passage. Furthermore, the probe can be more coaxially aligned, partially owing to special fluoroscopic guidance systems and newer guiding catheter techniques, making it more advantageous than wire-dissected planes.

A new generation of hollow fiber catheter, the Halocath (Trimedyne), is being evaluated for use in the larger arteries that may present inflow problems for a graft. It features a fused quartz lens that distributes 100% of the holmium laser energy to create a path greater than the 3.0 mm diameter of the probe. While the design retains the central 0.035 inch guidewire channel, the lens configuration reduces the number of fibers in the bundle, increasing flexibility.

For graft laser recanalization, the 2.5 mm Spectraprobe-Max is placed at the occlusion, activated for 2-3 seconds and then passed into the arterial segment below. Once the lesion has been opened, a guidewire is easily passed to facilitate further treatment.

Balloon dilatation. Traditional balloon angioplasty is an effective means of dealing with compliant anastomotic stenoses that have been cleared of thrombus by lytic therapy. However, the recurrence rate following balloon dilation alone is very high because the underlying condition has not been addressed.

Atherectomy. Either as sole therapy or as an ancillary procedure, atherectomy can sometimes be valuable in graft salvage. Using the Simpson device (Atherocath, Devices for Vascular Intervention, Redwood City, CA) as a biopsy instrument, recurrent lesions can be biopsied to determine the histopathologic etiology. In this manner, the presence of intimal proliferation or fibrosis, or both, can be ascertained, and the extent of the process in both the graft neointima and the native vessel can be determined.

Among the other atherectomy devices, the transluminal endarterectomy catheter (TEC, Interventional Technologies, San Diego, CA) can provide satisfactory debulking of soft plaque stenoses and thrombotic material, but the excisions are not consistent and it does not perform well with calcified tissue. For hard plaque, rotational atherectomy with the Rotablator (Heart Technology, Belleview, WA) works far better but can produce hemoglobinuria. Furthermore, both of these devices require a lumen for wire guidance.

For wire-resistant occlusions, the Trac-Wright (formerly Kensey device) (Dow Corning Wright, Arlington, TN) high-speed drill is the only atherectomy device that can bore through calcified plaque, but the device is hard to control, and the small channel it creates necessitates subsequent balloon dilation. Indeed, given the current technology, most atherectomies must be accompanied by dilation.

Stent Implantation. Despite the success in opening occluded grafts and removing thrombus and neointima with today's new technology, restenosis remains a problem, particularly when recoil and fibrotic lesions are encountered.

Stents, which have become a prime component in the battle to overcome restenosis, may also prove helpful to graft salvage by ensuring inflow and maintaining anastomotic integrity following an intervention (our references). In the iliac arteries, we now use stents routinely after opening occluded arteries[9].

Theoretically, the same rationale that led to our use of stents in the iliac system should apply to the superficial femoral artery. However, early experience in Europe has shown that the stents behave differently when placed below the inguinal ligament and exhibit a greatly reduced patency rate. Nevertheless, this is an area that needs to be explored, particularly in any stenoses that demonstrate abnormal dilation characteristics (e.g., resistance, recoil) or dilation failure (e.g., persistent filling defect, dissection, thrombosis, or occlusion). The use of stents in grafts is undergoing evaluation at this time, and our initial experiences have been encouraging (Fig. 4)[10].

The Palmaz balloon-expandable stent (Johnson & Johnson Interventional Systems, Warren, NJ) for the peripheral vessels is a stainless steel tube designed with multiple rows of staggered rectangular slots that assumes a diamond shape when expanded, reducing to 10% the amount of metal in contact with the luminal surface. Because of its longitudinal rigidity, the Palmaz stent is best suited for straight vessels and end-to-end anastomoses. For aortoiliac applications, the premounted, 3 mm by 3 cm stent (0.015 mm thick) is expanded to a ratio of 6:1 by an 8 mm by 3 cm balloon delivered through a 9F Pinnacle sheath (Terumo, Medi-tech, Watertown, MA) over an Amplatz 0.035 inch super stiff wire (Medi-tech).

The Strecker stent (Medi-tech) is a tubular stent of knitted tantalum wire 0.1 mm in diameter. It is radially and longitudinally flexible and somewhat elastic. It becomes up to 3 cm long when deployed and comes in diameters ranging from 5-8 mm that are expanded by 5F balloons delivered through 8

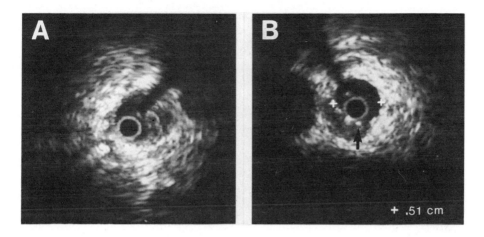

Fig. 4. Proximal anastomotic stenosis with lesion recoil in a PTFE femoropopliteal graft was treated with the Strecker stent when repeated dilations failed to produce an adequate lumen. This 2-dimensional intravascular ultrasound (IVUS) shows the stent (arrow shows a stent strut) in apposition to the graft wall.

or 9F sheaths. The flexibility of this stent makes it particularly useful for delivery through curved arteries, implantation overlying the graft-artery junction in end-to-side anastomoses, and in vessels subject to flexion from adjacent joints or structures, such as the common femoral and popliteal arteries. Currently, this stent is awaiting approval for clinical investigation in the U.S., so it is restricted to compassionate use only.

In the area of procedural monitoring, the importance of ultrasound imaging cannot be underestimated in today's vascular procedures[12]. Preoperatively, duplex scanning provides good quantification of a lesion, its characteristics and the impact on flow. These ultrasound studies of plaque morphology are becoming ever more important in the selection of an appropriate interventional device. For example, if dense calcium is present, the lesion may not be amenable to laser therapy at all.

Intraprocedurally, intravascular ultrasound scanning (IVUS) is invaluable for both preprocedural evaluation and post-interventional assessment. Anastomotic sites and inflow lesions are interrogated routinely with a 20 or 30 Mhz intravascular ultrasound (IVUS) catheter [6F Diasonics (Milpitas, CA) or 8F Cardiovascular Imaging Systems (Sunnyvale, CA), respectively] for 2-dimensional imaging. Three-dimensional reconstruction is achieved with a real-time processing system (Image Comm Systems, Inc., Santa Clara, CA).

IVUS provides baseline luminal dimensions pre- and post-angioplasty (intraluminal cross-sections and arterial circumferences) along with precise determination of graft-artery architecture and pathology. In most cases, the

IVUS examination following balloon dilation plays a significant role in determining the need for stenting (Fig. 5).

Of all the assessment modalities, however, angioscopy is the most important when dealing with occluded femoropopliteal bypass grafts. Direct visualization of lesion pathology, particularly at the anastomotic suture lines, and estimation of thrombosis and its removal are fundamental to procedural progress. The 1.5 to 3.0 mm disposable angioscopes can be connected to high-quality medical video color monitors with hard copy documentation available through video recorders.

Standard monitoring equipment is also used in a unique fashion to measure pressure differentials across proximal inflow lesions and stenotic anastomoses. Employing a special 5F wire-guided, radiopaque-tipped catheter (Medi-tech) placed retrograde across the lesion, the exact proximal origination point of the gradient is determined by pulling the catheter back through the lesion and noting the level at which the radial artery and catheter pressures began to differ. Complete abolition of the gradient is the only end point for a satisfactory recanalization in native iliac artery disease and aortoiliac and even femoropopliteal graft retreatment. Failure to achieve this goal is another important criterion for stent implantation.

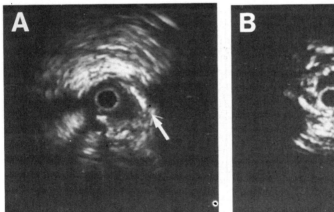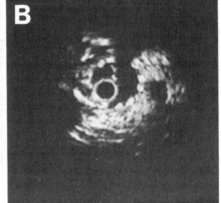

Fig. 5. (A) After balloon dilation in a superficial femoral artery, a dissection plane (arrow) was seen to move in the real-time scan, dictating stent implantation. (B) With the stent in place, the lumen is supported and the dissection plane is tacked up against the vessel wall.

APPROACHES TO RECURRENT GRAFT DISEASE

Our present approach to treating infrainguinal graft occlusion typically begins with thrombolysis followed by one or more of these endovascular techniques to address the cause of the occlusion and salvage the conduit. The selection process matches the etiology of the recurrence and specific lesion pathology to the capabilities of the device, as outlined above.

Treating femoropopliteal graft outflow occlusions is dependent on the type of graft and the lesion pathology at the distal anastomosis. For the typical prosthetic graft, once access at the proximal anastomosis is achieved (surgically in the case of proximal involvement or percutaneously with a 9F sheath insertion if no disease is present), a 0.035 inch hydrophilic guidewire (Glidewire, Medi-tech) is passed through the distal lesion to facilitate thrombectomy, atherectomy, and/or balloon dilation. If the distal occlusion is resistant, the 2.5 mm Spectraprobe-Max can be used, delivering pulsed holmium energy to open a channel for subsequent wire passage and dilation with 5 or 6 mm balloons.

If lesions in the runoff vessels are also noted on post-recanalization angiography, balloon dilation of these small vessels can open distal circulation. Laser angioplasty of small caliber distal vessels is not appropriate with the current technology.

Infrainguinal saphenous vein grafts are best salvaged by the adjuvant use of thrombolysis with balloon angioplasty; stents may also be useful here. However, acute occlusions less than 6 weeks old are generally the result of technical errors that need surgical correction.

Situations exist in which an occluded graft cannot be opened and the claudication becomes debilitating or the extremity is in jeopardy. Occasionally, it is possible to open the original superficial femoral artery using laser technology. This is particularly applicable if the proximal portion of the SFA is patent, thus permitting percutaneous access and laser probe insertion. Although the long-term patency associated with this technique is limited, it can be very useful in critical situations.

ROLE OF POST-PROCEDURE ANTICOAGULATION

The benefit of post-procedural heparinization has become controversial of late. We use a 1000 unit/hr heparin IV drip (to maintain the activated coagulation time above 200 seconds) for 24-48 hours only in cases of complex or long lesions.

There has also been some discussion about the advantages of using warfarin during the healing process. Again, we are unsure as to the benefits, but we have added warfarin (doubling the partial thromboplastin time for six months) to the post-treatment drug regimen consisting of aspirin (325 mg/day) and dipyridamole (75 mg tid).

THE FUTURE OF GRAFT INTERVENTIONS

A variety of new modalities is now available both for assessment and intervention of infrainguinal recurrent disease and failed reconstructions. It can be stated empirically that most of these devices have demonstrated satisfactory performance in the larger peripheral arteries. We must look at intraluminal graft recanalization as a new era in interventional therapy and, as these tools undergo modification, newer and more efficacious models will be forthcoming.

The demand for this technological development is very real. The results of infrainguinal bypass surgery are not nearly as good as the literature might suggest. Moreover, graft occlusion is a common phenomenon and one that frequently leads to a less than ideal outcome. Even if there are major limitations to the endovascular devices currently being applied in this arterial location, these tools offer a viable alternative (and sometimes the only alternative) to salvage a limb. If they are utilized in the proper framework, they can be extremely useful.

REFERENCES

1. Baker WH, Hadcock MM, Littooy FN: Management of polytetrafluoroethylene graft occlusions. *Arch Surg,* 1980;115:508-13.
2. Bergan JJ, Moore WS, Haimovici H: Reoperations for early and late occlusive complications of arterial surgery. In: Haimovici H, Callow AD, DePalma RG, Ernst CB, Hollier LH (eds.): Vascular Surgery: Principles and Techniques, Norwalk, CT, Appleton & Lange, 1989, pp. 575-90.
3. Bergan JJ, Veith FJ, Bernhard VM, et al: Randomization of autogenous vein and polytetrafluoroethylene grafts in femoral-distal reconstruction. *Surgery,* 1982;92: 921-30.
4. Calligaro KD, Friedell ML, Rollins DAL, Semrow CM, Buchbinder D: A comparative review of in situ versus reversed vein grafts in the 1980s. *Surg Obstet Gynecol,* 1991;172:247-52.
5. Callow AD: Current status of vascular grafts. *Surg Clin N Am,* 1982;62:501-513.
6. Charlesworth PM, Brewster DC, Robison JG, Hallet JW: The fate of polytetrafluoroethylene grafts in lower limb bypass surgery: a six year follow-up. *Br J Surg,* 1985;72:896-9.
7. Courtney DF, Flinn WR, McCarthy WJ, Yao JST, Bergan JJ: Factors contributing to success and failure of femorotibial bypass grafts. *World J Surg,* 1988;12:768-76.
8. Cranley JJ: Revascularization of the femoropopliteal arteries using saphenous vein, polytetrafluoro-ethylene and umbilical vein grafts. *Arch Surg,* 1982;117: 1543-50.
9. Diethrich EB: Endovascular stents in occlusive vascular disease. In: Proceedings of the Second World Week of Professional Updating in Surgery of the University of Milan, Montorsi W (ed.), Bologna, Italy, Monduzzi Editore, 1990, pp. 449-452.
10. Diethrich EB, Ravi R: Intraluminal stent implantation for the treatment of aortic graft stenosis. *J Invasive Cardiol,* 1991;3:165-167.
11. Diethrich EB, Santiago O, Bahadir I: Laser-assisted angioplasty in the treatment of prosthetic graft stenosis. *Angiology,* 1991;42:576-80.
12. Diethrich EB, Ivens Ferraz D, Bahadir I, Santiago O: Intravascular ultrasound imaging: use in peripheral laser-assisted angioplasty. *J Intervent Cardiol,* 1990; 3:145-155.
13. Echave V, Loornick A, Haimov M, Jacobson JH: Intimal hyperplasia as a complication of the use of the polytetrafluoroethylene graft for femoral-popliteal bypass. *Surgery,* 1979;87:791-798.
14. Fogel MA, Whittemore AD, Couch NP, Mannick JAA: A comparison of in situ and reversed saphenous vein grafts for infrainguinal reconstruction. *J Vasc Surg,* 1987;5:46-52.
15. Grimley RP, Obeid ML, Ashton F, Slaney G: Long term results of autogenous vein bypass grafts in femoropopliteal arterial occlusion. *Br J Surg,* 1972;66:723-6.
16. Haimovici H, Veith FJ: Femoropopliteal arteriosclerotic occlusive disease. In: Haimovici H, Callow AD, DePalma RG, Ernst CB, Hollier LH (eds.): Vascular Surgery: Principles and Techniques, Norwalk, CT, Appleton & Lange, 1989, pp. 474-500.
17. Hall JV, Rostad H: In situ vein bypass in the treatment of femoropopliteal atherosclerotic disease: a ten year study. *Am J Surg,* 1978;136:158-61.

18. Hiatt JG, Raviola C, Baker JD, Busuttil RW, Machleder HI, Moore WS: The limitations of predictability of success of femoral-popliteal bypass grafts. *J Vasc Surg,* 1984;1:617-22.
19. Kacoyanis GP, Whittemore AD, Couch NP, Mannick JA: Femoro-tibial and femoro-popliteal bypass vein grafts. *Arch Surg,* 1981;116:1529-34.
20. Koyanagi N, Muto Y, Yang Y, DuPree J, Wendler FW, Matsumoto T: Argon laser thrombectomy of the polytetrafluoroethylene graft. *Contemp Surg,* 1989; 34:13-17.
21. Leather RP, Shah DM, Karmody AM: Infrapopliteal arterial bypass for limb salvage: increased patency and utilization of the saphenous vein used "in situ". *Surgery,* 1981;90:1000-8.
22. Muto Y, DuPree JJ, Duemler S, Yang Y, Koyanagi N, Cuffari WJ, Matsumoto T: Effects of argon laser on vascular materials. *J Vasc Surg,* 1988;7:562-7.
23. Painton JF, Avellon JC, Plecha FR: Effectiveness of reoperation after late failure of femoropopliteal reconstruction. *Am J Surg,* 1978;135:235-237.
24. Quinones-Baldrich WJ, Martin-Paredero, V, Baker D, Busuttil RW, Machleder HI, Moore WS: Polytetrafluoroethylene grafts as the first choice arterial substitute in femoropopliteal revascularization. *Arch Surg,* 1984;119:1238-43.
25. Schulman ML, Badhey MR, Yatco R, Pillari G: An 11-year experience with deep leg veins as femoro-popliteal bypass grafts. *Arch Surg,* 1986;121:1010-15.
26. Seeger JM, Abela GS, Klingman N: Laser radiation in the treatment of prosthetic graft stenosis. A preliminary study of prosthesis damage by laser energy. *J Vasc Surg,* 1987; 6:221-225.
27. Taylor LM, Phinnet FS, Porter LM: Present status of reversed vein bypass for lower extremity revascularization. *J Vasc Surg,* 1986;3:288-97.
28. Taylor RS, McFarland RJ, Cox MI: An investigation into the causes of failure of PTFE grafts. *Eur J Vasc Surg,* 1987; 1:335-343.
29. Tilanus HW, Obertop H, van Urk H: Saphenous vein or PTFE for femoropopliteal bypass. *Ann Surg,* 1985;202:780-2.
30. Veith AJ, Gupta SK, Ascer E: Femoral, popliteal and tibial occlusive disease. In: Wilson SE, Veith FJ, Hobson RW, Williams RA (eds.): Vascular Surgery: Principles and Practices, New York, McGraw-Hill Book Company, 1987, pp. 353-75.
31. Veith FJ, Gupta SK, Ascer E, et al: Six-year prospective multicenter comparison of autologous saphenous vein and expanded polytetrafluoroethylene grafts in infrainguinal arterial reconstruction. *J Vasc Surg,* 1986;3:104-14.
32. Veith FJ, Gupta S, Daly V: Management of early and late thrombosis of expanded polytetrafluoroethylene (PTFE) femoropopliteal bypass grafts: favorable prognosis with appropriate reoperation. *Surgery,* 1980;87:581-587.
33. Whittemore AD: Failure of peripheral arterial reconstruction. *Acta Chir Scand* Suppl 1988;550:74-80.

Secondary Follow-Up in Infrainguinal Area

G. Bracale, B. Bernardo, B. Perretti, O. Filice and A. Vosa

*Department of Vascular Surgery, II School of Medicine,
University of Naples, Italy*

Failure of a vascular procedure in infrainguinal area constitutes a frequent problem in vascular surgery; most patients return to their preoperative status or deteriorate, thereby facing limb loss.

The presence of technical errors, poor runoff, the development of vein graft stenosis and the progression of atherosclerosis are all major causes of graft occlusion, occurring in three distinct time periods: immediate (<1 month), early (<1 year), late (>1 year)[8].

Many patients require a re-do procedure: thrombectomy, revascularization or amputation. Secondary bypasses are always below the knee, often on a single tibial vessel and almost need the use of prosthetic matherial. By recent reports, the results of re-do surgery in these patients are indeed poor, with 3-year patency and limb-salvage rates in the range of 30% to 40%[1,6,11,12,15,16].

Also and overall in re-do surgery for infrainguinal area, early and late failures are often preceded by the development of graft-threatening lesions (intrinsic stenosis, inflow or outflow stenosis). Szilagyi, in his famous report published in 1973[21] found significant structural defects in 32,7% of reversed vein grafts at a mean follow-up of 5 years.

It's universally accepted that the correction of graft threatening lesions before thrombosis can result in long-term patency and is usually accomplished with a relatively minor procedure[3,4,9,19,22,24].

These data clearly distress the importance of an accurate routine post-operative surveillance to detect correctable lesions before graft occlusion. Although the criteria for graft revision may vary, depending on the pathological findings, its location or individual preference of surgeons, all recommend correction of occlusione lesions associated with recurrent ischemia. Re-do surgery in asymptomatic patients is more controversial, but many reports have shown that often a postimplantation lesion can result in graft thrombosis without premonitory ischemic symptoms.

The concept of serial detailed postoperative surveillance is overall important in secondary follow-up, because of the higher risk of limb-loss after graft occlusion.

TECHNIQUES OF GRAFT SURVEILLANCE

The diagnosis of correctable lesions before graft occlusion can salvage 80% of graft with impeding failure and improve overall graft patency by 15%-20%[4,7,23,25].

Many methods have been reported to assess graft function and detect failure threatening (Table 1):

- *clinical assessment:* deterioration of walking perimeter, recurrent ischemic symptoms;
- *Doppler evaluation:* waveform analysis, segmental systolic arterial pressures, ankle/ brachial index (ABI);
- *spectral analysys;*
- *serial duplex scanning:* morphological and haemodynamic evaluation, measurement of graft flow velocity (GFV);
- *color-doppler flow imaging;*
- *arteriography* (conventional, DSA-A, DSA-V).

Table 1 - Reported series of vein graft surveillance

Method	Occlusions %	Total lesions	Inflow %	Outflow %	Stenosis %
ANGIOGRAPHY					
Szilagyi [21]	31	23	not reported		20
CLINICAL ASSESSMENT + ABI (<15% previous examination)					
Sladen [20]	21	19	not reported		19
Berkovitz [7]	24	21	5	4	12
DUPLEX SCANNING (GVF <45 cm/sec; GVF ratio)					
Cullen [10]	27	35	6	3	22
Bandyk [4]	7	22	0,5	2	20
Grigg [14]	15	30	not reported		24
Mills [18]	5	13	5	8	6
COLOR-FLOW DUPLEX SCANNING					
Londrey [17]	—	20	not reported		—

Follow-up protocols must identify graft at risk for thrombosis without causing unnecessary interventions. Because of its invasivity and attendant risk, angiography is an unsatisfacory method for routine serial assessment of infrainguinal revascularizations. Thus, noninvasive haemodynamic testing has assumed an important role in lower extremity bypass graft evaluation.

We adopt a secondary follow-up at 1 month after the discharge, every 6 months for the first 2 years and yearly thereafter, in order to high occurence of failure in the first year after surgery due to myointimal hyperplasia. Such protocol monitors the haemodynamics of the limb and of the graft: goal is to identify abnormal but patent grafts. When the occlusive lesions are associated with a low-flow state in the graft (decrease in GFV <45 cm/sec.) or symptoms of limb ischemia, graft revision is recommendend if the lesion is correctable.

Because clinical assessment and standard noninvasive laboratory testing (ABI) aren't able to recognize failing graft before occlusion[23], according to Bandyk[5] we adopt this protocol:

a) Measurement of resting limb arterial pressure at ankle (ABI) by c.w. doppler

b) Doppler spectral analysis of graft blood flow patterns with calculation of peak systolic blood flow velocity in the graft (GFV)

c) Duplex-scanning or color-doppler flow-imaging (from 1990). ·

ANKLE/BRACHIAL SYSTOLIC INDEX (ABI)

Segmental systolic pressures and ABI evaluation are sensitive and accurate in detecting haemodynamically significant changes in arterial circulation of the limb.

Major limitations of this method are inability to localize the occlusive lesion and the failure to identify not significant stenosis or bypasses with poor outflow and low-flow that are at high risk for sudden thrombosis.

The ABI is considered abnormal when is decreased by more than 10% to 15% from the previous examination and constitutes indication to duplex-scan exploration and, if according, to angiography. The ABI is a very important accompanying test to the duplex scan. Green[12] reports that when ABI is normal and duplex scan is abnormal the risk of graft occlusion is 4% over the next 3 months; in presence of reduction >10% of ABI with duplex scan abnormal, the risk up to 66% (Table 2).

Table 2 - Value of ABI + duplex-scan in evaluating risk of infrainguinal graft occlusion

ABI + Duplex-scan	occlusion
Normal ABI	1,5%
Normal ABI/Normal duplex	0%
Abnormal ABI (<10%)	11%
Abnormal duplex/Normal ABI	4%
Abnormal duplex/Abnormal ABI	66%

SPECTRAL ANALYSYS

A decrease in ABI >0,15 or GVF >30 cm/sec from previous examination promptes diagnostic studies to locate a stenotic or occlusive lesion intrinsic to graft or to native above and belove vessels. Until 1990, all these suspected patients were evaluated by angiography; after this time, the work up includes duplex scanning or color-doppler flow imaging of the entire by-pass and inflow/outflow vessels.

DUPLEX SCANNING/COLOR-DOPPLER FLOW IMAGING

Several reports have distressed the role of serial duplex scanning to assess vein graft function and detect failing grafts[3,10,14].

Bandyk, first[2], reported the value of duplex-derived peak systolic GFV (graft flow velocity) measurements and showed that a low GFV <45 cm/sec was associated with impeding graft failure. Other detailed duplex methods have been used to localize graft stenosis like duplex examination of the entire graft with determination of sequential velocity ratios (V2:V1) by comparing peak flow measurements in adiacent 2 cm graft segments. A V2:V1 ratio >3:2 corresponding to a 50% increase in GVF, has been considered significant and correlates with a lesion reducing the lumen by 20%.

Several reports have demonstered that duplex scanning is more reliable in identification of failing vein grafts than is ABI determination. Its application is founded on following assumptions:

1. to recognize bypass graft and arterial native anatomy by their echogenic characteristics

2. vessel lumen narrowings produces frequency shifts thar are predictive of the severity of stenosis

3. accurate calculation of blood flow velocity (GFV)

4. detection of graft occlusion or graft aneurysmal dilatation by the combined use of imaging and velocity waveform analysis

5. early diagnosis of stenosis in grafts patent but at risk of occlusion.

In evaluating a infrainguinal bypass by duplex scanning several questions

must be investigated:
- inflow assessment (aorto-iliac vessels)
- determination of GFV
- detection of intrinsic abnormalities in the graft (stenosis, aneurysm)
- outflow assessment
- anastomosis (myointimal hyperplasia)
- functional resistance of the runoff vessels.

Although clear advantages over ABI and angiography for post-operative bypass surveillance, duplex scanning presents some limitations:
- difficult in case of obesity or anatomic variations
- strong dependance from operator knowledge
- difficult approach for peroneal bypass.

Recently, several reports have emphasized the use of color-doppler flow imaging in infrainguinal bypass grafts[17,20]. Color is used to real-time differentiate flow direction as well as to determinate flow velocity, thus eliminating the need for multiple velocity samples throughuot the graft.

In our early experience, by using a Apogee CX Interspec instrument with 7,5 MHz sector probe, we have scanned 35 infrainguinal bupass grafts evaluating occurrence of:
- stenosis (myointimal hyperplasia, intrinsic stenosis due to valvular fibrosis, atherosclerotic lesions in inflow and outflow vessels)
- residual fistulas (for in situ procedures)
- aneurysmal dilatations (expecially for Dardik grafts replacements) (Fig.1).

The examination consists of imaging the entire graft, measuring diameter and GFV in the proximal and distal anastomosis as well as in all cases of increased velocity by color flow imaging. It's easy to identify a stenosis by an abrupt virage of color from red to withe; occurrence of blue or black pixels in a sample area is indicative of turbolence, characteristic of a stenosis or AV fistula. To differentiate a stenosis from a AV fistula (in situ procedures) following criteria have been observed:

1. Stenosis:　　> peak systolic velocity
　　　　　　　　< diameter
　　　　　　　　abrupt color change

2. AV fistula:　> velocity in the proximal portion
　　　　　　　　< velocity in the distal portion (due to decreased outflow resistance).

Grigg and Sladen[14,20] have proposed to use "duplex velocity ratio" (increase in velocity within an aera of stenosis relative to normal graft) to classify the degree of stenosis:
DVR 2: mild stenosis (40%)
DVR 3: moderate stenosis (60%)
DVR >3: high grade stenosis (>60%)

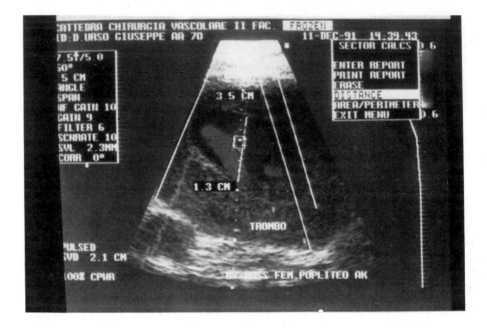

Fig. 1. Color-doppler flow imaging examination in patients operated on AK femoro-popliteal by pass with Dardik Biograft in 1984. Increasing swelling of thigh at level of proximal anastomosis. Figure shows an aneurysmal dilatation of prosthesis (max diameter: 3,5 cm.) with an inner thrombus (thrue lumen: 1,3 cm.) Color shifts in blue are indicative of internal turbolence due to high grade dilatation

CONCLUSIONS

In order to relatively poor results of re-do surgery for infrainguinal graft occlusions, has been universally accepted the importance of detection and correction of graft-threatening stenosis before occlusion. Clinical assessment and c.w. doppler evaluation have been shown to be relatively insensitive for detecting these preocclusive lesions. In our experience, duplex scanning and color-doppler flow imaging have demonstered an high-grade accuracy as a surveillance method. The speed and relative ease of examination make it an ideal method for following infrainguinal bypasses.

REFERENCES

1. Ascer E, Collier P, Gupta SK, Veith FJ Reoperation for polytetrafluoroethylene bypass failure: the importance of distal outflow site and operative technique in determining outcome *J Vasc Surg,* 1987;5:298-310
2. Bandyk DF Postoperative surveillance of femoro-distal grafts: the application of echo-Doppler (duplex) ultrasonic scanning In: Bergan JJ, Yao JST, EDS Reoperative arterial surgery. Orlando: Grune & Stratton, 1986:59-79

3. Bandyk DF, Kaebnick HW, Stewart GW, Towne JB Durability of the in situ saphenous vein arterial bypass: a comparison of primary and secondary patency *J Vasc Surg,* 1987;5:256-66
4. Bandyk DF, Schmitt DD, Seabrook GR, Adams MB, Towne JB Monitoring functional patency of in situ saphenous vein bypasses: the impact of surveillance protocol and elective revision *J Vasc Surg,* 1989;9:286-94
5. Bandyk DF, Bergamini TM, Towne JB, Schmitt DD, Seabrook GR Durability of vein graft revision: the outcome of secondary procedures *J Vasc Surg,* 1991;13:200-10
6. Bartlett ST, Olinde AJ, Flinn WR, et al. Reoperative potential of infrainguinal by-pass: long-term limb and patient survival *J Vasc Surg,* 1987;5:170-9
7. Berkowitz HD, Hobbs CL, Roberts B, et al. Value of routine vascular laboratory studies to identify vein graft stenosis *Surgery,* 1981;90:971-9
8. Bracale GC, Bernardo B, Porcellini M (1991) Ultrastructural changes of arterialized vein grafts. In: Vein graft in vascular surgery, edited by D'Addato M, Stella A, pp 11-20. Ed. Grasso, Bologna, Italy
9. Cohen JR, Mannick JA, Couch NP, Whittemore AD Recognition and management of impending vein-graft failure *Arch Surg,* 1986;121:758-9
10. Cullen PJ, Lehay AL, Ryan SB, McBride KD, Moore DY, Shanik GD The influence of duplex scanning on early patency rates of in situ by-pass to the tibial vessels *Ann Vasc Surg,* 1986;1:340-6
11. Dennis JW, Littooy FN, Greisler HP, Baker WH Secondary vascular procedures with polytetrafluoroethylene grafts for lower extremity ischemia in a mail veteran population *J Vasc Surg,* 1988;8:137-42
12. Green RM, Ouriel K, Ricotta JJ, DeWeese JA Revision of failed infrainguinal bypass graft: principles of management. *Surgery,* 1986;100:646-53
13. Green RM, McNamara J, Ouriel K, DeWeese JA Comparison of infrainguinal graft surveillance techniques. *J Vasc Surg,* 1990;11:207-15
14. Grigg MJ, Nicolaides AN, Wolfe JHN Femoro-distal vein by-pass graft stenosis. *Br J Surg,* 1988;75:737-40
15. Harris RW, Andros G, Salles-Cunha SX, Dulawa LB, Oblath RW, Apyan RL Alternative autogenous vein grafts to the inadequate saphenous vein. *Surgery,* 1986;100:822-7
16. Harris RW, Andros G, Salles-Cunha SX, Dulawa LB, Oblath RW, Apyan RL Totally autogenous venous composite by-pass grafts. *Arch Surg,* 1986;121:1128-32
17. Londrey GL, Hodgson KJ, Spadone DP, Ramsey DE, Barkmeier LD, Sumner DS Initial experience with color-flow duplex scanning of infrainguinal by-pass grafts *J Vasc Surg,* 1990;12:284-90
18. Mills JL, Harris JE, Taylor LMJr, Beckett WC, Porter JM The importance of routine surveillance of distal bypass grafts with duplex scanning: A study of 379 reversed vein grafts *J Vasc Surg,* 1990;12:379-89
19. Sladen JG, Gilmoure JL Vein graft stenosis: characteristics and effects of treatment. *Am J Surg,* 1981;141:549-53
20. Sladen JG, Reid JDS, Cooperberg PL, et al Color flow duplex screening of infreinguinal grafts combining low-and high-velocity criteria *Am J Surg,* 1989;158:107-12
21. Szilagyi DE, Elliott JP, Ageman JH, et al. Biological fate of autogenous vein implants as arterial substitute: clinical, angiographic and hystopathologic observations in femoro-popliteal operations for atherosclerosis *Ann Surg,* 1973;178:232-46
22. Turnipseed WD, Acher CW Postoperative surveillance: an effective means of detecting correctable lesions that threaten graft patency *Arch Surg,* 1985;120:324-8
23. Veith FJ, Weiser RK, Gupta SK, et al. Diagnosis and management of failing lower extremity arterial reconstruction prior to graft occlusion *J Cardiovasc Surg,* 1984;25:381-4
24. Whittemore AD, Clowes AW, Couch NP, Mannick JA Secondary femoropopliteal reconstruction *Ann Surg,* 1981;193:35-42
25. Wolfe JHN, Thomas ML, Jamieson CW, et al Early diagnosis of femoro-distal graft stenoses *Br J Surg,* 1987;74:268-70

Subject Index